Tsutsugamushi Disease

Tsutsugamushi Disease

Edited by Akiyoshi Kawamura, Jr./Hiroshi Tanaka/Akira Tamura

UNIVERSITY OF TOKYO PRESS

Dedicated to the nineteen late Tamiyaians, Drs. Takeo Tamiya, Taiichi Ito, Kohei Toyokawa, Hikozaemon Hazato, Masami Kitaoka, Masao Teshigawara, Tadashi Yamamoto, Noboru Higashi, Tadashi Kugoh, Kaoru Okubo, Shigehiro Katsura, Masaichi Hashimoto, Kiyoshi Oikawa, Fumihiko Shimizu, Kiyotoshi Kaneko, Kazuo Katsuta, Teruhiko Tsukamoto, Hiromu Takahashi, Tsuyoshi Iida; and to my father Rinya Kawamura.

ISBN 4–13–067104–9
ISBN 0–86008–512–0
Printed in Japan

Contents

Editors

Akiyoshi Kawamura, Jr., M. D., D. M. Sc.
Professor Emeritus, University of Tokyo, Tokyo, Japan

Hiroshi Tanaka, M. D., D. M. Sc.
Professor Emeritus, University of Tokyo, Tokyo, Japan and JICA Chief Advisor, Institute for Medical Research, Kuala Lumpur, Malaysia

Akira Tamura, D.M. Sc.
Professor, Department of Microbiology, Niigata College of Pharmacy, Niigata, Japan

Contributors

Kiyoshi Asanuma	Honorary Member, National Science Museum, Tokyo, Japan (3–4, 4–4)
Yumiko Furuya	Researcher, Division of Virology, Kanagawa Prefectural Public Health Laboratory, Yokohama, Japan (1–5, 3–8, 4–7, 6–2e, 6–2f, 6–3a, 6–3b)
Ikuo Kaiho	Researcher, Division of Virology, Public Health Laboratory of Chiba Prefecture, Chiba, Japan (1–5, 2–6, 2–10, 3–1, 4–7, 6–2a, 6–2c, 6–2g, 6–2h)
Akiyoshi Kawamura, Jr.	Professor Emeritus, University of Tokyo, Tokyo, Japan (Preface, 1–1, 1–2, 1–3, 1–4, 1–5, 1–6, 2–2, 2–5, 2–10, 3–1, 3–2, 3–3, 3–4, 3–5, 3–6, 3–7, 3–8, 4–1, 4–2, 4–3, 4–4, 4–5, 4–6, 4–7, 5–1, 5–2, 6–1, 6–2, 6–3)
Michisato Murata	Chief, Laboratory of Experimental Animals, Jichi Medical School, Minamikawachi, Tochigi, Japan (1–1, 1–2, 1–4, 2–2, 2–6, 2–10, 3–3, 3–7, 4–7, 6–1a, 6–1b, 6–1d, 6–2b)
Sadao Nogami	Associate Professor, Department of Medical Zoology, School of Veterinary Medicine, Nihon University, Fujisawa, Kanagawa, Japan (1–3, 3–4, 3–5, 3–6, 3–7, 3–8, 4–7, 6–2d)
Norio Ohashi	Research Associate, Department of Microbiology, Niigata College of Pharmacy, Niigata, Japan (2–1, 2–2, 2–3, 2–4, 2–5, 2–6, 2–7, 2–8)
Mamoru Takahashi	Kawagoe Agricultural Senior High School, Kawagoe, Saitama, Japan (1–5, 3–4, 3–5, 3–8, 4–1, 4–2, 4–3, 4–4, 4–5, 4–6, 4–7, 5–1, 5–2)

Akira Tamura	Professor, Department of Microbiology, Niigata College of Pharmacy, Niigata, Japan (2–1, 2–2, 2–3, 2–4, 2–5, 2–6, 2–7, 2–8, 2–9, 2–10, 4–7, 5–1, 6–1, 6–2, 6–3)
Hiroshi Tanaka	Professor Emeritus, University of Tokyo, Tokyo, Japan and JICA Chief Advisor, Institute for Medical Research, Kuala Lumpur, Malaysia (1–6, 3–4, 4–1, 4–2, 4–3, 4–4, 4–5, 4–6, 4–7, 5–1, 5–2, 6–1, 6–2, 6–3)
Hiroshi Urakami	Associate Professor, Department of Microbiology, Niigata College of Pharmacy, Niigata, Japan (2–1, 2–2, 2–3, 2–4, 2–5, 2–6, 2–7, 2–8, 4–7, 5–1)
Yoshiya Yoshida	Chief, Division of Virology, Kanagawa Prefectural Public Health Laboratory, Yokohama, Japan (1–5, 2–10, 3–1, 3–3, 3–8, 4–7, 6–2e, 6–2f, 6–3a, 6–3b)

(The numbers in parentheses refer to the chapters and sections for which each contributor was responsible.)

Preface

The history of Tsutsugamushi disease research is now 100 years old; during this time there have been four major phases, marking turning points in the research. For many years, it was known that a disease occurred after people were bitten by Kedani mites in summer at river terraces on the northern coast of the Sea of Japan. The disease had a very high fatality rate and had been greatly feared by the inhabitants of the region. Baelz and Kawakami (1879) first scientifically described the clinical picture of this disease as an acute infection. However, they did not support the concept of mites as disease vectors. With this report as the turning point, research enthusiasm heightened in Japan, and the disease was subsequently determined to be transmitted by trombiculid mites. Debates at scientific meetings were extremely fierce until the pathogen was identified as a rickettsia, by Nagayo *et al.* in 1930. This period in the research, which lasted approximately 50 years, was the first phase. Toward the end of this period, R. Kawamura (1926, 1930) described this disease for a worldwide audience not only as a disease entity endemic in Japan, but as an infectious disease that was of keen interest in general, noting epidemiology, clinical course, pathology, and the vector, trombiculid mites. With the exception of his statement regarding the causative agent, the descriptions are still useful today.

In the meantime, outside Japan, there were sporadic reports of a disease similar to Tsutsugamushi disease in Southeast Asia and in the islands of the southwestern Pacific. As these areas became the battlefields of World War II, soldiers from both sides were plagued with the totally unexpected Tsutsugamushi disease. It has been said that, in the Allied forces, the number of Tsutsugamushi disease patients surpassed the number of direct casualties due to the war. Initiated by the Australian forces, and followed by United States and British forces, expert teams were organized to cope with Tsutsugamushi disease. As a result, research on this disease progressed by leaps and bounds, and concomitantly, it was brought to the forefront as an extensive endemic disease in Asia and the southwestern Pacific regions. However, on the Japanese side, which met with military defeat, virtually no measures were taken against the disease. Therefore, the principal role in the research of this disease shifted from Japan to the United States and Great Britain.

The above period comprised the dramatic second phase, which lasted 15 years. The third phase encompassed the subsequent 30 years to 1975. In particular, the United States stationed research teams comprising Army and Navy physicians and scientists in Japan, Thailand, Malaysia, Taiwan, and the Philippines for continued research. Meanwhile, in Japan, there was an outbreak of Tsutsugamushi disease among soldiers of the United States forces during maneuvers in the foothills of Mt. Fuji. Triggered by this incident, the existence of Tsutsugamushi disease from autumn to winter was confirmed, in addition to the summer disease counterpart occurring along the northern coast of the Sea of Japan. Subsequently, occurrences of this disease were also confirmed in other areas in Japan, in Tsurumi in Yokohama City and in Izu Shichito Islands (where it was known as Shichito fever). Furthermore, a Tsutsugamushi disease rickettsia was isolated from rodents in other islands of the Japanese archipelago, Shikoku and Hokkaido. This led to a nationwide survey and research on trombiculid mites by teams centered around that of Sasa *et al.* (1956), and developments were made in Tsutsugamushi disease research by Fukuzumi (1950), Kawamura (1952), Kitaoka (1953), and others.

Fortunately, during this research phase, the United States government supported the research group represented by Emeritus Prof. T. Tamiya, with grants implemented from 1954. Although a few influential scientists in the field did not participate, a majority of the Japanese researchers joined the research team and undertook a nationwide survey and research on Tsutsugamushi disease in Japan during the period of the grant, which lasted until 1960. Their achievements were published in 1962 as a monograph entitled *Recent Advances in Studies of Tsutsugamushi Disease in Japan* (edited by Tamiya). This book still serves as a source of valuable data on Tsutsugamushi disease research. Subsequently, the United States government signed separate research contracts with Drs. M. Kitaoka and K. Asanuma, and research continued, centered around the establishment of methods for the diagnosis of Tsutsugamushi disease and investigations of rickettsial transmission to trombiculid mites. However, in the meantime, the number of Tsutsugamushi disease patients in Japan had rapidly decreased, and the disease even seemed to have disappeared. On the other hand, no significant change occurred in the number of patients infected in the Southeast Asian region, and research groups centered around the United States Army recorded steady advances, in particular, in the laboratory rearing of trombiculid mite colonies and the typing of rickettsial strains.

The fourth phase of research into this disease is the period from 1975 to the present. The situation has evolved to the stage such that Tsutsugamushi disease should not be regarded only as a typical acute fever endemic in Asia; rather it should be acknowledged that a considerable number of fevers of unknown origin in endemic foci are Tsutsugamushi disease without typical symptoms. This fact should be translated into a strong warning to local physicians and public health officials. In order to cope with the situation, it is necessary to popularize the diagnostic techniques and make treatment available to everyone. This is one of the major objectives of the authors in the publication of this book. In the background of this situation are the findings that the rickettsial strains that cause Tsutsugamushi disease are extremely heterologous, and immunity against them is not lasting. Consequently, reinfections and repeated reinfections are quite common in endemic foci. The situation is further complicated by the fact that rickettsial pathogenicity in humans and mice displays a spectrum of virulence, posing a serious risk of contracting Tsutsugamushi disease in endemic sites.

However, research on Tsutsugamushi disease has now resulted in the development of techniques based on cellular and genetic engineering, together with techniques that have led to the rearing of trombiculid mite colonies. Consequently, researchers now have adequate means to cope with the challenges they face.

The second objective of this book is to review the progress in research made chiefly by our group, subsequent to the abovementioned monograph edited by Tamiya. Tsutsugamushi disease, which once seemed about to disappear in Japan, has continued to occur nationwide, except in Hokkaido, since 1975, as was predicted by one of the authors (A. Kawamura, Jr.). It has also occurred in Korea since 1985, at an incidence more than two-fold higher than that in Japan. In China, Tsutsugamushi disease was identified around 1950 in the southwestern region, occurring during approximately the summer season. Despite a subsequent decrease in incidence in China (except Hainan Island), as occurred in Japan, the disease has been on the increase in China since the 1980s. Especially noteworthy is the finding that as many as 30–50% of the population are seroepidemiologically antibody-positive healthy persons. A new autumn-to-winter type Tsutsugamushi disease, like that found in Korea, has been occurring since 1986 in Shandong Province, north of the Yangzi river. The recent increase in the number of patients in Japan, Korea, and China cannot be attributed solely to our heightened awareness of Tsutsugamushi disease.

While editing this monograph, Tamura *et al.* (1995) proposed that the species of *R. tsutsugamushi* be transferred from genus *Rickettsia* to genus *Orientia*, newly established by them, by reason of differences in (1) morphological and chemical structures of the outer envelope of this organismus; (2) homology of species-specific protein; (3) reactivity to varied antibiotics; and (4) the 16S rRNA gene sequence. Since it takes several years for a proposed generic name to be accepted generally, *Rickettsia tsutsugamushi* is used as a species name in this monograph.

The collaborating researchers, who are introduced in the List of Contributors, have divided the writing of this volume according to their areas of expertise. The principal contributing authors are A. Kawamura, Jr., and H. Tanaka, who take responsibility for overseeing the whole volume; A. Kawamura, Jr., Preface and Chapters 1 and 3; A. Tamura, Chapters 2 and 6; H. Tanaka and M. Takahashi, Chapters 4 and 5. Other contributors are K. Asanuma, Y. Furuya, I. Kaiho, M. Murata, S. Nogami, N. Ohashi, H. Urakami, and Y. Yoshida.

The authors would like to express their heartfelt gratitude to the members of the former Tamiya research group, and to Ms. E. Hamao, Ms. M. Fushitani, and Ms. S. Schmidt of the International Publications Department, University of Tokyo Press, for their immense help in preparing this book for publication.

Tokyo, April 1995

Tsutsugamushi Disease

1

Tsutsugamushi Disease — An Overview

1. Introduction

Tsutsugamushi disease is an acute infectious disease that occurs when humans are bitten by larval trombiculid mites harboring the etiological agent *Rickettsia tsutsugamushi*. Typical symptoms include fever, headache, rash, eschar, and lymphadenopathy. Atypical symptoms are also frequently found in sites endemic for *R. tsutsugamushi*-harboring trombiculid mites, and it has been shown that mildly pathogenic *R. tsutsugamushi* also results in abortive or inapparent infections. Chloramphenicol and the tetracycline antibiotics have demonstrated marked therapeutic efficacy and lead to a complete cure. However, it is unfortunate that fatalities, though rare, occur each year due to the erroneous choice of antibiotics resulting from ambivalent diagnoses. Such diagnoses are due to the heterogeneity of *R. tsutsugamushi* strains being so wide that interstrain cellular immunity cannot cope with it; it is therefore not uncommon for subjects to have reinfections or repeated reinfections in endemic foci. Secondly, there are variations in *R. tsutsugamushi* pathogenicity to humans; even today, ignorance prevails as to proper diagnostic methods, and proper treatments remain unrecognized. As long as Tsutsugamushi disease is a common regional disease widely distributed from Southeast Asia to the regions of the southwest Pacific, physicians and health care administrators in the endemic foci should be aware of these facts.

2. Historical Background

As stated in the Preface, there have been four major phases to date in the history of Tsutsugamushi disease research. The first phase was from ancient times until the time when the pathogen *Rickettsia* was identified. The first record of a febrile disease thought to be Tsutsugamushi disease appeared in China in 313 A.D., when it was described by Hong Ge in a clinical manual of the time called "Zhouhofang," along with the morphology of the vector mites. In 610, Yuan-Fang Chao described the epidemiology, clinical course, and treatment of the disease in a poem which is medically accurate even today. In 1596, a well-known Chinese physician, Shi-Zhen Li, described the characteristics of the disease in a book entitled "Ben Cao Gang Mu." Thus, it is evident that the presence of a Tsutsugamushi-like disease had attracted attention in China since ancient times. Despite this fact, investigative research on this disease finally began in China in earnest only in 1942 (Fan *et al.*, 1987).

Meanwhile, in Japan in the early nineteenth century, it was recorded that a serious febrile disease occurred after people were bitten by Kedani (mites) in midsummer at river terraces on the coast of the Sea of Japan, in Niigata, Yamagata, and Akita Prefectures. The disease was feared by the inhabitants of the area. The first scientific clinical report of this disease was made in 1879 by Baelz and Kawakami, who did not support the concept of mites as disease vectors. With this report as a turning point, many scientists in Japan began intensive studies of the disease, and great advances were thus made in research regarding the clinical course, epidemiology, and pathology of the disease; trombiculid mites were subsequently identified as vectors. Above all, the scientists' desire to be the first to discover the pathogen resulted in a fierce competition. In 1930, Nagayo *et al.* inoculated material containing the pathogen into the anterior chamber of a rabbit eye, allowed a large number of the pathogenic rickettsiae to grow in the cells of Descemet's membrane, and passaged them, positively identifying rickettsiae as the pathogens of Tsutsugamushi disease. They published their findings, naming the pathogen *Rickettsia orientalis* Nagayo, Tamiya, Mitamura *et* Sato, 1930. In opposition, Ogata presented a different story, and Bergey's Manual finally adopted the name *Rickettsia tsutsugamushi* starting with the 6th edition, based on the judgment of C.B. Philip (1948b). Regarding the circumstances during this period, we discuss, in Section 6 below, the questions that arose with respect to the rules of nomenclature. This dispute aside, there was marked progress in experimental techniques until the causative agent of

Tsutsugamushi disease was determined. At one time, monkeys exhibiting symptoms similar to those of humans were used exclusively as experimental animals. Ogata and Unno (1929) first used an intratesticular inoculation method in a rabbit, followed by the above-mentioned method of inoculation into the anterior chamber of a rabbit's eye. Finally Ogata *et al.* (1932) developed a method of intraperitoneal inoculation in mice, which is indispensable for *R. tsutsugamushi* research even today. The impact of the use of mice as experimental animals on *R. tsutsugamushi* research was immeasurable, and the achievement of the Ogata group is worthy of special mention. Of note also was the introduction of Tsutsugamushi disease to the world through two publications, one in English and one in German, in which the clinical course, epidemiology, pathology, and the vector trombiculid mites were described by the author's father, R. Kawamura (1926, 1930). Other than the theory of causation, much of the data are still useful today, and they served as important references, especially during World War II, when battlefields were the infective areas of Tsutsugamushi disease. In these publications, the mites *Leptotrombidium pallidum* were suggested to be the vector of Tsutsugamushi disease in Japan during non-summer season transmission, in addition to the Tsutsugamushi disease vector *L. akamushi* in the summer. This was a keen observation for the time.

Meanwhile, outside Japan, there were successive reports of the presence of a disease similar to Tsutsugamushi disease: in 1902 in Delhi and Sumatra, in 1908 in eastern Taiwan and the Philippines, in 1910 in North Queensland, Australia, in 1915 in Saigon, Indochina, and Peninsular Malaya, in 1930 in New Britain, in 1933 in Burma, in 1935 in New Guinea, and in 1939 in Java; but fatality was low, and the disease did not attract attention as did the Tsutsugamushi disease occurring in Niigata, Yamagata, and Akita Prefectures, Japan (Hatori, 1919–20; Kawamura, 1926; Ogata, 1958). In addition, with some exceptions, studies of Tsutsugamushi disease in Japan suddenly decreased after the pathogen had been determined. Furthermore, with the effects of the war between Japan and China that began in 1937 and of World War II from 1941, Tsutsugamushi disease research in Japan was neglected.

However, the above-mentioned infective sites for Tsutsugamushi disease, Southeast Asia and the southwestern Pacific regions, became principal battlefields during World War II. Both the Japanese and the Allied forces were plagued not with malaria, which had been anticipated, but with a totally unexpected ailment, Tsutsugamushi disease. There is no accurate record from the defeated Japanese forces, but it has been reported that, in the Allied forces, the number of victims of battlefield diseases, especially of Tsutsugamushi disease, surpassed the number of direct casualties due to the war (Philip, 1948a; Philip and Kohls, 1945). The number of patients recorded was upward of 10,241 and deaths numbered upward of 394. The average fatality was 3.85%, but this varied greatly by region; 27.5% and 35.3% were the highs in Goodenough Island and Finchhaven of New Guinea, respectively, and 1.5% and 0.6% were the lows in Embilipitiya, south of Ceylon, and in Biak and Owi Islands, north of Western New Guinea, respectively.

Among the Allied forces, Australia first hurriedly organized an expert team to cope with Tsutsugamushi disease in early 1943, followed by the United States in October 1943 and the British in February 1944. These intensive studies filled the research void and became a springboard for further research on this disease (Audy, 1949; Audy *et al.*, 1947; Blake *et al.*, 1945; Kohls *et al.*, 1945; McCulloch, 1946; Philip, 1948a; Philip and Kohls, 1945; Philip *et al.*, 1946). The second phase of research ends here, during this phase, the major achievement was the development of the complement fixation test as a diagnostic technique for Tsutsugamushi disease, using Cox-Craigie type antigens obtained from *R. tsutsugamushi* cultured in an embryonated egg yolk sac (Craigie, 1945). This test had come to play a major role in the diagnoses, replacing the previously used Weil-Felix reaction (Bengtson, 1945, 1946).

The next phase of research was the period from the end of World War II to the time of the introduction of cellular and genetic engineering as experimental methods, in 1975. After the end of the war, the United States stationed Tsutsugamushi disease research teams in the areas in which an occupying force was stationed in Japan, Taiwan, the Philippines, Malaysia, and Thailand, for continued research. In the autumn of 1946, a group of soldiers of the United States forces stationed in Japan were afflicted with Tsutsugamushi disease during maneuvers in the foothills of Mt. Fuji. Several years later, Tsutsugamushi infections occurred among United States Marines in the same region. In addition, the Tsutsugamushi disease that emerged in Japan from autumn to early winter was confirmed to be a different type from the Tsutsugamushi disease that occurred in the summer along the northern coast, along the Sea of Japan. Sakita (1934) had already reported Tsutsugamushi disease in the Mt. Fuji region in 1933; in the autumn of 1937, R. Kawamura had also encountered a disease which could only be Tsutsugamushi disease in Enzan, Yamanashi Prefecture (R. Kawamura, personal communication, 1946). However, hindered by the fixed idea that the disease did not exist in areas other than river terraces along the northern coast facing the Sea of Japan, neither case was pursued. The United States forces reports of the disease occurring in the foothills of Mt. Fuji stimulated Japanese researchers, and the occurrence of Tsutsugamushi disease from autumn to early winter was confirmed at Tsurumi in Yokohama City, in the Izu Shichito Islands (where it was known as Shichito fever), in the Boso Peninsula in Chiba, and in the Izu Peninsula (Tamiya, 1962). At the same time, a team led by Sasa conducted an extensive nationwide survey and research into trombiculid mites in Japan (Sasa,1956); and Fukuzumi, Kitaoka, Kawamura A. Jr., and others (Tamiya, 1962) successfully isolated *R. tsutsugamushi* in succession from both patients and wild rodents in the area where infections occurred. For this research series in Japan, where research funds were scarce after the war, fortunately, the United States government supported Emeritus Professor T. Tamiya with a research grant from 1954 to 1960. The team organized during the period accumulated enormous amounts of survey and research data, including a survey of patients nationwide, determination of the *R. tsutsugamushi* harboring rate among field rodents, data on the growth of *R. tsutsugamushi*, establishment of purification and diagnostic techniques, seroepidemiological studies, a survey of trombiculid mites and their seasonal prevalence, and searches for *R. tsutsugamushi* carrier trombiculid mites. The results of these studies were published as a monograph (Tamiya, 1962). The data contained in that publication are relevant even today and are widely used. During this period, techniques were developed for culturing *R. tsutsugamushi* and for its partial purification, using a cation exchange resin (Amberlite XE-64) and 8% KCl treatment (Kawamura, 1962; Yamamoto *et al.*, 1958). Shishido (1962a) modified these techniques for the diagnosis of Tsutsugamushi disease and carried out the typing of *R. tsutsugamushi* isolates, using modified complement fixation test antigens. The trombiculid mites were also investigated, and the transmissibility of Tsutsugamushi disease, the bearing rates of *R. tsutsugamushi*, and other factors were examined. These findings have greatly influenced subsequent studies.

After evaluating the achievements of the Tamiya group, the United States government signed additional contracts for separate research on Tsutsugamushi disease carried out by two groups, represented by Drs. M. Kitaoka and K. Asanuma. Their major achievements included: (1) the establishment of methods for the diagnosis of Tsutsugamushi disease and the typing of *R. tsutsugamushi* isolates by complement fixation test and immunofluorescence (Iida *et al.*, 1966a, 1966b; Shishido, 1962a, 1964; Shishido *et al.*, 1967); in particular, the establishment of a novel immunofluorescence technique using an improved labeling technique, purified labeled antibodies, and improved fluorescence microscopes (Kawamura, 1969), the confirmed isolation of *R. tsutsugamushi* soluble antigens (Shishido *et al.*, 1969), and the isolation and maintenance of mildly pathogenic *R. tsutsugamushi* using nude mice (Murata and Kawamura, 1977); (2) the determination of *R. tsutsugamushi* carrier trombiculid mite species and their predilection for humans, and the determination of *R. tsutsugamushi*-harboring rate for each species (Asanuma, 1983); and (3) investigation of the possibility of *R. tsutsugamushi* transmission from *R. tsutsugamushi*-infected animals (mice, wild rodents) to mites and subsequent transmission to the next generation (Miura and Kawai, 1968; Toyokawa, 1972). Details of these achievements will be presented in Chapters 2 through 5 of this book.

While this research was unfolding at a somewhat leisurely tempo, the number of Tsutsugamushi disease patients in Japan was rapidly decreasing, and the disease even seemed to be disappearing for some period. However, not much change occurred in the number of patients infected in the Southeast Asian region, and, based on a number of grounds, one of the authors had been asserting in the late 1950s that Tsutsugamushi disease would again occur in Japan (Kawamura, 1958; Kawamura and Takigami, 1957; Kawamura and Tanaka, 1988; Kawamura *et al.*, 1980; Rapmund, 1984). As discussed below, Tsutsugamushi disease began to increase suddenly in Japan from about 1975 and in Korea from about 1985 (Chang *et al.*, 1990; Kawamura and Tanaka, 1988; Ree *et al.*, 1991c). Meanwhile, during this period, the United States Army research group established laboratory-reared colonies of *R. tsutsugamushi*-positive and -negative *L. fletcheri*, and *L. arenicola,* and demonstrated that *R. tsutsugamushi* could be vertically transmitted in mites and, moreover, that the larvae produced were all females. This research group conducted *R. tsutsugamushi* transmission experiments using these colonies (Rapmund, 1984; Traub *et al.*, 1975). In addition, they made steady progress in the typing of *R. tsutsugamushi* strains isolated from humans, wild rodents, and trombiculid mites and in the direct typing of *R. tsutsugamushi* in trombiculid mites (Elisberg *et al.*, 1967, 1968, 1978; Shirai *et al.*, 1979b, 1981b, 1981d, 1982a, 1982b, 1982c). Host resistance to experimental *R. tsutsugamushi* infections was analyzed in a mouse model by Osterman's group and others (Osterman, 1985; Tringali *et al.*, 1983). Details of these studies will be presented in later chapters.

The period from 1976 to the present represents the fourth phase of Tsutsugamushi disease research in Japan. Tsutsugamushi disease has reappeared rapidly, nationwide, since 1975. However, coincidentally, various experimental techniques have been devised for Tsutsugamushi disease research, and astonishing progress is being made concurrently, due to what one may call a revolution in microbiological research, *i.e.*, cellular and genetic engineering, fields which were just emerging in the 1970s. This subject will be discussed in depth in Section 5 below. In *R. tsutsugamushi* research, developments have occurred in rapid succession; these include an isolation technique for *R. tsutsugamushi* mildly pathogenic to mice, an *R. tsutsugamushi* purification technique, preparation of monoclonal antibodies, the development of indirect immunoperoxidase techniques, the elucidation of *R. tsutsugamushi* type-specific antigens and their genes, and the detection of *R. tsutsugamushi* DNA, using the polymerase chain reaction (PCR) or nested PCR, in which parts of the gene sequence are used as primers. Further, a large number of laboratory-reared colonies of *R. tsutsugamushi*-positive and -negative vector trombiculid mites have been established and maintained. Research on Tsutsugamushi disease is now flourishing. Moreover, one may say that the Kawamura research group in Japan is at the forefront of the research in this field.

3. Seasonal Prevalence of the Disease in Japan and Neighboring Countries

a. Tsutsugamushi disease in Japan: New perspectives

Rickettsia tsutsugamushi, the etiologic agent of Tsutsugamushi disease, has been isolated from wild rodents and certain species of trombiculid mites found over wide areas of the Pacific and Asia, as far west as Afghanistan. In Japan, Tsutsugamushi disease in humans is a rather localized endemic disease with seasonal occurrence. Occasionally, endemic areas, or so-called hot spots, change from one place to another. The prevalent season and the severity of the disease also vary by locality.

These findings cannot be explained by the difference in strains of *R. tsutsugamushi* or by differences in the species of vector mites. It is also known that the high-risk areas in which rickettsia-positive trombiculid mite colonies are found change over a period of time, and in some instances, even naive areas are converted to hot spots. Therefore, the questions that remain are how and where *R. tsutsugamshi* is maintained during interepidemic periods, and how the foci of infective vector mites develop.

In Japan, there are two types of Tsutsugamushi disease: the classical Tsutsugamushi disease, transmitted by *Leptotrombidium akamushi*, and a newer type, transmitted by *L. pallidum* or *L. scutellare*. The classical type occurs only in the summer, when temperatures are above 25°C, in areas along river banks in northern coastal regions facing the Sea of Japan, as found in Niigata, Yamagata, and Akita Prefectures. This summer-type disease was the only one recognized until 1946.

The new type of Tsutsugamushi disease was first recognized after the end of World War II, when American troops on maneuvers in the foothills of Mt. Fuji in October 1946 and 1948 contracted a febrile disease which was diagnosed as Tsutsugamushi disease by complement fixation test. Since 1951, areas endemic for this new type of Tsutsugamushi disease have been found successively in the Izu Shichito Islands (part of greater Tokyo, where the disease is known as Shichito fever), the Izu Peninsula in Shizuoka Prefecture, the Boso Peninsula in Chiba Prefecture, Kagawa Prefecture (where the disease is known as Umayado fever), and other areas (Tamiya, 1962) (Fig. 1).

This new type of the disease is transmitted by *L. pallidum*, which appears twice a year from late spring to early summer and from autumn to early winter, or by *L. scutellare*, which appears in autumn to winter, when the temperature reaches 18–20°C. The clinical symptoms of this type of the disease are mild, similar to those generally known in other countries.

L. scutellare-borne Tsutsugamushi disease (Shichito fever) prevailed on the Izu Shichito Islands from 1951 through 1953 during the autumn to winter season. Symptoms were mild and *R. tsutsugamushi* was easily isolated from humans and wild rodents, and rarely from trombiculid mites. After 1955, except for a few spo-

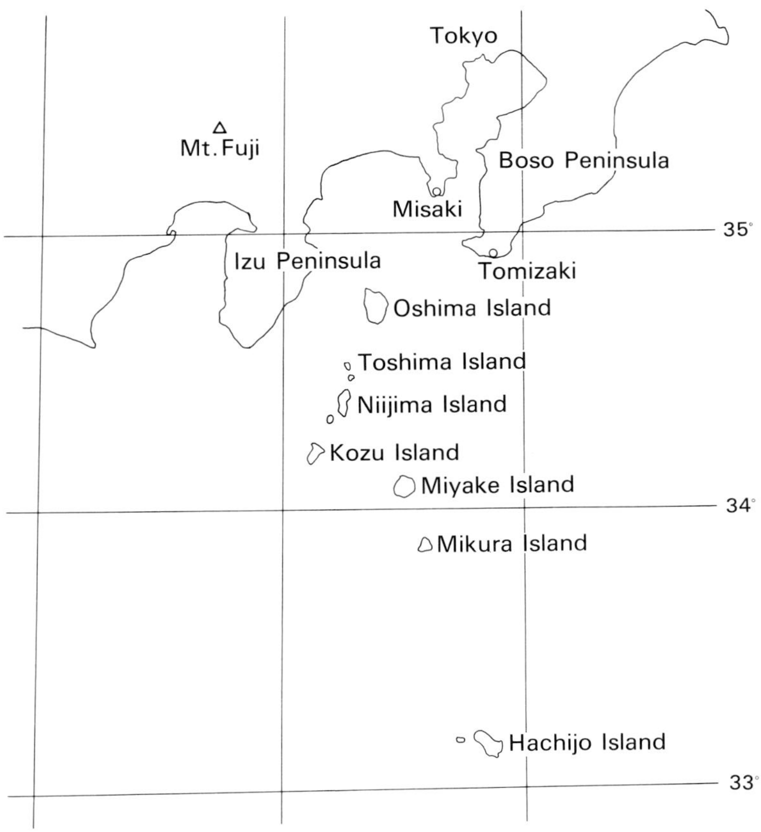

Fig. 1. Izu Shichito Islands

Table 1. Incidence of Shichito Fever Patients from 1951 to 1981

Year	Island Population in 1951	Hachijo 13,000	Miyake 6,500	Oshima 1,300	Mikura 360	Niijima 600	Toshima 380	Total
1951		285	18	24				327
1952		109	31	50		28		218
⋮	rapidly disappeared							
1964					1			1
⋮								
1974				7				7
1975				9				9
1976			8	19				27
1977			3	5		9		17
1978				4		3		7
1979				10		8		18
1980			8	5				13
1981		1	10	16		21		48

radic cases, the endemicity of Shichito fever subsided, and our repeated attempts to isolate *R. tsutsugamushi* from field rodents and vector chiggers were unsuccessful during the period 1956 to 1958, as shown in Table 1 (Kawamura and Tanaka, 1988; Kawamura *et al.*, 1980).

Based on records of earlier outbreaks of Shichito fever-like disease in 1918 and 1935, a periodic epidemic pattern occurring at intervals of 15–25 years was postulated by Kawamura, who suggested in the late 1950s (Kawamura, 1958; Kawamura and Takigami, 1957) that there would be such outbreaks in future. As anticipated from this forecast, Shichito fever began to reappear on Oshima Island in 1974 and on Miyake Island in 1976 (Kawamura *et al.*, 1980). In this outbreak on Miyake Island, only 12 cases were confirmed by our studies from 1976 to 1977, whereas the total number of cases in previous outbreaks had been approximately 560. Despite all our efforts to isolate rickettsiae from rodents and trombiculid mites on Miyake Island during this period, we were successful in isolating only one strain, an avirulent strain of *R. tsutsugamushi* Karp type, using athymic nude mice derived from a seronegative *Rattus norvegicus*. This strain was not pathogenic to conventional hairy mice and could be maintained only in nude mice (Kawamura *et al.*, 1980). These findings suggested that, in nature, the percentage of field rodents and trombiculid mites harboring virulent *R. tsutsugamushi* was generally low.

The seroepidemiology of field rodents on Miyake Island was studied by indirect immunofluorescence from 1977 to 1980, and it was found that positivity in these animals increased rapidly, from 0% (0/25) in January 1977 to 83.3% (15/18) in November 1978. Thereafter, positivity remained at about 50%. Thus, it is possible that field rodents may have been infected at high rates with *R. tsutsugamushi* during these four years (Kawamura *et al.*, 1980). In 1978, the seropositivity of the inhabitants of Miyake and Toshima Islands was surveyed from May through October; it was found to be 26.1% (42/161) and 23.5% (23/98), respectively. The antibody titer was low (< 1:160), and no difference was noted between the male and female populations. Moreover, none of these seropositive subjects had a history of Shichito fever. These findings indicate that approximately one-quarter of the population on both islands may have had inapparent infection with avirulent *R. tsutsugamushi* (Kawamura *et al.*, 1980).

From 1965 to 1974, the incidence of both types of Tsutsugamushi disease decreased in Japan (Figs. 2 and 3). The declining incidence of classical Tsutsugamushi disease was considered to be due mainly to changes in the vegetation, plant cultivation, and terrain conditions, and to improvement of the environment at river banks where the disease was endemic. A typical example of such changes, resulting in the disappearance of trombiculid mites, was seen at an area in

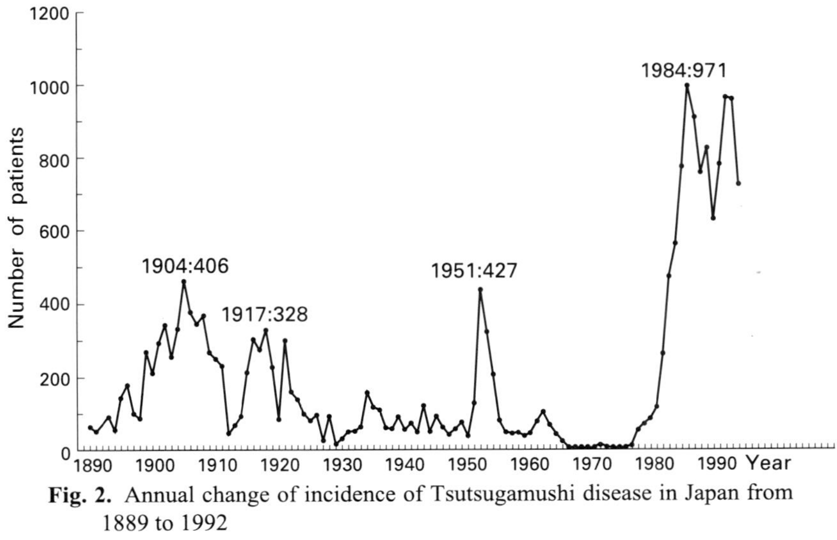

Fig. 2. Annual change of incidence of Tsutsugamushi disease in Japan from 1889 to 1992

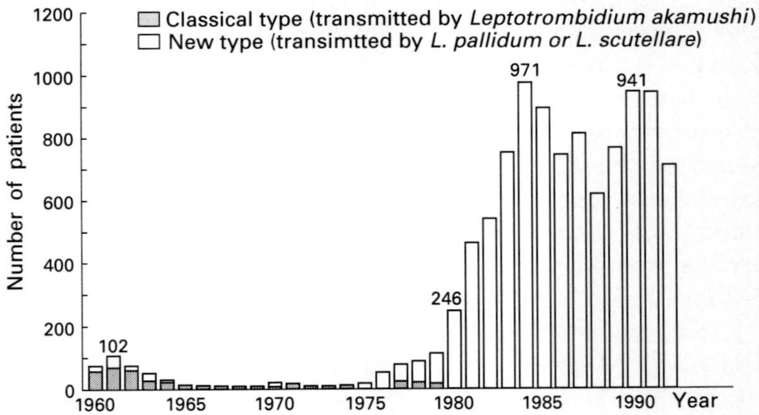

Fig. 3. Annual change of incidence of classical and new types of Tsutsugamushi disease in Japan (since 1960)

Niigata Prefecture that had been a high-risk area in the past. Nevertheless, the decrease in the incidence of the new type of Tsutsugamushi disease could not be explained only by such environmental changes. Since 1974, there has been a remarkable resurgence in the number of reported cases of Tsutsugamushi disease involving Shichito fever in Japan after about 10 years of virtual absence, as shown in Figs. 2, 3 and Table 1 (Kawamura and Tanaka, 1988; Kawamura *et al.*, 1980; Rapmund, 1984). Figure 2 shows the annual change of incidence of Tsutsugamushi disease in Japan from 1889 to 1992. Prior to 1950, there were many peaks of incidence of the so-called classical type of Tsutsugamushi disease. A peak from 1951 to 1953 was caused by the outbreak of Shichito fever. After 1965, classical and new types of Tsutsugamushi disease declined, as mentioned above. Since 1976, there has been a remarked resurgence, with the incidence of Tsutsugamushi disease increasing to new recorded levels each year until 1984. The total number of patients from April 1984 to March 1985 was the maximum for this most recent outbreak (Kawamura and Tanaka, 1988; Rapmund, 1984). Figure 3 indicates the annual changes in the incidence of the classical and new types of Tsutsugamushi disease in Japan since 1960. During the latest resurgence of Tsutsugamushi disease, the majority of reported cases were obviously of the new type.

Table 2 indicates the monthly incidence of Tsutsugamushi disease

Table 2. Monthly Incidence of Tsutsugamushi Disease in Each Prefecture from April of 1984 to March 1985

Prefecture \ Year	1984									1985			
Month	4	5	6	7	8	9	10	11	12	1	2	3	Total
Aomori			1	1	1		1						4
Iwate				1									1
Miyagi					1			1					2
Akita		19	23	6	4	1	2	4	1				60
Yamagata		2	3				2						7
Fukushima				1			1		1		1		4
Ibaraki	1	2	1					1	1				6
Tochigi			1										1
Gumma		1				1	6	9	1				18
Saitama								1					1
Chiba		1					2	24	29	1	1		58
Tokyo								4	13	3			20
Kanagawa							5	10	1				16
Niigata	1	36	34		4	2	1	3					81
Toyama			1				1	15					17
Fukui								1					1
Nagano		2	4	2		1	1	(1)8	2				20
Gifu		1	2					33	17				53
Shizuoka		1					3	5	3			1	13
Aichi		1						3					4
Mie								1					1
Shiga													
Kyoto		1			1			2					4
Hyogo									1				1
Shimane													
Hiroshima													
Kochi													
Saga		1					1	2	1				5
Nagasaki					2		2	6					10
Kumamoto								2	2				4
Oita								2	4	1			7
Miyazaki							12	108	31	4	2		157
Kagoshima	8	5	8	6	4	1	4	104	221	28	5	1	395
Total	10	73	78	17	17	6	44	349	329	37	9	2	971

( ): Number of deaths.

in each prefecture during the period from April 1984 to March 1985, this period coinciding with the Japanese fiscal year 1984. This period shows the peak incidence more clearly than reporting by the calendar year, because the incidence increases in October, reaches a peak in November and December, and decreases sharply by March every year. Each year there are two apparent peaks of incidence of Tsutsugamushi disease; one from late spring to early summer, and the other from autumn to early winter. These periods correspond to the season in which *L. pallidum* and *L. scutellare* appear. The recent resurgence in disease incidence is not thought to be related to an increased population of new young susceptibles, or to an extraordinary multiplication of field rodents, or to the restricted use of mitecides and insecticides, or to the misapplication of antibiotics. It is most likely that the remarkable resurgence is related to an increase in the number of vector mite colonies that carry *R. tsutsugamushi*. However, there is no good explanation as to how these foci of infective vector mites develop (Kawamura and Tanaka, 1988).

To resolve these problems, it is necessary to analyze the transmission dynamics of *R. tsutsugamushi* in vector mite foci and to diagnose Tsutsugamushi disease in humans correctly using immunological methods. Studies of the dynamics of *R. tsutsugamushi* transmission in vector chiggers have been performed by research groups in Malaysia since 1969 (Rapmund, 1984; Rapmund *et al.*, 1969) and now are being conducted by our group (Takahashi *et al.*, 1988b). Biotechnological approaches to the investigation of *R. tsutsugamushi* have recently been developed by American and Japanese research groups; these approaches include the production of monoclonal group- and strain-specific antibodies against rickettsia (Eisemann and Osterman, 1985; Murata *et al.*, 1986), rickettsial antigen production and purification (Takahashi *et al.*, 1985; Tamura *et al.*, 1982), analysis of the polypeptide composition and strain- and group-specific antigenic components of rickettsia (Eisemann and Osterman, 1985; Hanson, 1985; Tamura *et al.*, 1985), and purification of a type-specific antigen (TSA) of rickettsia and the molecular cloning and sequence analysis of the gene encoding TSA of *R. tsutsugamushi* (Oaks *et al.*, 1987; Ohashi *et al.*, 1989, 1990a, 1992a; Stover *et al.*, 1990a). It is anticipated that the results of the above biotechnological approaches will serve as the basis of defined serological methods for the routine diagnosis of Tsutsugamushi disease that will be simple and rapid. The immunoperoxidase test (Suto, 1982; Yamamoto and Minamishima, 1982) and indirect immunofluorescence (Kawamura and Aoyama, 1983) were recommended by a meeting of the Task Force of WHO, Regional Office for the Western Pacific, held in Okinawa on 24 November 1986, not only for the detection of *R. tsutsugamushi* antibody but also for the differentiation of immunoglobulin class (Regional Office for the Western Pacific of WHO, 1987).

b. Tsutsugamushi disease in neighboring countries

Korea

After the first report of eight cases of Tsutsugamushi disease among United Nations Army soldiers in Korea in the period 1951–1953, there were no reported cases for more than 30 years, until 1985, when 64 cases were reported. Since 1985, the number of cases reported yearly has been 460 in 1986, 992 in 1987, 832 in 1988, 1,365 in 1989, 1,301 in 1990, and 2,166 in 1991. Most cases were found in October (33.9%) and November (59.7%). Cases were reported throughout the country, including Cheju Island, the highest number occurring in the two southernmost provinces; Kyongsangnam-do (19.4%) and Chollanam-do (14.3%), followed by Chollabug-do (12.0%) and Chungeheongnam-do (12.5%). All endemic areas are in the plain region of the Korean Peninsula (Ree *et al.*, 1991c; Ree's personal communication to Kawamura, 1993). To date, the *R. tsutsugamushi* strains isolated in Korea have been divided into three types, using monoclonal antibodies. The Karp and Gilliam types were found mostly in the middle of the Korean Peninsula, and the Boryong strain type, which seems to belong to a new local type closely related to the Karp type, was found in the south (Chang *et al.*, 1990).

In order to determine the vector species of Tsutsugamushi disease in Korea, 2,466 chiggers were individually examined for *R. tsutsugamushi* by indirect immunofluorescence. Two of 447 *L. pallidum* mites were found to be positive (0.4%), and 6 of 1,142 *L. scutellare* mites were positive (0.5%). *L. pallidum* is the predominant species and is distributed throughout the Korean Peninsula, except for the southern part. *L. pallidum* started appearing in September, showed a large peak in October–November (83.2%) and a small peak in April–May (9.2%), and almost disappeared in winter and summer. *L. scutellare*, on the other hand, is distributed at high density in the southern part of the Korean Peninsula and Cheju Island. This species started appearing in September (1.4%), showed a prominent peak in October (81.7%), sharply decreased in November (16.6%), and disappeared thereafter (Ree *et al.*, 1991a, 1991b; Ree's personal communication to Kawamura, 1993).

People's Republic of China (*Fan* et al., *1987*)
As stated in the Historical Background section above, the existence of Tsutsugamushi disease has been known in China since ancient times. However, the first actual recorded cases of Tsutsugamushi disease in China were two patients in 1942 in Kunming, Yunnan Province, confirmed through use of the Weil-Felix test and by elevated agglutinating antibodies against *Proteus* OX-K. *R. tsutsugamushi* was successfully isolated in 1948 from patients in Guangdong Province, and 26 cases were confirmed in 1949. In 1952, the vector trombiculid mites were identified as *L. deliense*. Subsequently, *R. tsutsugamushi* was isolated from Tsutsugamushi disease patients in eight southeastern and southwestern provinces, and the disease was clinically observed in four other provinces. Between 1952 and 1954, there was an outbreak of more than 500 cases in Guangzhou (Canton), where the fatality rate was as high as 5.4%.

However, the incidence of Tsutsugamushi disease in southwestern China then rapidly decreased, with a small number of patients reported in 1981–1984. However, on Hainan Island, Tsutsugamushi disease actually continued to occur, with the number of patients exceeding 10,000 between 1956 and 1985. Seroepidemiological studies of the residents of Hainan Island, using the complement fixation reaction, identified 52.5% as antibody-positive in 1983 and 31.8% in 1984. These patients were distributed over the entire island, and *R. tsutsugamushi* was isolated from patients in all parts of the island. Similar seroepidemiological results were found in 1986 in Sha Wan County of the Xinjiang Uygur Autonomous Region, where as many as 36.1% of normal, healthy people were antibody-positive, as determined by indirect immunofluorescence. These results suggest the presence of atypical Tsutsugamushi disease due to reinfections or multiple infections, based on the heterogeneity of *R. tsutsugamushi* and inapparent infections of weakly pathogenic *R. tsutsugamushi*, in addition to typical Tsutsugamushi disease.

In Fujian Province in the southeastern region of China, outbreaks of Tsutsugamushi disease were observed beginning in 1951, and *R. tsutsugamushi* was isolated from patients, field rodents, and trombiculid mites. A similar phenomenon was observed in Zhejiang Province, also, beginning in 1954. In addition, in 1951, Tsutsugamushi disease was reported for the first time in the Guangxi Zhuang Autonomous Region, 75% of the cases occurring in June–August. The time of the outbreak was similar to that in other regions: beginning in May, peaking in June–July, and abating in August.

However, Hainan Island is an exception, cases being found year-round, as in Southeast Asia. The above-mentioned time of outbreak also approximately coincides with the time of *L. deliense* emergence. However, patients in Fujian Province who became symptomatic during the *L. deliense*-free period may possibly have been exposed to *L. scutellare* as the vector, whose mite is found during the same period. The majority of vector mites responsible for Tsutsugamushi disease in Zhejiang Province are believed to be *L. gaohuensis*. The *R. tsutsugamushi* types isolated in Fujian Province were Karp, Gilliam, Karp-Gilliam mixtures, and TA 716.

At about the time of resurgence of Tsutsugamushi disease in Korea, beginning in 1985, the first occurrence of Tsutsugamushi disease in Shandong Province was reported in 1986. There had been suspected cases in the past, but these were the first definitive cases. Patients became symptomatic in September, with the peak number of cases (84.6%) occurring in October. The vector is likely to have been *L. pallidum*.

Taiwan

In 1908, a febrile disease with a rash, which was endemic in the eastern region of Taiwan, was reported as a Tsutsugamushi disease-like ailment; in 1914 it was confirmed to be Tsutsugamushi disease. Due partly to the fact that Taiwan was under Japanese domination at the time, comparative studies with classical Japanese Tsutsugamushi disease were conducted, and a low fatality (approximately 3%) was verified (Hatori, 1919–20; Kawamura, 1926; Morishita, 1934). Subsequently, the Pescadores in Taiwan attracted attention as an isolated island group where the incidence of the disease was high (Yamamiya and Honda, 1933).

Currently, the annual incidence of the disease in Taiwan is more than 100, and the vector trombiculid mite for Tsutsugamushi disease in the plains, including the isolated islands of the Pescadores, is principally *L. deliense*, as it is in Southeast Asia. However, in the mountainous and forested areas, *L. scutellare* and *L. pallidum* have also been collected, and their involvement as vectors is notable (Otsuru, 1992). The typing of 49 *R. tsutsugamushi* strains isolated from humans, trombiculid mites (*L. deliense*), and field rodents in the Pescadores by direct immunofluorescence showed 46.9% TA716 and 34.7% Karp + TA716 mixture, resembling the findings in Fujian Province, China (Shirai *et al*., 1982b). In subtropical and tropical regions, such as Southeast Asia and the western Pacific, as in Taiwan and on Hainan Island, Tsutsugamushi disease occurs virtually all year around. The vectors will be described in later chapters.

4. Variations in Disease Severity

a. Fatality

Prior to the introduction of antibiotics in 1950, classical Tsutsugamushi disease in Japan was often fatal: in Niigata Prefecture, fatality was 31.9% in the period 1903–1948; in Akita Prefecture, 36.8% in the period 1915–1917, and 21.1% in the period 1920–1950; and in Yamagata Prefecture, 40.1% in the period 1913–1949. The number of patients was high in Niigata but low in Yamagata (Kawamura, 1926; Tamiya, 1962). However, beginning in 1950, with the exception of deaths due to misdiagnoses (the majority of these being due to the new type of Tsutsugamushi disease), there were no further fatalities.

Tsutsugamushi disease fatality in the Pescadores, Taiwan, was low in the pre-1950 years, being approximately 3% (Yamamiya and Honda, 1933). Fatality in the Allied forces in World War II battlefields in Southeast Asia and the western Pacific averaged 3.85%, with highs of 27.5% and 35.5% in some places and lows of 1.5% and 0.6% in others; there were marked regional variations (Philip, 1948a). In the People's Republic of China, the fatality of Tsutsugamushi disease prior to the use of antibiotics was as high as 5.4% in some areas like Guangzhou (Fan *et al*., 1987).

To summarize, Tsutsugamushi disease-related fatality prior to the introduction of antibiotics varied widely, depending on the locality. This phenomenon is assumed to be due to variation in the pathogenicity of *Rickettsia tsutsugamushi* in humans. Compared to classical Tsutsugamushi disease, the new types of Tsutsugamushi disease, such as Shichito fever in Japan, generally display mild symptoms (see Chapter 3) and are not fatal, provided that suitable treatment is given. However, it is noteworthy that the *R. tsutsugamushi* strain which causes Tsutsugamushi disease in humans but has low pathogenicity in mice is still widely endemic (see Chapters 2 and 3).

b. Reinfection

R. tsutsugamushi strains are extremely heterogeneous. Consequently, even cellular immunity cannot cope with the entire range of strain differences, and it is not uncommon for subjects to have reinfections of Tsutsugamushi disease three times or more in highly endemic areas with dense populations of *R. tsutsugamushi*-positive mites. For example, in one area highly endemic for classical Tsutsugamushi disease in Japan (Niigata Prefecture), the reinfection rate in 104 cases was 29.8%, and the rate of reinfection three or more times was 4.8% (Tamiya, 1962). Similar rates were seen in Tsutsugamushi disease cases in the Chinese military garrisoned in the Pescadores, Taiwan, in 1976–1977; of 103 patients, 78 were primary infections and 25 were reinfections. In addition, during the course of subsequent investigations, 14 cases of single or multiple reinfections were found in these two groups, but all patients were asymptomatic (Bourgeois *et al.*, 1982).

c. Inapparent infection

Some strains of *R. tsutsugamushi* are obviously weakly pathogenic to humans, and even when humans are infected, no reaction other than an immune response occurs, and infections can be demonstrated only serologically. As noted above, this phenomenon is different from reinfection or repeat infections of *R. tsutsugamushi* that are asymptomatic. In 1960, Shishido (1962b) measured, by means of complement fixation, anti-*R. tsutsugamushi* antibody levels in school children from Hachijo Island, Izu Shichito. Although more than 5 years had elapsed since an epidemic outbreak of Shichito fever, 45/100 (45%) seropositive subjects were detected. Of these 45, only 4 had a history of Shichito fever. In the autumn of 1959, there were a few cases of Tsutsugamushi disease among infantrymen of the Japanese Self-Defense Forces stationed at the foot of Mt. Fuji at the Fuji School. During this period, 10 of 148 infantrymen who visited the medical services office with a so-called common cold showed a seropositive reaction for anti-*R. tsutsugamushi* antibody by complement fixation. These cases may have been, in a strict sense, either very mild or abortive cases of Tsutsugamushi disease.

Seroepidemiological studies were conducted, using indirect immunofluorescence, in examining the subjects of a repeat epidemic of Tsutsugamushi disease that began in 1976 on Miyake Island, Izu Shichito. These studies were also conducted to examine the general population of Toshima Island, where no incidence had previously been reported. The results from both islands demonstrated that approximately one-quarter of the inhabitants were positive for anti-*R. tsutsugamushi* antibodies. Moreover, interviews of all persons with positive serologies revealed that none of them had a history of Shichito fever, and none had symptoms of the disease in the previous 2 years (Kawamura *et al.*, 1980). Fan *et al.* (1987) reported a similar phenomenon in their seroepidemiological studies of Hainan Island inhabitants using the complement fixation reaction. They found that in 1983, 52.5% of the population were positive for anti-*R. tsutsugamushi* antibodies; in 1984, 31.8% were positive. In addition, in a seroepidemiological study of healthy individuals in the Xinjiang Uygur Autonomous Region conducted in 1986, using an indirect immunofluorescence assay, they found that 36.1% of this population were seropositive. These results may be interpreted as being due to variations in pathogenicity to humans rather than to the heterogeneity of *R. tsutsugamushi*.

d. Low pathogenicity of Rickettsia tsutsugamushi

In mice, it is relatively easy to isolate *R. tsutsugamushi* from Tsutsugamushi disease patients exhibiting typical symptoms. The majority of *R. tsutsugamushi* isolates are frequently highly pathogenic to mice. However, many *R. tsutsugamushi* researchers have found empirically that there are *R. tsutsugamushi* strains that cannot be isolated and passaged in mice, as they do not exhibit typical disease pattern in mice even though they are pathogenic to humans. In addition, some strains of *R. tsutsugamushi* have been confirmed to have low pathogenicity and to manifest as inapparent infections in humans, as described above (Fan *et al.*, 1987; Kawamura *et al.*, 1980; Shishido, 1962b). The mechanism that underlies *R.*

tsutsugamushi pathogenicity in humans and mice is not known. To elucidate this mechanism it is necessary to analyze the different levels of pathogenicity exhibited by *R. tsutsugamushi* in humans and mice.

With regard to host factors, there are mouse strains that are naturally susceptible or resistant to *R. tsutsugamushi* infection, and it has been shown that this natural resistance is controlled by the *Ric* gene (Groves and Osterman, 1978; Groves *et al.*, 1980). Consequently, it is conceivable that susceptible mouse strains could be used to isolate *R. tsutsugamushi*. However, this would exclude the isolation of *R. tsutsugamushi* strains that have low pathogenicity in mice, as stated above. In order to overcome this problem, Kobayashi *et al.* (1978) used cyclophosphamide, an immunosuppressive agent, in mice at the time of isolating *R. tsutsugamushi* and succeeded in isolating *R. tsutsugamushi* that had low pathogenicity to mice. They also reported that it was possible to passage these *R. tsutsugamushi* strains as long as cyclophosphamide was used. This method contributed to the successful isolation, in Miyazaki Prefecture, of the Irie and Hirano strains, which have low pathogenicity in mice although they produce typical symptoms of Tsutsugamushi disease in humans.

The use of cyclophosphamide was also a key to the successful isolation of the Shimokoshi strain (Niigata Prefecture) (Tamura *et al.*, 1984) and the Kawasaki (Miyazaki Prefecture) (Yamamoto *et al.*, 1986), and Kuroki (Miyazaki Prefecture) (Yamamoto *et al.*, 1989) strains, which are genotypically different from the three existing prototypes of *R. tsutsugamushi* described in Chapters 2 and 3. The significance of the isolation of these three new strains is further enhanced by the fact that they were added to the previous three prototype strains to make the six prototype strains used for *R. tsutsugamushi* typing in Japan. Incidentally, these *R. tsutsugamushi* strains with low pathogenicity in mice are easy to maintain since they grow in cell cultures at a level similar to that of a highly pathogenic *R. tsutsugamushi*. In addition, athymic nude mice were used to restore the pathogenicity of *R. tsutsugamushi* which had been attenuated as a consequence of repeated passages in yolk sac or mice (Murata and Kawamura, 1977). Nude mice have also been proven to be very useful for isolation and passage of *R. tsutsugamushi* having low pathogenicity to normal mice (Kawamura *et al.*, 1980). The important problem remaining is the isolation of *R. tsutsugamushi* strains that exhibit only inapparent infections in humans and totally lack pathogenicity in mice. It may be necessary to isolate *R. tsutsugamushi* in larval trombiculid mites directly using cell cultures and to materially identify the factors that determine pathogenicity.

5. Biotechnological Approaches to the Investigation of *Rickettsia tsutsugamushi* and Its Transmission Dynamics

In Japan, nationwide outbreaks of Tsutsugamushi disease began again in 1974, occurring in rapid succession. Coincidentally, at about that time, novel experimental methods were being introduced for *R. tsutsugamushi* studies by research groups in both the United States and Japan; in particular, biotechnological approaches such as cell engineering and genetic engineering were used.

Meanwhile, with the establishment of laboratory colonies of the vector mites, the research achievements were astonishing. The research focused on the elucidation and typing of *R. tsutsugamushi* heterogeneity at the molecular level and on analysis of the interaction between *R. tsutsugamushi* and the vector mites.

a. Isolation of R. tsutsugamushi *with mild pathogenicity to mice*

For the isolation of *R. tsutsugamushi* strains only mildly pathogenic to mice, various techniques were established to facilitate the isolation and passage of the pathogen; *e.g.*, an immunosuppressive agent, cyclophosphamide, was administered to conventional mice (Kobayashi *et al.*, 1978), or athymic nude mice were used (Kawamura *et al.*, 1980; Murata and Kawamura, 1977). These techniques led to the isolation of the Shimokoshi (Tamura *et al.*, 1984), Kawasaki (Yamamoto *et al.*, 1986), and Kuroki (Yamamoto *et al.*, 1989) strains, which would have been overlooked if conventional techniques had been used. These strains are genotypically different *R. tsutsugamushi* that are only mildly pathogenic to mice, although they are pathogenic to humans.

b. Culture of R. tsutsugamushi

The conventional method of culturing *R. tsutsugamushi* involved inoculation into the yolk sac of embryonated eggs. In 1959, a tissue culture technique was used to culture typhus group rickettsiae; since that time, this technique has also been used for the culture of *R. tsutsugamushi,* and it is now the principal technique. The cells predominantly used for culture are mouse fibroblast-derived L-929 cells (Tamura *et al.*, 1982; Urakami *et al.*, 1983) and the green monkey kidney cell-derived BS-Cl and BS-C40 cell lines (Tachibana *et al.*, 1982; Yamamoto *et al.*, 1986, 1989). No variation in growth was found among the *R. tsutsugamushi* strains. The majority of the *R. tsutsugamushi* strains used today are cloned by the plaque method.

c. Purification of rickettsia cells

Many techniques have been used to purify rickettsia cells to analyze the metabolic, chemical, and morphologic properties of *R. tsutsugamushi*. In the era when the source of rickettsia was yolk sac emulsion, various methods were used: a differential centrifugation-based ethyl-ether-water method (Cragie, 1945), a Celite treatment method (Bovarnick and Snyder, 1949), and a bovine serum albumin treatment method (Bovarnick and Miller, 1950); however, the anticipated objective was not achieved with *R. tsutsugamushi*. The cation exchange resin method (Amberlite XE-64) (Kawamura, 1962; Yamamoto *et al.*, 1958) then appeared, and this contributed to antigenic analyses and metabolic studies. However, only partial purification was achieved. After tissue culture became the source for *R. tsutsugamushi* growth, Shishido *et al.* (1969) succeeded in fractionating *R. tsutsugamushi* into particular antigens (type-specific antigens) and soluble antigens (group-specific antigens) for the first time, by carrying out density gradient centrifugation of ultrasonically disrupted material. However, the results suggested that *R. tsutsugamushi* was unlike other rickettsia species; common soluble antigens were present in extremely low quantities and antigenicity was controlled by type-specific antigens. As this procedure had a yield problem, density gradient centrifugation, using Renografin (Dasch and Weiss, 1977), which had produced favorable results in the purification of other rickettsiae, was used for the purification of *R. tsutsugamushi*. However, since the surface properties of *R. tsutsugamushi* differed from those of other rickettsiae species, it was difficult to separate *R. tsutsugamushi* from host cell components with Renografin. Taking the envelope adhesive nature of *R. tsutsugamushi* into consideration, Tamura *et al.* (1982) established a purification technique using density gradient centrifugation with Percoll. This technique resulted in the purification of type-specific antigens (TSA) of *R. tsutsugamushi* and made possible the elucidation of the genetic code and of the total amino acid sequences.

d. Introduction of monoclonal antibodies

Monoclonal antibodies to the respective different *R. tsutsugamushi* types contributed to the purification of type-specific antigens and their genetic analysis (Eisemann and Osterman, 1985; Murata *et al.*, 1986). Although the envelope polypeptides of *R. tsutsugamushi*, which corresponded to the findings of immunoblotting (Western blot analysis) performed with conventional antisera obtained from guinea pigs and rabbits (Iida *et al.*, 1966a; Murata *et al.*, 1986; Shishido, 1962a), could have been fractionated (Oaks *et al.*, 1987; Tamura *et al.*, 1985), the type-specific antigens were more precisely analyzed by using these monoclonal antibodies (Murata *et al.*, 1986).

e. Assay system

The immunofluorescence (IF) used for the diagnosis of Tsutsugamushi disease and for *R. tsutsugamushi* assays was improved so that there was less non-specific fluorescence (Kawamura, 1977; Kawamura and Aoyama, 1983; Murata and Kawamura, 1980). At the same time, the introduction of monoclonal antibodies enhanced the importance of this technique (Murata *et al.*, 1986). Further, an indirect immunoperoxidase (IP) reaction with higher sensitivity than immunofluorescence was developed and the Western blot assay was usefully employed (Suto, 1982; Yamamoto and Minamishima, 1982). IF and IP methods for the diagnosis of Tsutsugamushi disease were recommended by a WHO Task Force meeting (Regional Office for the Western Pacific, WHO, 1987), and the methods are also used for the differentiation of immunoglobulin class.

f. Structural proteins of R. tsutsugamushi

Studies of the purification of *R. tsutsugamushi* type-specific antigens and their genes have been advanced mainly by the Tamura (Tamura *et al.*, 1985) and Stover (Stover *et al.*, 1990a) groups; the discussion here is centered on the achievements of the former group. When *R. tsutsugamushi* grown in cell culture were harvested, purified by Percoll density gradient centrifugation, solubilized, and assayed by sodium dodecyl sulfate-polyacrylamide gel electrophoresis (SDS-

PAGE), approximately ten major polypeptides were found in the *R. tsutsugamushi* envelope. Of these, the 80-, 70-, 60-, 54- to 58-, and 46- to 47-kDa polypeptides were common to all *R. tsutsugamushi* strains. Quantitatively, the 54- to 58-kDa polypeptides constituted the largest amount, accounting for approximately 20% (Oaks *et al.*, 1987; Tamura *et al.*, 1985). However, the 54- to 58-kDa polypeptides exhibited *R. tsutsugamushi* strain-dependent electrophoretic variations; the Karp, Gilliam, Kawasaki, and Shimokoshi strains were 56 kDa, the Kato strain was 54 kDa, and the Kuroki strain was 58 kDa. When purified rickettsiae were labeled with ^{125}I, using lactoperoxidase, and developed with SDS-PAGE, the 80-, 56-, 46-, 43-, 39-, 35-, 28-, and 25-kDa polypeptides were labeled. As the 56-kDa polypeptides disappeared when the rickettsiae were treated with trypsin, it was determined that these polypeptides were on the surface (Tamura *et al.*, 1985). On the other hand, the 60-kDa polypeptides, which were not labeled with ^{125}I, occurred inside, and quantitatively constituted the second largest amount after the 54- to 58-kDa polypeptides. Stover *et al.* (1990b) cloned the gene coding for this polypeptide (Karp strain) and suggested that it was a stress protein, because of its high homology with the *Escherichia coli* heat shock protein 60-kDa family.

g. *Antigenic structure of* R. tsutsugamushi

The inter-strain relationship of the *R. tsutsugamushi* structural proteins described above as antigens can be most effectively analyzed by immunoblotting following SDS-PAGE. Results obtained by this technique, even with conventional antisera, confirmed that the type-specific antigens (TSA) of various *R. tsutsugamushi* were predominantly 54- to 58-kDa polypeptides, and the group-specific antigens were 70- and 46- to 47-kDa polypeptides. In particular, the 54- to 58-kDa polypeptides exhibited strong reactivity with homologous antibodies and weak reaction with heterologous antibodies (Oaks *et al.*, 1987; Tamura *et al.*, 1985). Analysis with monoclonal antibodies clearly confirmed these results that the 54- to 58-kDa polypeptides were type-specific antigens (Eisemann and Osterman, 1985; Hanson, 1985; Murata *et al.*, 1986). Eisemann and Osterman, in 1981 extracted SDS-PAGE-fractionated polypeptides and, using enzyme-linked immunosorbent assay (ELISA), detected six antigens. However, the relationship of these polypeptides with the polypeptides fractionated by Tamura's group is unknown. Hanson and Wisseman (1981) and Hanson (1984) extracted polypeptides from the three prototype *R. tsutsugamushi* strains using detergents and, following immunoprecipitation with antisera, assayed them with SDS-PAGE. They stained the antibodies and differentiated antibody-binding polypeptides; the Karp and Gilliam strains contained 63-, 60-, and 50-kDa polypeptides and the Kato strain, 63-, 58-, 57-, and 50-kDa polypeptides. These are probably equivalent to the results of Tamura *et al.* showing 60-, 54- to 56-, and 46-kDa polypeptides (Murata *et al.*, 1986; Tamura *et al.*, 1985). In particular, since Hanson's 60-kDa polypeptide showed heat modifiability, it may be considered identical to the 54- to 58-kDa polypeptides of Tamura *et al.* In addition, Oaks *et al.* (1989) reported the existence of a 110-kDa polypeptide, in addition to a 56-kDa type-specific antigen. By analyzing the Gilliam and Karp strains with polyclonal antibodies, Tamura *et al.* (1985) also found high molecular weight antigenic polypeptides. However, they stated that the determination of molecular weight was difficult, and since the quantity was small, they doubted that they were dealing with higher action as specific antigenicity than 54- to 58-kDa polypeptides (Tamura *et al.*, 1985).

h. Heat modifiability of R. tsutsugamushi *outer membrane polypeptides*

Urakami *et al.* (1986) found that changes occurred in the migratory patterns of polypeptides depending on the difference in SDS-PAGE solubilization conditions for purified *R. tsutsugamushi*, namely, changes from 43 to 46 and 56; 25 to 28; and 21 to 25 kDa. They reported that these polypeptides were heat modifiable and that their migratory distances were affected by heat treatment. Hanson (1984), as cited above, also described a 60-kDa polypeptide that showed heat modifiability.

i. Purification of 56-kDa type-specific antigen (TSA)

In order to purify the hydrophobic outer membrane polypeptides of purified *R. tsutsugamushi*, *i.e.*, type-specific antigens, Tamura's group (Ohashi *et al.*, 1989; Takahashi *et al.*, 1985; Tamura *et al.*, 1985) first solubilized many polypeptides other than the outer membrane polypeptides by treatment with an anionic detergent (sodium N-lauroyl sarcosinate: Sarkosyl, Nakarai Chemicals, Ltd., Kyoto,

Japan). They then recovered the outer membrane polypeptides as an insoluble fraction, solubilized them in a phosphate buffer containing SDS, filtered them through a gel filtration column for high-performance liquid chromatography (HPLC), and separated the 56-kDa polypeptide fraction recovered by HPLC on a reverse-phase column. The amino acid sequences of the respective 56-kDa polypeptides of the three prototype *R. tsutsugamushi* strains obtained as described above were elucidated to positions 34–35 from the N-terminal end. The homology of the amino acid sequences of the three strains was 74–88%.

j. Cloning of type-specific antigen (TSA) polypeptide genes and base sequence analyses

Ohashi *et al.* (1990a, 1992a) cloned the type-specific antigen (56-kDa) polypeptide gene, purified as described immediately above, as follows (the Gilliam strain is used in this example):

(1) Synthesize radio-labeled oligo-deoxyribonucleotides corresponding to the seven amino acids determined in the N-terminal sequence to produce probes.
(2) Extract DNA of the Gilliam strain, cut it with the restriction enzyme, *Hin*dIII, and electrophorese.
(3) Perform Southern blotting, using the probe from (1), and recover the 2.3-kb DNA fragment detected by the probe.
(4) Incorporate the above DNA fragment into pUC plasmid vector and transduce it into *Escherichia coli*.
(5) Select radioactive (+) clones from the transformants obtained by colony hybridization using the activated probe.
(6) After recovering the transduced 2.3-kb DNA from the clones, cut them with *Pst*I or *Dra*I.
(7) Subclone with M13mp18 or M13mp19.
(8) Determine the base sequence of the 2.3-kb DNA fragment.

The results obtained by this procedure confirmed the presence of a structural gene coding for the entire region of the 56-kDa polypeptide of the Gilliam strain in the 2.3-kb *Hin*dIII fragment. Further, using the activated *Hin*dIII fragment of the Gilliam strain as a probe, Ohashi *et al.* (1990a, 1992a) were able to clone 56-kDa genes from the DNA of other prototype strains, except for the Karp strain. The open reading frame of these genes consisted of 1563–1596 bp, which coded for 521–532 amino acids. Oaks's and Stover's groups

(Oaks *et al.*, 1987, 1989; Stover *et al.*, 1987, 1990a, 1990b) analyzed *R. tsutsugamushi* genes and cloned several of the antigenic polypeptide genes. However, there are virtually no other reports. The base sequences determined were only for the 60-kDa polypeptides (internal polypeptides, *E. coli* heat shock protein 60-kDa family) (Stover *et al.*, 1990b), the type-specific antigen (56 kDa) polypeptides of the Karp strain (Stover *et al.*, 1990a), and the type-specific antigen polypeptides of Ohashi *et al.* (1990a). In addition, Oaks *et al.* (1989) found eight *R. tsutsugamushi* polypeptides, of 110, 72, 58 (Ohashi's 60 kDa), 56, 47, and 20 kDa etc. that reacted with anti-*R. tsutsugamushi* rabbit serum expressed in the λgt11 library constructed from *R. tsutsugamushi* DNA fragments.

k. Homology of the 56-kDa base sequence and amino acid composition of the type-specific antigen polypeptides of the six type R. tsutsugamushi

Stover *et al.* (1990a) determined the genetic structure and the base sequence of the Karp strain. Combining these findings of Stover *et al.* with the findings for five other *R. tsutsugamushi* strains, Ohashi *et al.* (1992a), studied the base sequence homology of the genes and the amino acid composition of the type-specific antigen 56-kDa polypeptides in the six strains that now serve as *R. tsutsugamushi* standard types in Japan. They found that: (1) homology among the three strains, Gilliam, Karp, and Kuroki (Yamamoto *et al.*, 1989) was high; there was 86–89% base sequence homology and 81–82% amino acid sequence homology; (2) the Kawasaki strain (Yamamoto *et al.*, 1986) and the Gilliam strain showed 83% base sequence homology and 76.2% amino acid sequence homology; their homology with the four other strains was lower; (3) the Shimokoshi strain (Tamura *et al.*, 1984) showed 71–73% homology with the base sequences of all the other strains and 59–62% amino acid sequence homology (the lowest homology) with other strains; and (4) the Kato strain showed 75–79% base sequence homology and 66–72% amino acid sequence homology with strains other than the Shimokoshi strain. In other words, it was confirmed that the Gilliam, Karp, and Kuroki strains were closely related; the Kawasaki strain was close to the Gilliam strain but different from other strains, and the Shimokoshi strain was the most distantly related to other strains.

l. Detection of R. tsutsugamushi *DNA by polymerase chain reaction (PCR) and nested PCR*

It is laborious to chemically determine the type-specific antigen of individual *R. tsutsugamushi* isolates. However, it has become possible to detect *R. tsutsugamushi* DNA by the polymerase chain reaction (PCR) or by nested PCR, using a part of the base sequence of the 56-kDa genes characterizing type-specific antigens of the six strains as primers (Furuya *et al.*, 1991a, 1993). In other words, in practice it has become relatively simple to detect *R. tsutsugamushi* DNA in a patient's blood, in infected mouse material, or in vector trombiculid mites. This presents a useful tool for accurately diagnosing Tsutsugamushi disease, for typing *R. tsutsugamushi*, and for elucidating *R. tsutsugamushi* transmission.

m. Transmission dynamics

The recurrent outbreaks since 1974 of the once dormant Tsutsugamushi disease in Japan are related to an increase in *R. tsutsugamushi*-positive vector mite colonies. However, there is no explanation for the increase in these colonies. In order to solve this problem, the transmission dynamics of *R. tsutsugamushi* in the vector mite foci must be elucidated. It is necessary to experimentally analyze vertical transmission by establishing *R. tsutsugamushi*-positive and -negative colonies in a laboratory. The rearing of trombiculid mites in laboratories has been attempted for many years. The problems of rearing nymphae and adult mites have been solved, and many laboratory colonies of vector mites have been successfully established by United States research groups. Colonies of *Leptotrombidium fletcheri* (*R. tsutsugamushi*-positive and -negative) (Rapmund, 1984; Rapmund *et al.*, 1969), *L. arenicola* (*R. tsutsugamushi*-positive and -negative) (Rapmund *et al.*, 1972; Roberts and Robinson, 1977), *L. deliense* (*R. tsutsugamushi*-negative only) (Rai and Bandopadhyay, 1978) have been maintained in Malaysia, and transovarian transmission of *R. tsutsugamushi* has been confirmed. In addition, the findings that *R. tsutsugamushi*-positive mites in the colonies were all female is noteworthy. Traub *et al.* (1975) attached *R. tsutsugamushi*-negative trombiculid mites to *R. tsutsugamushi*-infected animals and reported that *R. tsutsugamushi* was transferred to mites and transmitted to the subsequent generation, even if very seldom, while, other researchers have all shown negative results (see Chapter 5). Five breeding colonies of Malaysian mites were supplied to Kawamura's group in Japan for maintenance and are being bred by Takahashi.

In Japan, Takahashi *et al.* (1988b) established laboratory colonies of *R. tsutsugamushi*-positive and -negative *L. pallidum* and carried out experiments to elucidate vector transmission. However, the *R. tsutsugamushi*-positive colonies contained approximately equal male-female populations. Takahashi *et al.* are also maintaining *R. tsutsugamushi*-negative *L. akamushi* colonies, and Kawamura's group is now breeding a total of eight colonies, including the above-mentioned five Malaysian colonies. The results of experimental *R. tsutsugamushi* infections, using these colonies, and the dynamics of *R. tsutsugamushi* transmission in mites are described in Chapter 5.

6. Discovery and Nomenclature of Causative Rickettsiae

The scientific name of the causative agent of Tsutsugamushi disease is *Rickettsia tsutsugamushi* (Hayashi, 1920) Ogata, 1931, as given in the Approved List of Bacterial Names (Skerman *et al.*, 1980), following the name used for the first time in the 6th edition of Bergey's Manual of Determinative Bacteriology (1948).

The Approved List of Bacterial Names (1980) and the latest edition of Bergey's Manual (Krieg and Holt, 1984), state that January 1, 1980, was agreed upon internationally as the new starting date for the priority of bacterial scientific names. There was much debate and discussion regarding the scientific name of *R. tsutsugamushi* before 1980; however, since then all such discussion has ceased. Highlights in the history of the discovery and naming of this causative agent are briefly recorded and reviewed in this section.

Bergey's Manual (7th ed., 1957) states that the specific name *R. tsutsugamushi* originates from *Theileria tsutsugamushi* Hayashi, 1920, despite Hayashi's descriptions and illustrations that clearly showed organisms belonging to the genus *Theileria* of order Piroplasmida Wenyon, 1926 in protozoan Sporozoa. Wolbach, cited in Blake *et al.* (1945), did not believe that Hayashi had ever seen the actual causative organism; Wolbach followed the methods that Hayashi had employed and concluded that Hayashi could not have demonstrated true rickettsiae by these methods. Most rickettsiologists now believe that the description given in Hayashi (1920) was not a description of *Rickettsia*, and that the organism was mistakenly termed *Theileria* in that paper.

Rickettsial organisms were clearly distinguished for the first time in a study by Ogata and Unno (1929), who injected the blood of a human patient into a rabbit testis and were successful in isolating, demonstrating, and successively transferring the causative organisms to the other testis. Although the paper was written in Japanese (and the information was not, therefore, widely disseminated) and no binomial scientific name was given, these investigators were the true discoverers of this causative agent of Tsutsugamushi disease. In 1927, Ogata had given material containing these causative agents to Nagayo and to R. Kawamura.

Nagayo *et al.* (1930) were successful in demonstrating the massive proliferation of the causative agents in Descemet's membrane of the anterior eye chamber of the rabbit, and they identified the organism as *Rickettsia* for the first time, describing the isolated agent by the scientific name *Rickettsia orientalis*.

Ogata (1931) described *Rickettsia tsutsugamushi*, and Kawamura and Imagawa (1931) described *Rickettsia akamushi*. Even though Ogata and Unno (1929) were the first discoverers of the causative agent, *R. tsutsugamushi* Ogata, 1931 is a synonym for *R. orientalis*, the same as *R. akamushi* Kawamura *et* Imagawa, 1931, in accordance with the International Code of Nomenclature.

Bergey's Manual (1948) was misleading and caused confusion in regard to the nomenclature of this rickettsia. The family Rickettsiaceae was not listed in the 5th edition of the Manual (1939) and appeared for the first time in the 6th edition (1948).

The 1948 description, which gave *Rickettsia tsutsugamushi* (Hayashi) Ogata, without referring to the years of publication, totally adopted the report of a member of the U.S. Armed Forces Health Services Staff who studied papers in Japan and interviewed the Japanese researchers concerned immediately after World War II in occupied Japan and arrived at his own conclusion, ignoring the principles of the International Code of Nomenclature and the opinions of the Japanese researchers. His report, described in a footnote in the 6th edition (1948), was misleading in regard to the scientific name of the *Rickettsia* that is a causative agent of Tsutsugamushi disease.

This footnote stated that *Theileria tsutsugamushi* Hayashi, 1920 was the first description of the causative agent of Tsutsugamushi disease, mainly because Hayashi in his report "On Rickettsia" (1924) expressed the opinion that his organism was a rickettsia, although he did not denote a binominal scientific name in that report. After comparative studies Hayashi later reached the conclusion (1932) that his rickettsia, *R. tsutsugamushi* of Ogata, and *Rickettsia orientalis* of Nagayo *et al.* referred to one and the same species. Ogata was identified as the first researcher who used the binomial name *Rickettsia tsutsugamushi*. Finally, this footnote stated that, under these conditions, the only valid name appears to be *Rickettsia tsutsugamushi*. When we read these descriptions now, we note that the international code contains no such effective rule where by two authors' names can be loosely used for a scientific name in that way.

In the 7th edition of Bergey's Manual (1957), the name was changed to *Rickettsia tsutsugamushi* (Hayashi, 1920) Ogata, 1931. This description correctly demonstrated that Hayashi had discovered the causative agent and Ogata had changed the generic name from *Theileria* to *Rickettsia*, as mentioned in the footnote in the 6th edition (1948). Nevertheless, there was no such interpretation or conclusion in the 6th edition (1948).

Even if Hayashi's description (1920) had been correct, when the genus was changed from *Theileria* to *Rickettsia*, only the first publication, which used *Rickettsia* as the generic name, should have been considered. In this case, *Theileria tsutsugamushi* Hayashi, 1920 should have been changed to *Rickettsia tsutsugamushi* (Hayashi, 1920) Nagayo *et al.*, 1930.

Nevertheless, since the name *Theileria tsutsugamushi*, is not regarded as the correct name for the true causative agent of Tsutsugamushi disease, it can be concluded, that the first valid description of the causative agent using the correct binomial scientific name was the one published by Nagayo *et al.* (1930).

The above evidence, presented chronologically, leads to the conclusion that the correct scientific name should have been *Rickettsia orientalis* Nagayo, Tamiya, Mitamura *et* Sato, 1930, if the International Code of Nomenclature of Bacteria (Lopage *et al.*, 1976) before 1980 is strictly followed without emotion or sentiment, even though moral issues remained unsettled between Nagayo *et al.* (1930) to Ogata (1931). It is regrettable that the first wrong description in 1948 was accepted, misused, and finally authorized in the Approved List in 1980.

2

Microbiological Aspects of *Rickettsia tsutsugamushi*

1. Structure of *Rickettsia tsutsugamushi*

a. Morphology

R. tsutsugamushi is an obligate intracellular parasite that multiplies in the host cell cytoplasm by binary fission. The rickettsiae are easily observed with a light microscope in specimens stained by a modification of the Giménez procedure or by Giemsa's stain (Fig. 1). Macchiabello staining, which is generally used for the observation of microbes in other species of the genus *Rickettsia*, is not recommended for *R. tsutsugamushi*, because the red color with basic fuchsin fades easily during the decolorization step in counter-staining.

The first electron microscopic observation of *R. tsutsugamushi* was reported in 1959 by Higashi, who observed rickettsiae multiplying in host cell cytoplasm and being released from the host cell sur-

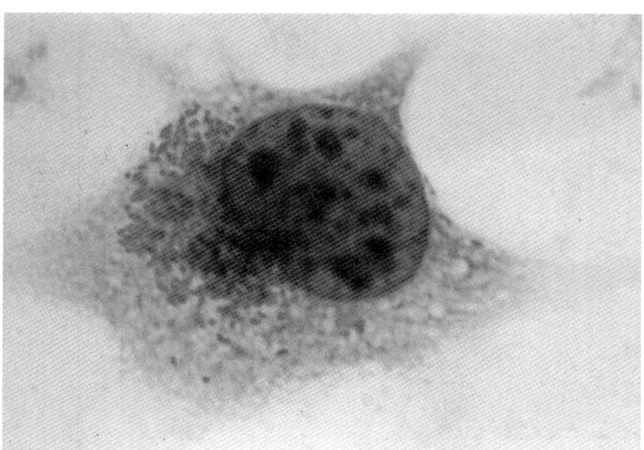

Fig. 1. *R. tsutsugamushi* seen in L cell culture by Giemsa staining

face. Subsequently, several investigators have reported on various aspects of electron microscopic observations of this rickettsia (Ewing *et al.*, 1978; Hase, 1983a, 1983b; Ito and Rikihisa, 1981; Rikihisa and Ito, 1980, 1981, 1982, 1983; Rikihisa *et al.*, 1979; Silverman and Wisseman, 1978; Tsuruhara *et al.*, 1982; Urakami *et al.*, 1982a, 1982b, 1983, 1984)

Figure 2 shows intracellular *R. tsutsugamushi* sectioned at the center along the long axis. The fundamental morphology of the rickettsia is similar to that of gram-negative bacteria, the organism is surrounded by a cytoplasmic membrane and a cell wall, showing a clear periplasmic space, where amorphous materials are seen. In the cytoplasm, the electron-dense ribosome-rich area and the less dense network area with DNA fibers are distinctive, but in general, no

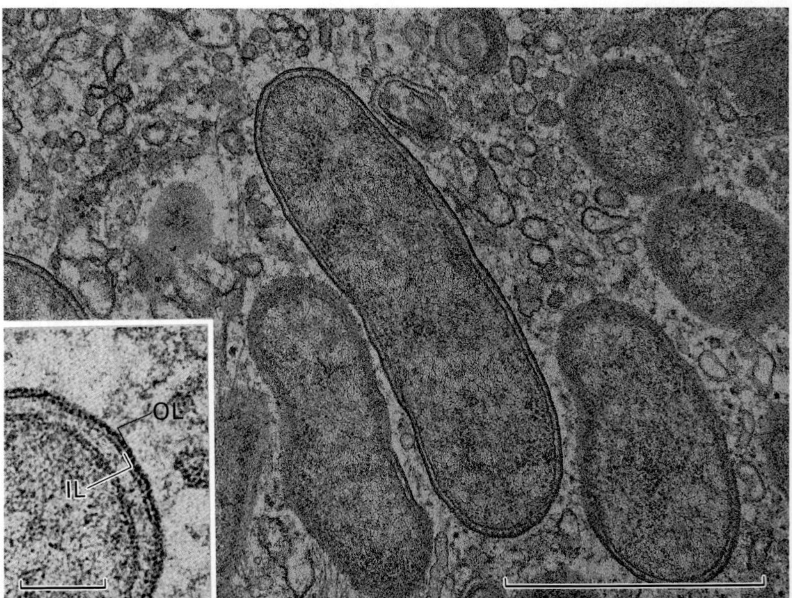

Fig. 2. a. Electron micrograph of thin section of a rickettsia observed in a cell at 72 h after infection. Bar indicates 1 μm.
b. Higher magnification of the rickettsial surface. OL: outer leaflet of cell wall; IL: inner leaflet of cell wall. Bar indicates 0.1 μm.

other characteristic structures are seen. Wright *et al.* (1984) observed tubular structures inside rickettsiae in the vector mite, but these structures are rarely observed in rickettsiae growing in cultured cells.

Generally *R. tsutsugamushi* is approximately 0.5 μm wide and 1.2 to 3.0 μm long. This size, estimated by electron microscopic observation, is a little larger than that of the typhus and spotted fever group rickettsiae, which range from 0.2 to 0.56 μm in width and 0.5 to 2.5 μm in length (Table 1) (Tamura *et al.*, 1990b). On light microscopic observations, however, *R. tsutsugamushi* seems to be smaller than other rickettsiae (Krieg and Holt, 1984). This discrepancy may be due to the presence of capsule layers that are recognized electron-microscopically on the surface of typhus and spotted fever-group rickettsiae but not on *R. tsutsugamushi*. Occasionally, extremely long forms of *R. tsutsugamushi*, several micrometers longer than those commonly seen, are seen in infected cells (Fig. 7c) (Urakami *et*

Table 1. Size of Rickettsiae in Ultrathin Sections

Species	Size (μm)		Host cell	References
	Width	Length		
R. prowazekii	0.35	0.9	L cells	Smirnova *et al.*, 1986
	0.45	1.5	CE cells	Silverman *et al.*, 1980
(in log phase)	0.32	1.4	CE cells	Wisseman *et al.*, 1976
(in stationary phase)	0.27	0.7	CE cells	Wisseman *et al.*, 1976
R. typhi	0.4	2.0	Louse	Ito *et al.*, 1978
	0.2–0.3	< 1.0	Yolk sac	Ito *et al.*, 1975
	0.3–0.45	< 2.5	Flea	Ito *et al.*, 1975
R. canada	0.4	1.6	Tick	Lyle and Burgdorfer, 1971
R. rickettsii	0.25–0.4[c]		CE cells	Silverman and Wisseman, 1979
	0.3[b]	0.5[b]	L cells	[a]
R. sibirica	0.5[b]	1.3[b]	L cells	[a]
R. rhipicephali	0.39–0.56	0.86–1.7	Tick	Hayes and Burdorfer, 1979
R. tsutsugamushi	0.5–0.6	1.5–1.6	L cells	Wright *et al.*, 1984
	0.6–0.8[c]	1.2–3.0[c]	BHK cells	Rikihisa and Ito, 1983
	0.5–0.7[b]	1.3–2.5[b]	L cells	Urakami *et al.*, 1984
	0.6[b]	1.3–2.5[b]	Mite	Urakami *et al.*, 1988b

[a] Unpublished data, Tamura's laboratory.

[b] Measured by the same observation methods.

[c] Measurement was done for the micrographs in the references.

al., 1984). These may be produced by a disorder in rickettsial cell division.

There are morphological differences in the cell walls among species of the genus *Rickettsia*. Silverman and Wisseman (1978) reported that the outer leaflet of the cell wall in the typhus and spotted fever group rickettsiae was thinner than the inner leaflet. However, in *R. tsutsugamushi*, the outer leaflet of the cell wall is thicker than the inner leaflet. This morphological difference in the cell wall may reflect different chemical structures in these microorganisms, as described below. A capsule-like layer is observed on the surface of the typhus and spotted fever rickettsiae (Anacker *et al.*, 1967; Hayes and Burgdorfer, 1979, 1982; Ito *et al.*, 1975, 1978; Popov and Ignatovich, 1976; Popov *et al.*, 1986; Silverman and Wisseman, 1978; Silverman *et al.*, 1978), and an electron lucent halo zone is observed around these rickettsiae growing in the host cells (Hayes and Burgdorfer, 1979, 1982; Ito *et al.*, 1975, 1978; Lyle and Burgdorfer, 1971; Popov *et al.*, 1986, 1987; Silverman *et al.*, 1987). In *R. tsutsugamushi*, however, the capsule-like layer is not clear, and the halo zone around the intracellular rickettsiae is not recognized, although Silverman and Wisseman (1978) suggested the presence of a capsule-like layer on the surface of *R. tsutsugamushi* in electron-microscopic observations of antibody-treated rickettsiae. *R. tsutsugamushi* is surrounded by a very soft and fragile outer envelope, and is disrupted easily by osmotic shock (Takahashi *et al.*, 1985). In cell-free suspension, the rickettsiae are round (Tamura *et al.*, 1982), while they are rod- or coccobacillus-shaped at the growing stage in the host cell cytoplasm (Urakami *et al.*, 1984). This property clearly distinguishes them from other species of rickettsiae. The difference in fragility may also reflect differences in the chemical structure of the cell walls, as discussed below.

b. *Chemical composition*

In rickettsiae of the typhus and spotted fever groups and in *Coxiella burnetii*, lipopolysaccharide (LPS) and its components have been isolated and the LPS ladder pattern has been observed on polyacrylamide gel electrophoresis (PAGE) analysis (Amano and Williams, 1984b; Amano *et al.*, 1984; Baca and Paretsky, 1974; Schramek and Mayer, 1982; Schramek *et al.*, 1977). Further, the presence of muramic acid and diaminopimelic acid was demonstrated in the typhus group rickettsiae (Allison and Perkins, 1960; Myers *et al.*, 1967) and in *C. burnetii* (Amano and Williams, 1984b), suggesting the presence of peptidoglycan in these rickettsiae. However, Amano *et al.* (1987) found that *R. tsutsugamushi* lacked muramic acid, glucosamine, heptose, 3-deoxy-D-mannooctulosonic acid (KDO), and hydroxy fatty acids, which are the general components of peptidoglycan or LPS. Furthermore, in the proteinase K-digestion of whole rickettsiae, no LPS-like bands were seen on PAGE analysis (Amano *et al.*, 1987). These lines of evidence lead to the conclusion that *R. tsutsugamushi* lacks both peptidoglycan and LPS in the cell wall. This conclusion coincides well with evidence that *R. tsutsugamushi* is completely resistant to the beta-lactam antibiotics (Miyamura *et al.*, 1989), which inhibit bacterial peptidoglycan synthesis, whereas these antibiotics disturb the growth of other rickettsiae, such as *R. prowazekii* and *R. rickettsii* (Wisseman *et al.*, 1974, 1982). The differences in the morphology and fragility of the cell wall between *R. tsutsugamushi* and other species of the genus *Rickettsia* may also reflect these differences in the chemical structure among these rickettsiae. Additionally, the lack of LPS supports the finding that treatment of *R. tsutsugamushi* with periodate does not alter its antigenic properties in the neutralization test of infectivity with immune sera (Hanson, 1985).

Sodium dodecyl sulfate (SDS)-PAGE of purified *R. tsutsugamushi* lysates (Tamura *et al.*, 1985) reveals as many as 30 polypeptide bands (Fig. 3a, b). The major polypeptides are designated as 110, 80, 70, 60, 56, 46, 42, 35, 28, and 25 kDa from their mobility on the PAGE analysis. These polypeptides, except for the 70 and 60 kDa, are labeled by the surface radioiodination method, indicating that they are located on the rickettsial surface. The 56-kDa polypeptide is present in the largest amounts. This polypeptide is an immunodominant antigen showing type-specific antigenicity (Ohashi *et al.*, 1988), and is easily digested by treatment of intact rickettsiae with trypsin (Tamura *et al.*, 1985), indicating that it is located in the outermost layer. There are minor differences in the polypeptide patterns in PAGE among antigenically different strains, *i.e.*, the Gilliam, Karp, Kato, Shimokoshi, Kawasaki, and Kuroki (Fig. 3b). For example, the 56-kDa band in the strains appears in the 54-kDa region in the Kato strain and in the 58-kDa region in the Kuroki strain, and the 46-kDa band in the Karp strain is located in

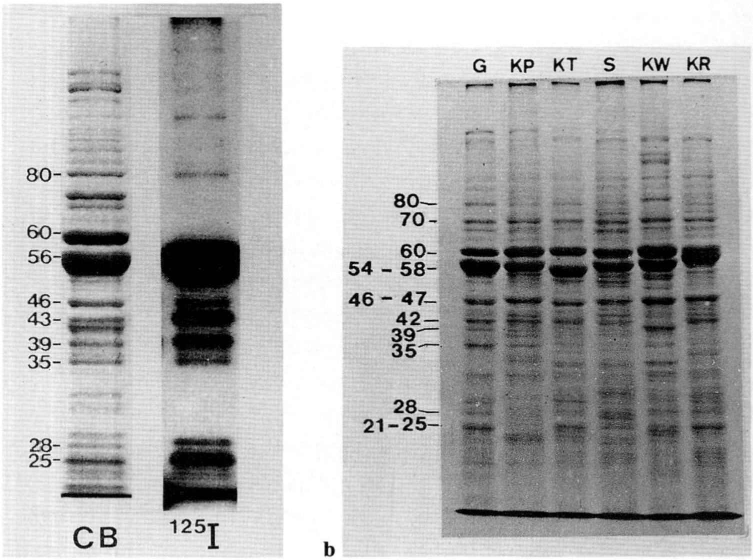

Fig. 3. a. SDS-PAGE pattern of radioiodinated polypeptides in rickettsiae (Gilliam strain). The left and right columns show the pattern of Coomassie blue staining and the autoradiogram, respectively. The numbers on the left side indicate the molecular size (in kDa) of the bands which were determined in comparison with the migrations of standard proteins.

b. SDS-PAGE patterns of antigenically distinctive strains of *R. tsutsugamushi* (Coomassie blue staining). G: Gilliam; KP: Karp; KT: Kato; S: Shimokoshi; KW: Kawasaki; KR: Kuroki. The numbers on the left side are the same as those in panel a.

the 47-kDa region. However, the overall patterns of polypeptides on PAGE are similar in the different antigenic type strains. Three polypeptides, 56, 28, and 25 kDa, are heat-modifiable and are located in the 43-, 25-, and 21-kDa regions on PAGE analysis when the rickettsial sample is solubilized at less than 50°C (Urakami *et al.*, 1986). When the sample is solubilized in buffer without 2-mercaptoethanol (2-ME), the 46-kDa polypeptide is located in the 43-kDa region on PAGE analysis, suggesting that it contains intramolecular S-S bonds (Urakami *et al.*, 1986). It is possible that the 56-kDa polypeptide may form dimers or oligomers in the intact rickettsiae, since on PAGE analysis, the bands in the more than 100-kDa region in samples solubilized in buffer without 2-ME move to the

56-kDa position after treatment with 2-ME (Urakami *et al.*, 1986).

The 60-kDa polypeptide is located inside the rickettsial cells, but sometimes shows antigenicity in acute infection in humans (Ohashi *et al.*, 1988) and animals (Hanson, 1985). The antigenicity is group-specific (Ohashi *et al.*, 1988). Stover *et al.*, (1990b) cloned and sequenced the gene encoding this protein, and found a common amino acid sequence with heat-shock proteins of other bacteria and the stress protein promoter locus upstream of the start codon.

The 25- and 47-kDa polypeptides located on the rickettsial surface show subgroup-specific and group-specific antigenicity, respectively (Ohashi *et al.*, 1988; Tamura *et al.*, 1985). The 70-kDa polypeptide shows group-specific antigenicity (Tamura *et al.*, 1985), but its localization in the rickettsiae is obscure.

The genomic size of the genus *Rickettsia* is in the range of 1.1 – 1.5×10^9 dalton which corresponds to about 2000-kb pairs (Myers and Wisseman, 1980, 1981; Myers *et al.*, 1979, 1980). Recent pulse field gel electrophoresis analysis of genomic DNA in *R. tsutsugamushi* indicates that the size ranges from 2400- to 2700 -kb pairs for the various strains (Shimada *et al.*, 1994). The guanine and cytocine (G + C) contents of the DNA of these microbes in the genus *Rickettsia* have been determined by Tm (melting temperature) assay, density measurement, and high-performance liquid chromatography (HPLC) methods (Table 2). The G + C contents of DNA from six

Table 2. Comparison of G + C Contents in Rickettsial DNA

Rickettsiae		Source of	G+C contents			
Species	Strains	purified rickettsia	From density	From Tm	HPLC assay	References
Typhus group						
R. prowazekii	Madrid E	Yolk sac	30.3±0.4	29.3±0.9		a
		Human		28.5		b
	Breinl	Yolk sac	29.7±0.3	29.0±0.8		a
		Human		29.0		b
	Burundi	Human		29.7		b
	Flying squirrel	Flying squirrel		29.5		b
R. typhi	Wilmington	L cells	30.8±0.7	29.5±0.5		a
		Yolk sac	29.8±0.3	29.0±0.3		a
		Rat		29.0		b

	Pakistan	Rat		28.5		b
	Ethiopian	Rat		29.0		b
R. canada	McKiel	Yolk sac	30.3±0.1	29.3±0.2		a
Spotted fever group						
R. rickettsii	Bitterroot	Yolk sac	32.4±0.1	33.2±0.5		a
		L cells			32.1±0.0	c
	R	Yolk sac	32.9±0.7	32.0±0.5		a
R. conori	Malish	Yolk sac	33.3±0.3	32.9±0.9		a
	Simko	Yolk sac		33.4±0.2		d
R. akari	MK	Yolk sac	32.4±0.4	33.2±0.8		a
		L cells	32.2±0.1			a
R. sibirica	Barbash	Yolk sac		32.5±1.0		d
Scrub typhus group						
R. tsutsugamushi	Karp	L cells			30.5±0.0	c
	Gilliam	L cells			30.0±0.1	c
	Kato	L cells			29.7±0.0	c
	Kawasaki	L cells			29.7±0.4	c
		Vero cells			29.5±0.0	c
	Kuroki	Vero cells			29.3±0.0	c
	Shimokoshi	L cells			28.1±0.7	c
		Vero cells			28.5±0.1	c

a Tyeryar *et al.*, 1973 b Myers and Wisseman, 1980 c Kumura *et al.*, 1991 d Schramek, 1974.

antigenic variants of *R. tsutsugamushi*, Gilliam, Karp, Kato, Shimokoshi, Kawasaki, and Kuroki strains, are in the range of 28.5–30.0% (Kumura *et al.*, 1991). This value is close to that of the typhus group rickettsiae (29.0–30.3%), and is a little lower than that of the spotted fever group microbes (32.2–33.3%). DNA-DNA hybridization tests between DNA from *R. tsutsugamushi* and DNA from the other species of the genus *Rickettsia* has not yet been reported.

2. Proliferation in Animals and Cells

a. Animals

Successful infection in the anterior chamber of the eye (Nagayo *et al.*, 1930) and in the testis (Ogata and Unno, 1929) in rabbits led to the discovery of *Rickettsia tsutsugamushi* as the infectious agent of Tsutsugamushi disease in 1929/30. Soon thereafter, various animals — rabbits, guinea pigs, rats, and monkeys — were used for laboratory experiments and for the preparation of antisera (Tamiya, 1962). In particular, the finding that mice were highly sensitive to this rickettsia (Ogata *et al.*, 1932) contributed greatly to the progress of research on this organism. Subsequently, many investigators used mice not only for the passage of rickettsiae but also for the isolation of rickettsiae from patients or from the natural animal hosts. For infecting mice, rickettsiae are usually inoculated by intraperitoneal (i.p.) or subcutaneous (s.c.) injection, i.p. injections (generally 10^2–10^5 MLD_{50}) being more sensitive than the s.c. injection (Shishido *et al.*, 1958).

When rickettsiae were injected i.p. to mice, the organisms were observed in smears of peritoneal exudate, liver, spleen, kidney, and lung stained by Giemsa (Ogata *et al.*, 1932) and by direct immunofluorescence (Kundin *et al.*, 1964). Murata *et al.* (1985) examined in greater depth, by direct and indirect immunofluorescence, the sites of rickettsial growth in hairy DDD mice and BALB/c (*nu*/*nu*) nude mice at stages when symptoms were maximal after i.p. or s.c. injections with three standard strains, Gilliam, Karp, and Kato.

After i.p. injection, the greatest numbers of rickettsiae were detected in and around the mesothelial and inflammatory cells of these peritoneal smears. The numbers of rickettsiae were greater in nude mice than in DDD mice (Fig. 4, Series 1-A, 1-B). On cryostat organ sections of DDD mice, the growth of many rickettsiae was clearly observed in the inflammatory cells adhering around the capsule of liver, spleen, and kidney, but rickettsial growth was not detected in the parenchymal cells of these organs (Fig. 4, Series 2-A, 2-B, 2-C). On organ sections of BALB/c (*nu*/*nu*) mice, a certain degree of rickettsial growth was observed in the inflammatory cells attached to the organs, but growth was less in the Kupffer cells of the liver, in the endothelial cells of the spleen sinus, and in the lymph node sinus (Fig. 4, Series 3-A, 3-B, 3-C).

On the other hand, s.c. injection of the same amount of rickettsiae into both nude and hairy mice resulted in enlargement of the spleen and lymph nodes, but there was little viscous ascites and little rickettsial growth in mesothelial cells. On organ sections of nude mice, a large number of rickettsiae are observed in the Kupffer cells of the liver, in the endothelial cells of the spleen sinus, and in the lymph node sinus (Fig. 4, Series 4-A, 4-B, 4-C). In contrast, there was some rickettsial growth in the same organ cells of s.c. infected hairy mice. These profiles of rickettsial distribution were clearer in nude than in hairy mice.

Similar results were seen in nude mice which had received specific antibody i.p. and had been challenged i.p. with rickettsiae 6 h later (Fig. 4, Series 5-A, 5-B, 5-C). In each case, no difference was observed among the strains examined. The differences between results with i.p. and s.c. injections may be due to the differences in the pathway taken by the rickettsiae to reach the target cells. On i.p. injection, rickettsiae may immediately invade intraperitoneal mesothelial and inflammatory cells *in situ* and grow rapidly, resulting in the death of the mice, probably due to the rickettsial toxin (see Chapter 3), before the parenchymal cells are damaged. On s.c. injection, in contrast, rickettsiae seemed to be carried by lymphatic vessels to the regional lymph nodes, where the organisms multiplied and were transferred to the target organs.

Mice injected once i.p. with highly virulent rickettsial strains generally showed manifestations of disease such as ruffled fur and enlarged abdomen. If these manifestations did not occur after an injection, they did occur after several blind passages by injection with 10% liver and spleen homogenate. The mice usually died within 10 to 21 days after injection.

However, Kobayashi *et al.* (1978) demonstrated *R. tsutsugamushi* strains that showed low virulence in mice. Mice injected with these strains showed no symptoms, and rickettsiae were not generally seen in the peritoneal smears. These low-virulent strains have been successfully grown in mice treated with immunosuppressive agents such as cyclophosphamide. Kawamura *et al.* (1980) also recognized strains that showed low virulence to mice; they used athymic nude mice for rickettsial isolation.

The procedures for rickettsial isolation in cyclophosphamide-treated mice are as follows. Samples containing rickettsia — *e.g.*, a blood clot of an infected patient — harvested before antibiotic treatment are homogenized in sucrose phosphate buffered glutamic acid (SPG) solution [0.003 M KH_2PO_4, 0.0072 M K_2HPO_4, 0.004 M L-glutamic acid, 0.218 M sucrose; pH7.0 (Bovarnick *et al.*, 1950)], and the homogenates are injected i.p. into mice. The mice are then injected i.p. with cyclophosphamide (0.2 mg/g body weight) 1, 2, and 4 days after being injected with the rickettsial sample.

If the mice are healthy, an additional injection of the drug is given 7 days after infection. On days 10–14 after infection, the mice are sacrificed, and the peritoneal smears, stained by Giemsa or by immu-

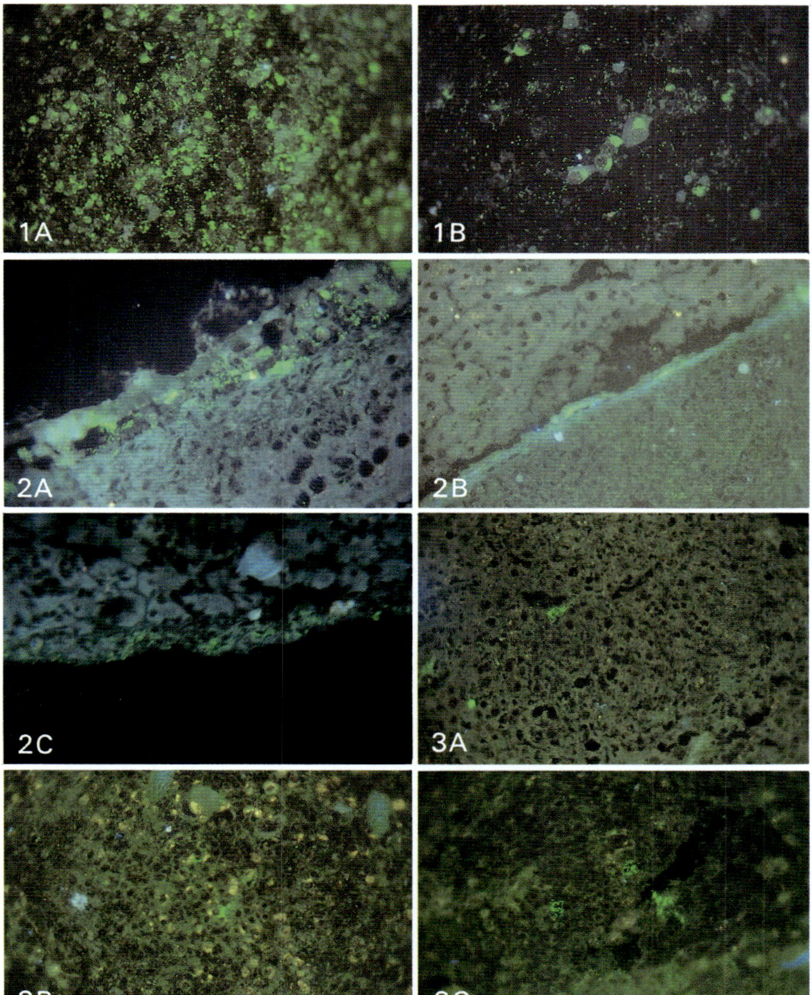

Fig. 4. Observations of *R. tsutsugamushi* in infected hairy DDD or BALB/c (*nu*/*nu*) mice by direct or indirect immunofluorescence. The photographs of series 1 are the observation of smeared cells by direct immunofluorescence and those of series 2–5 are the observation of cryostat sections by indirect immunofluorescence. Magnification of all figures is ×280.

Series 1. Mesothelial smears of BALB/c (*nu*/*nu*) (1-A) and DDD (1-B) mouse which had been infected intraperitoneally with Kato strain. A large number of rickettsiae are observed in and around mesothelial cells. A larger number of rickettsiae are seen in 1-A than in 1-B.

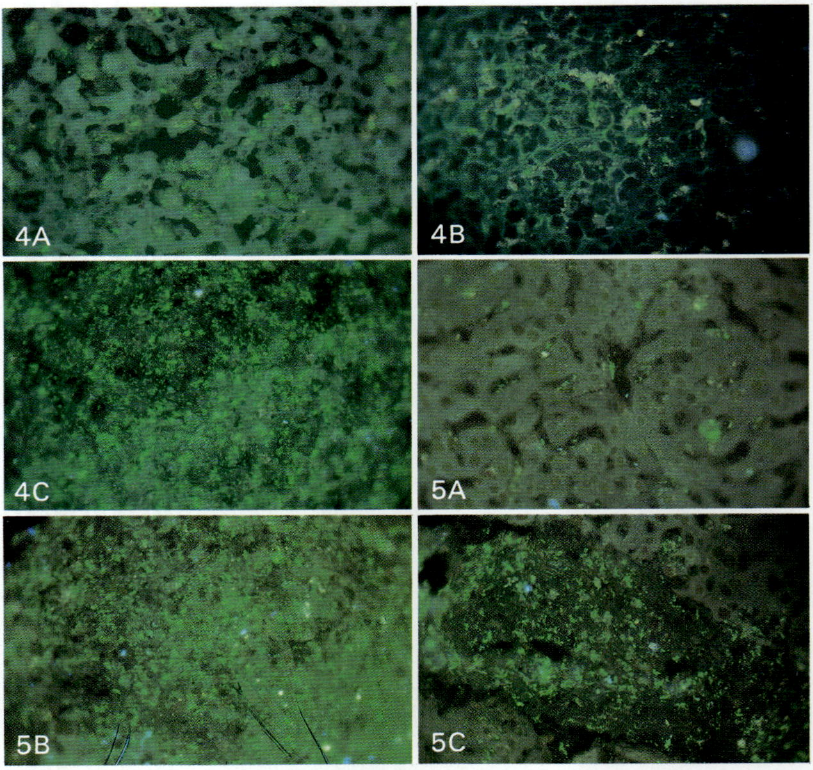

Series 2. Sections of liver, spleen, and kidney of a DDD mouse which had been infected intraperitoneally with Kato (2-A, 2-B) and Karp (2-C) strains. A large number of rickettsiae are mainly found in inflammatory cells attached to liver (2-A), liver and spleen (2-B), and kidney (2-C) capsules.

Series 3. Sections of liver (3-A), spleen (3-B), and lymph node embedded in liver (3-C) of a BALB/c (*nu*/*nu*) mouse which had been infected intraperitoneally with Gilliam strain. Growth of *R. tsutsugamushi* is observed in a few Kupffer cells (3-A), in endothelial cells of spleen sinus (3-B), and in lymph node sinus (3-C).

Series 4. Sections of liver (4-A), spleen (4-B), and lymph node embedded in liver (4-C) of BALB/c (*nu*/*nu*) mouse which had been infected subcutaneously with Miyake strain (Karp type). This strain was avirulent for DDD mice, but virulent for nude mice having a MLD_{50} titer of $10^{-5.2}$. A large number of rickettsiae are observed in Kupffer cells of the liver (4-A), in endothelial cells of spleen sinus (4-B), and in lymph node sinus (4-C).

Series 5. Sections of liver (5-A), spleen (5-B), and lymph node embedded in liver (5-C) of a BALB/c (*nu*/*nu*) mouse which had been administered anti-Karp antibody intraperitoneally and challenged intraperitoneally with Miyake strain after 6 h. A bright fluorescence is observed in Kupffer cells in liver (5-A), in endothelial cells of spleen sinus (5-B), and in lymph node sinus (5-C).

nofluorescence, are observed microscopically. If rickettsiae are not observed in the smear, the liver and spleen homogenates are injected to other mice for blind passage. The percentage of rickettsial isolation from patients with Tsutsugamushi disease is 90% or higher when these cyclophosphamide-treated mice are used (Yamamoto, 1988; Yamamoto *et al.*, 1989) (see Chapter 6).

b. Embryonated chicken eggs

R. tsutsugamushi can be grown by inoculation into the yolk sac of 5- to 7-day-old embryonated chicken eggs, similarly to other members of the genus *Rickettsia*. Four to 7 days after inoculation, yolk sacs are harvested from eggs, just before the death of the embryo, and rickettsiae in the yolk sac smears are observed microscopically by Giménez staining or immunofluorescence.

If necessary, blind passages of infected yolk sac homogenate are performed. While this cultivation method may be useful for the large-scale production of rickettsiae, it is not now generally used, since cultured cells are used more frequently for the laboratory maintenance of this rickettsia. Furthermore, in many cases, chickens receive feed containing antibiotics, and rickettsial growth is occasionally suppressed when eggs from these chickens are used by chance.

c. Cultured cells

R. tsutsugamushi is cultivated in primary cultured cells of chicken embryos and established cell lines such as HeLa, Vero, BHK, McCoy, and L. The growth rate of rickettsiae in each cell line differs depending on rickettsial strains. Therefore, cell selection is usually required before a rickettsial strain is cultivated.

After 1 to 2 h incubation of cells with rickettsial inoculum, the inoculum is removed and the cell layer is cultivated in fresh cell-maintenance medium at 35–37°C. The rickettsial growth in stained cell smears is observed microscopically at 2-day intervals, and, if necessary, the culture medium is occasionally changed, and cultivation is continued until massive rickettsial growth is observed in the cells.

To enhance rickettsial adsorption to cells, rickettsial samples are inoculated onto a cell layer on the flat bottom of a tube, and the tube is centrifuged at 200–300 × *g* for 30 min.

For large-scale cultivation of rickettsiae, it is preferable to use cells in suspension. L cells are commonly used for this purpose. Cells are spun down by centrifugation, mixed with rickettsial inoculum, at 10^7 cells per ml, and incubated at 37°C for 1–2 h for rickettsial adsorption to cells. The cells are then recovered by centrifugation and incubated, at 10^5 cells per ml, in fresh medium for cell maintenance until massive rickettsial growth is observed microscopically in the cell smears.

d. Determination of rickettsial infectivity in cultured cells

Plaque assays have been used generally for the titration of *R. tsutsugamushi* infectivity on monolayer cultures of chicken embryo cells (McDade and Gerone, 1970; Woodman *et al*., 1977), X-ray irradiated L-929 cells (Oaks *et al*., 1977), and the mouse embryo cell line, C3H/10T1/2 clone 8 (Hanson, 1987).

Tamura *et al.* also observed plaque formation on a UV-irradiated L cell monolayer (unpublished data). Briefly, they suspended L cells in phosphate buffered saline (PBS) in a Petri dish, irradiated the cells under a UV lamp at 30-cm distance for 30 sec, and seeded the cells in fresh dishes to form a monolayer. After adsorption of rickettsiae to cells, the cell layer was overlaid with 2 mm, in depth, of agar-containing medium and incubated in a 5% CO_2 atmosphere. Seven days after the first overlay, the same amount of agar-containing medium was overlaid again upon the first agar medium, and after 17 days, cells were stained with a third overlay medium that contained neutral red.

The plaque was 0.5–1.0 mm in diameter. A linear relation between the rickettsial concentration and the plaque count was observed, indicating that this plaque formation is useful not only for rickettsial infectivity assay but also for clone purification of the rickettsia.

This plaque forming assay for the determination of rickettsial infectivity requires 2–3 weeks. However, a simple and rapid method for the determination of infectivity was proposed by Tamura and Urakami (1981). These investigators suggested that, since the progeny of rickettsiae produced in the primary infection are released from the host culture cells 4 days or later after infection, secondary infection to the cells has not yet occurred in 3-day culture. Therefore, the infected cell counts in a 3-day culture correspond to the rickettsial concentration in the inoculum used.

In practice, their method consists of 4- to 5-fold serially diluted rickettsial samples inoculated onto cell layers on glass cover slips in a Leighton's tube. After 3-day incubation, the cells are fixed and stained by Giemsa, and the ratio of infected cells to the total number of cells is determined microscopically. The counts of infected cells are proportional to the dilution of the rickettsial inoculum in cultures with less than 50% cell infection.

3. Multiplication Cycle in the Host Cell

As stated earlier, *Rickettsia tsutsugamushi* is an obligate intracellular parasite that propagates in host cell cytoplasm by binary fission. Multiplication of this microorganism can be divided into three phases: (1) adsorption to and penetration of the host cell, (2) intracellular multiplication, and (3) release from the host cell.

These phases of multiplication have been observed electron microscopically (Tamura, 1988a; Urakami *et al.*, 1982a, 1982b, 1983, 1984). Several stages of rickettsial multiplication in L cell culture, observed in specimens of prepared at various intervals after infection, are shown in Figs. 5–9. The entire growth cycle of the rickettsia obtained by these observations is summarized in Fig. 10.

a. Penetration of rickettsia into the host cell

The first step in the penetration of rickettsia into the host cell is the attachment of the rickettsia to the host cell surface (Figs. 5a and Fig. 10, step 2). No action of the host cell can be seen at this stage. This attachment may constitute a reaction between the attachment site (ligand) on the rickettsial surface and receptors on the host cell membrane. When intact rickettsiae were treated with trypsin before inoculation, they did not attach to the cell surface, indicating that the ligands on the rickettsial surface were removed or destroyed by the enzyme.

Comparison of polypeptide composition in the rickettsia before and after trypsin treatment by polyacrylamide gel electrophoresis (PAGE) showed the disappearance of three polypeptides, 54–56 kDa, 35 kDa, and 21–25 kDa in size, all these being constituents of the rickettsial surface. This finding suggests that one of these polypeptides may play a role as a ligand of the rickettsia.

The next step in penetration is the formation of projections at the site of rickettsial attachment to the cell surface (Fig. 5b and Fig. 10,

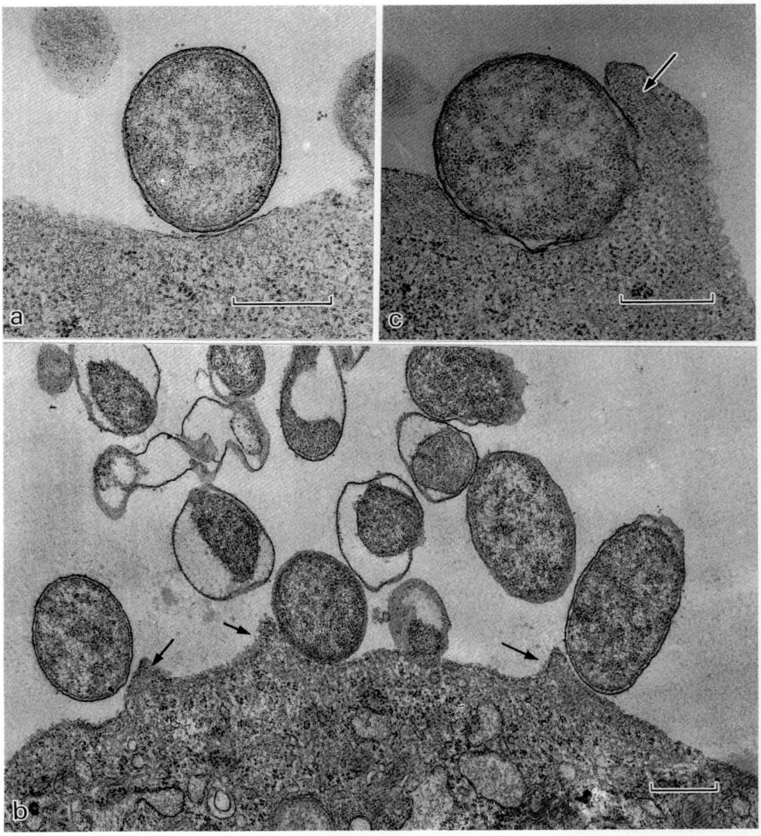

Fig. 5. Rickettsiae seen on the host cell surface in specimens prepared at 20 min (a and b) and 40 min (c) after infection

a. A rickettsia just attached to a host cell surface. No response of the host cell has been detected yet.
b. Formation of projections (arrows) at the attachment sites of the rickettsiae. Although heavily plasmolyzed rickettsiae are seen apart from or attached to the cell surface, it should be noted that the formation of a projection is seen only at the sites to which the morphologically intact rickettsiae adhere.
c. A rickettsia in the process of being phagocytosed. Microfilamentous structure (arrow) is seen in the projection.

step 3), indicating the initiation of phagocytosis. The formation of projections was seen at the attachment sites of morphologically intact rickettsiae only. Plasmolyzed rickettsiae or those killed by UV irradiation attached to the cell membrane but did not induce the for-

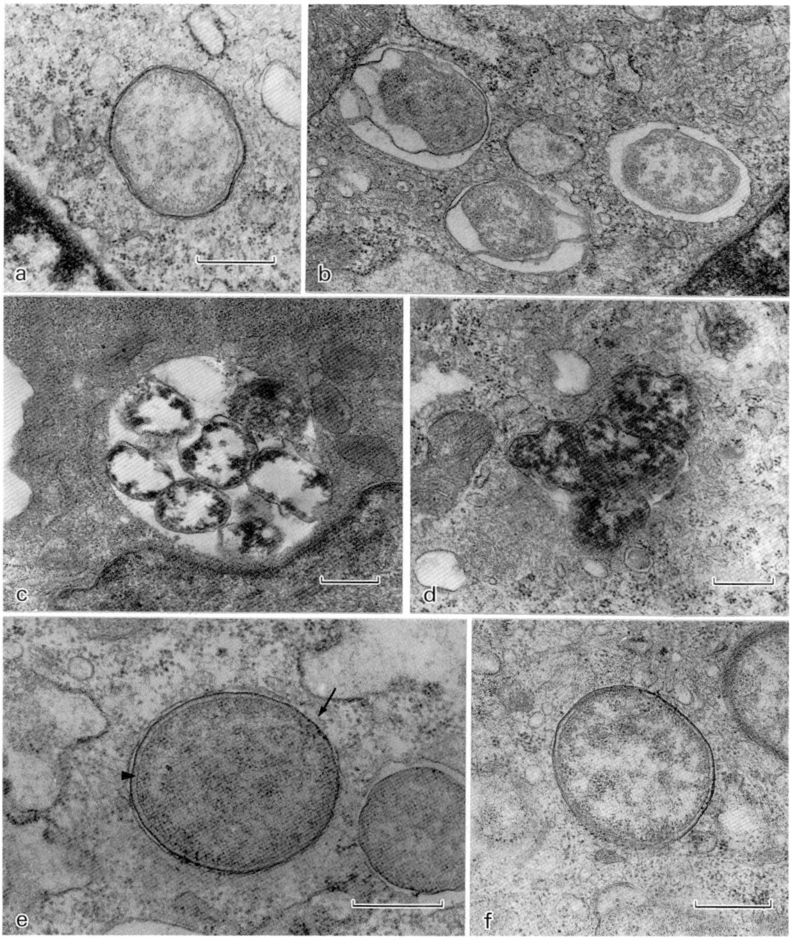

Fig. 6. Rickettsiae seen in the host cell cytoplasm in specimens prepared at 40 min after infection. Bars correspond to 0.5 μm.

a. A rickettsia enclosed tightly by the phagosomal membrane.
b. Rickettsiae in loose phagosome. Three rickettsiae are seen, and two of them show heavy plasmolysis.
c. A large loose phagosome containing several rickettsiae. The interior of these microorganisms is heterogeneous and granular.
d. A large phagosome containing several rickettsiae which are deformed and depressed.
e. A rickettsia surrounded by a partially disintegrated phagosomal membrane. The phagosomal membrane (arrowhead) is not seen at the portion indicated by the arrow.
f. A rickettsia in the cell cytoplasm free from the phagosomal membrane.

mation of projections. This suggests that rickettsiae must be intact to induce phagocytosis and that UV-sensitive factor(s) in the rickettsia may participate in this process.

In the progressive stage of phagocytosis, the cell surface is invaginated and an enlarged projection engulfs the microorganism (Fig. 5c and Fig. 10, step 4). Microfilament-like structures are observed in the projection. The host cell membrane lies closely along the surface of the rickettsia, leaving only a narrow space, 30 nm or less. The inclusion of a single rickettsia was frequently observed, while the inclusion of several rickettsiae together was rare.

The rickettsia is then taken into a phagosome of the host cell cytoplasm. In the cytoplasm, two kinds of phagosomes, tight and loose, are usually seen. In the tight phagosome, the membrane tightly encloses a rickettsia, leaving a narrow space of 30 nm or less between the phagosome membrane and the rickettsial outer envelope (Fig. 6a and Fig 10, step 5). The loose phagosome envelopes the rickettsia loosely, leaving a space of 0.1–0.5 μm (Fig. 6b and Fig. 10, step 6). Rickettsiae in the loose phagosome often show partial or extreme plasmolysis. Since heavily plasmolyzed rickettsiae are not phagocytosed and all rickettsiae in the process of being phagocytosed are surrounded tightly by the host cell membrane, as described above, the rickettsiae just after being phagocytosed would be in tight phagosomes. Therefore, these loose phagosomes may be derived from tight phagosomes after phagocytosis, and the plasmolyzed and deformed rickettsiae in the loose phagosome may be in the process of being inactivated and digested by lysosomes.

In the host cell cytoplasm, large phagosomes containing several rickettsiae were sometimes observed (Fig. 6c,d and Fig. 10, step 7). In these phagosomes, the rickettsiae were deformed and depressed and the rickettsial interior was heterogenous and granular, indicating that the organisms were inactive. The phagocytosis of multiple rickettsiae was rarely observed, suggesting that these large phagosomes may have been produced by the fusion of loose phagosomes.

In the tight phagosomes, the rickettsiae were morphologically intact, and partial disappearance of the phagosome membrane was frequently observed (Fig. 6e and Fig. 10, step 8). In the region of the discontinued membrane, the phagosome membrane was not seen, even on inclined goniometric observations. This may indicate the mechanism whereby rickettsiae escape from the phagosome into the cell cytoplasm. This partial degradation of the phagosome membranes was seen only in the tight phagosomes containing morphologically intact rickettsiae, not in the loose phagosomes surrounding degraded rickettsiae.

Figure 6f shows an intracytoplasmic rickettsia free of the phagosome membrane (corresponding to Fig. 10, step 9). A few of these intracytoplasmic rickettsiae were seen in the specimens 10 min after infection; more were seen in 20 min, and many in 40 min, indicating that the entire process of penetration was accomplished within 10–20 min. Rikihisa *et al.* (1979) and Rikihisa and Ito (1980, 1982, 1983) showed a similar mechanism of phagocytosis and penetration in cultured polymorphonuclear leucocytes.

Purified naked rickettsiae that are not covered with the host cell membrane enter host cells as described above; however, another penetration mode, in which the rickettsia is surrounded by the host cell cytoplasmic membrane just after release from the infected cell (Fig. 10, step 16), has been observed *in vivo*, by Ewing *et al.* (1978). As shown in Fig. 10, steps 18 and 19, the rickettsia, still enclosed by the host cell membrane, was phagocytosed in a phagosome of the other cells, following which the host cell membrane surrounding the rickettsia and the newly covered phagosome membrane fused together, resulting in the release of the rickettsia into the host cell cytoplasm (Fig. 10, step 20).

Phase contrast microscopic photography, performed at intervals of 1–3 min, has shown that in infected cells in intact cell culture, there was direct cell-to-cell transport of a rickettsia to a neighboring cell (Tamura *et al.*, unpublished data). In this case, an intracellular rickettsia pushed out of the host cell membrane from inside to outside, and the tip of the cell membrane that covered the rickettsia fused with the tip of a projection on a neighboring cell, resulting in the rickettsia entering the cytoplasm of the neighboring cell.

Thus, as described here, there are several mechanisms whereby rickettsiae penetrate the host cell. In all cases, the active participation of both the rickettsia and the host cell may be involved. Various matters, however, still require clarification; these include the identification and characterization of the rickettsial ligand and the host cell receptor, the factor(s) that induce phagocytosis, and the lytic factor(s) in the phagosome membrane that allow rickettsial escape from the phagosome.

b. Intracellular multiplication

The process whereby the rickettsia penetrates the host cell cytoplasm takes 10–20 min, as mentioned above; however, the intracellular multiplication process is relatively slow, and observations were made in specimens prepared at daily intervals. Twenty-four hours after infection, a small number of rickettsiae were found in the cytoplasm of sectioned cells. Most rickettsiae at this stage contained inner structures less electron-dense than those seen at a later stage of infection (Fig. 7a). The proportion of these less electron-dense rickettsiae to the electron-dense organisms decreased with time, indicating that the less dense rickettsiae may represent a form of lag phase. The less electron-dense rickettsiae were enveloped by a cell wall and cytoplasmic membrane identical to those of the dense rickettsiae, but the inside contained fewer ribosomes.

The rickettsiae multiplied by binary fission, forming a constriction at the middle of the long axis (Fig. 7b and Fig 10, step 10). Forty-eight to 72 h after infection, there was an apparent increase in the number of rickettsiae in the cell cytoplasm (Fig. 10, step 11). Most rickettsiae were 1.2–2.5 μm in length, but abnormally long organisms (10–15 μm) were sometimes seen in the cell cytoplasm, coexisting with normal sized rickettsiae or, occasionally, forming clumps (Fig. 7c). These long rickettsiae may be produced as a result of the blockage of binary fission by an unknown mechanism.

The site of rickettsial multiplication was usually in the host cell cytoplasm, but intranuclear rickettsiae were observed in a few cases (Fig. 10, step 12) (Urakami *et al.*, 1982b). These rickettsiae may have entered the nucleus during the process of cell mitosis.

c. Release from the host cell

In specimens prepared 72 h after infection, many rickettsiae were seen just under the host cell membrane, and most of them were pushing the host cytoplasmic membrane from the inside to the outside (Fig. 8a and Fig. 10, steps 13–15). This is similar to the budding process in enveloped viruses, and this stage of rickettsiae is referred to as budding rickettsiae. The direction in the budding process was not consistent: some rickettsiae budded perpendicularly and some horizontally to the rickettsial long axis. At this budding stage, rickettsiae in the process of binary fission were sometimes observed (Fig. 8b and Fig. 10, step 15).

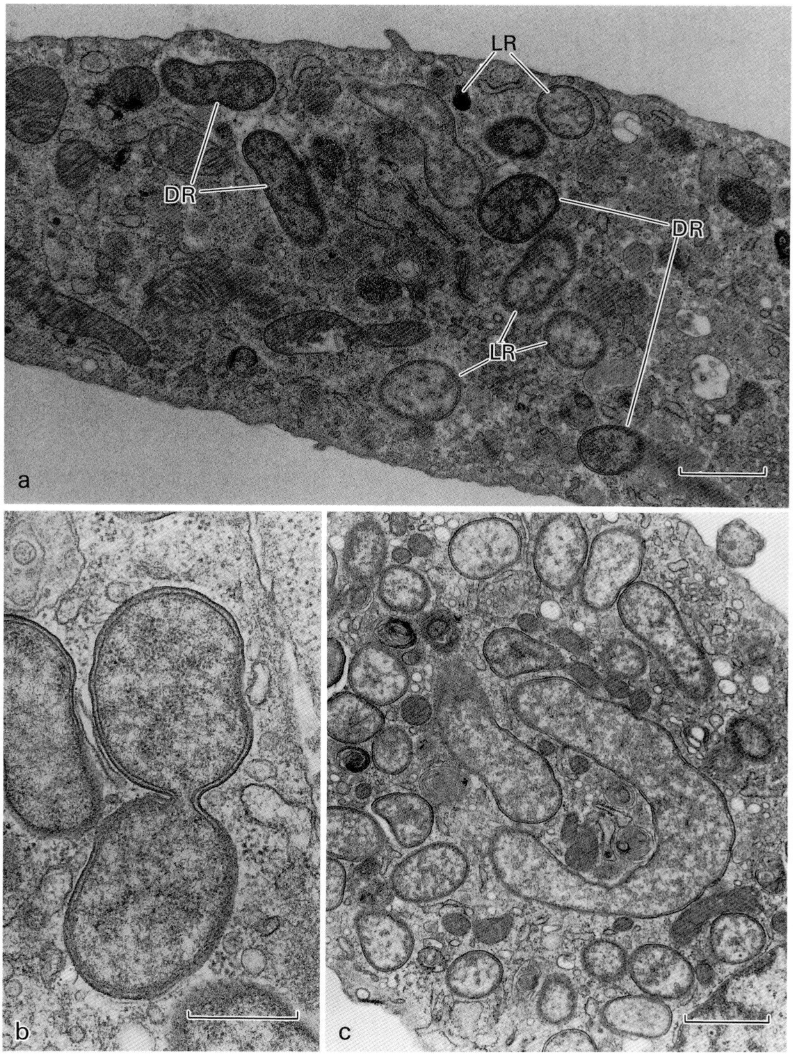

Fig. 7. Rickettsiae multiplying in host cell cytoplasm

a. Electron-dense (DR) and -less dense (LR) rickettsiae seen in a specimen at 48 h of infection. Bar indicates 1.0 μm.
b. Rickettsia in the process of binary fission in a specimen at 72 h of infection. Bar corresponds to 0.5 μm.
c. Abnormally long rickettsiae seen in a thin-sectioned cell at 96 h of infection. Bar indicates 1.0 μm.

Groups of budding rickettsiae were clearly seen on the cell surface by scanning electron microscopy (Fig. 8c). The infectivity in the culture fluid did not increase sharply even at this stage, indicating that these budding rickettsiae may be retained for a relatively long period *in situ*, resulting in their accumulation on the cell surface. The budding rickettsiae were always observed on the surface of host cells containing a number of intracellular rickettsiae, indicating that infection with, and multiplication of, this microorganism in cells was inevitably followed by the budding process.

The rickettsiae at the budding stage may be detached from the cell surface at the site of the constricted cell membrane by means of a mechanical shock or some other mechanism. The rickettsiae thus released (Fig. 10, step 16), which are covered with the host cell membrane, may enter neighboring cells directly (Fig. 10 steps 18 to 20), or alternately the outer host cell membrane may be slipped off (Fig. 10, step 17), leaving the naked rickettsiae (Fig. 10, step 1) to invade other cells.

Seventy-two hours after infection, the outer and inner leaflets of the nuclear membrane of the host cell separated, resulting in the formation of vacuoles. These vacuoles increased in size, becoming as large as the nucleus 96–120 h after infection (Fig. 9a, b). At this later stage of infection, the host cells were round and the cytoplasmic membrane had disappeared in some cells, resulting in the release of naked rickettsiae from the cells into the culture fluid (Fig. 9c and Fig. 10, step 21).

Hase (1983a, 1983b) proposed a discontinuous morphological change in the intracellular multiplication stage of *R. tsutsugamushi* involving the formation of rickettsial progeny by the differentiation of the granular cytoplasmic portion enclosed by a newly assembled rickettsial membrane. However, these processes have not been confirmed by other investigators.

d. Growth curve

A growth curve drawn by determining rickettsial infectivity in culture fluid and in cells (Urakami *et al.*, 1984) is shown in Fig. 11. Intracellular infectivity increased logarithmically between 24 and 72 h after infection, with a two-fold increase of the population every 9 h. The stationary phase was seen 96 h after infection. An apparent increase of infectivity in the culture fluid was observed 72 h after

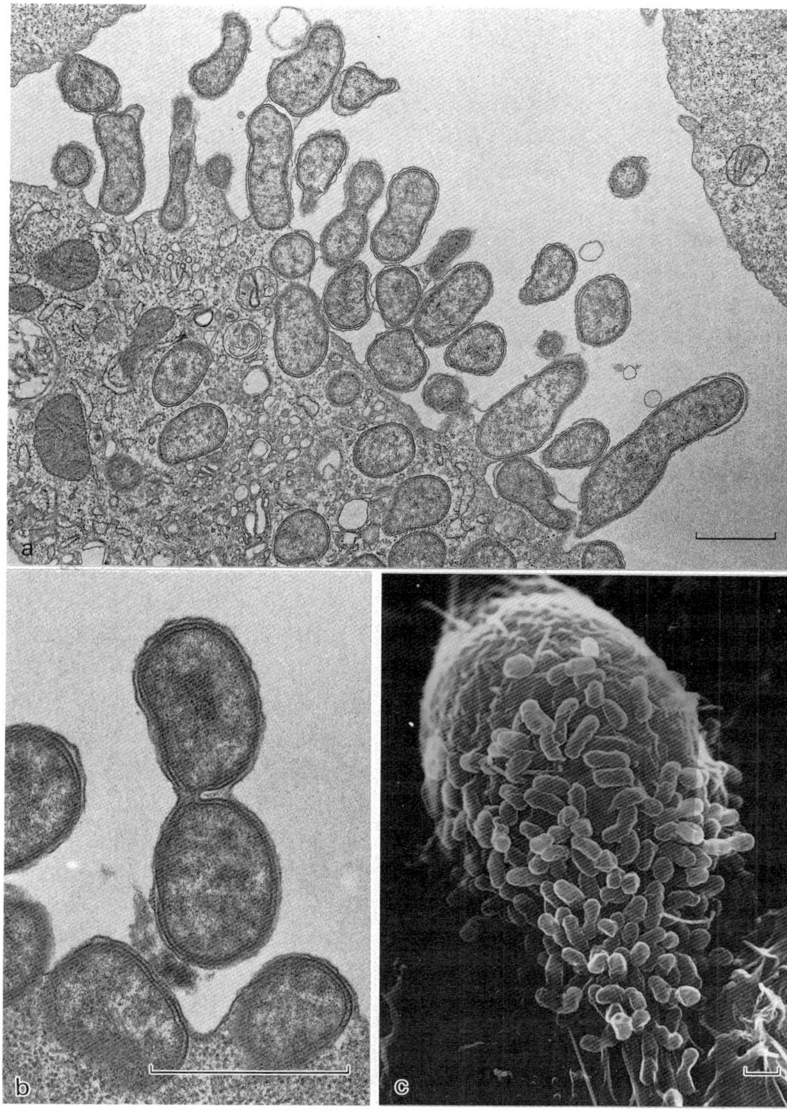

Fig. 8. Rickettsiae in the process of releasing from host cells. Bars indicate 1.0 μm.

a. Budding rickettsiae seen at the periphery of a cell at 72 h of infection.
b. Binary fission of rickettsiae in the budding process.
c. Scanning electron micrograph of budding rickettsiae seen on the cell surface at 72 h of infection.

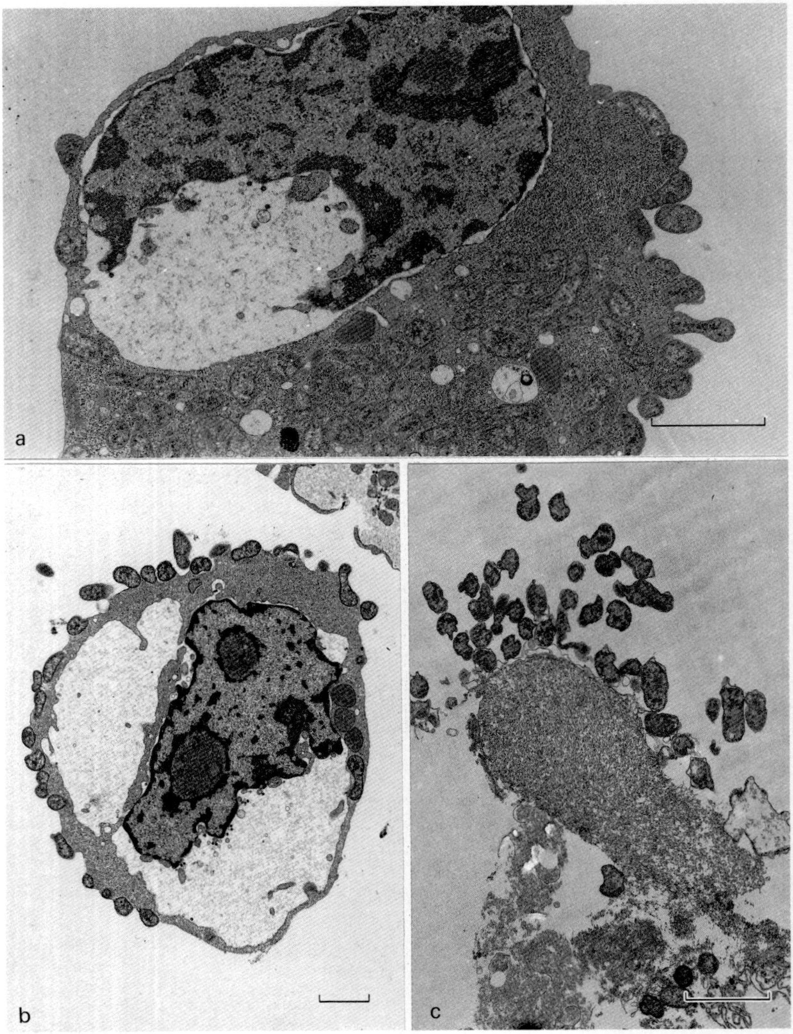

Fig. 9. Formation of vacuole between the outer and inner leaflets of the nuclear membrane seen at 96 h of infection (a); the enlargement of vacuole and rounding of cells seen at 120 h of infection (b); and cell lysis observed at 120 h of infection (c). Bars indicate 2.0 μm.

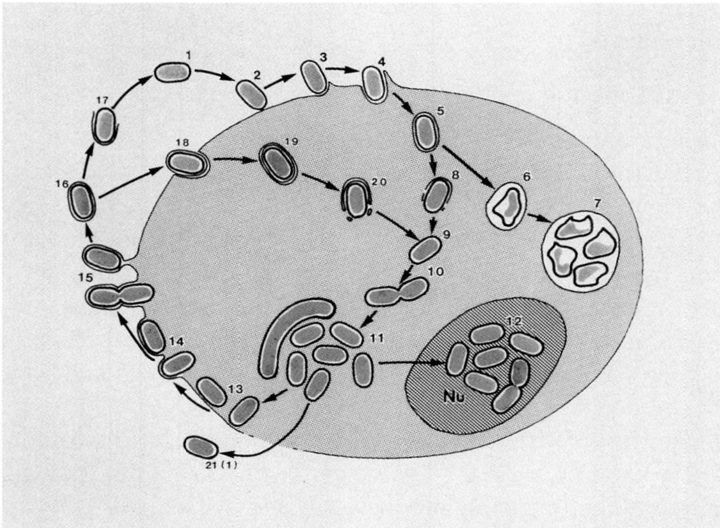

Fig. 10. A diagram of the growth cycle of *R. tsutsugamushi*. Numbers indicate steps in rickettsial multiplication. Nu: nucleus.

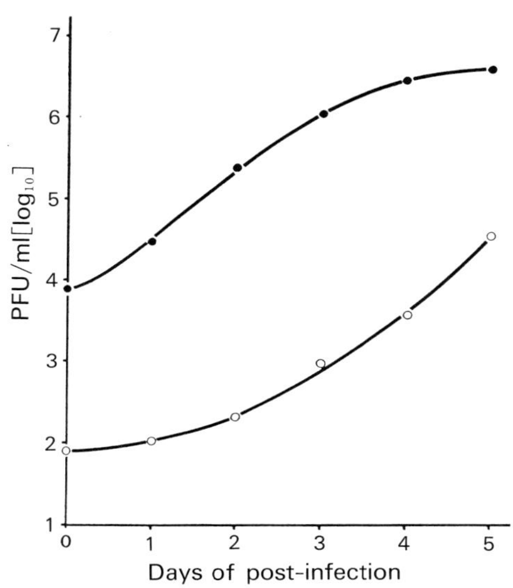

Fig. 11. Growth curve of rickettsiae in L cell culture. Titers are shown as plaque-forming units (PFU) per ml of the original culture volume. Closed circle: cell-associated titer; open circle: titer in culture fluid.

infection, but the titers were always 10^2 or 10^3 times lower than intracellular titers.

4. Purification

a. *Purification of* Rickettsia tsutsugamushi

Several methods have been reported for the purification of microbes in the genus *Rickettsia* from infected materials. Rickettsiae inactivated by a low concentration of formaldehyde or by ultraviolet irradiation have been used as starting materials for the study of their antigenic, chemical and/or morphological properties (Anacker *et al*., 1974; Palmer *et al*., 1974). To purify viable rickettsiae, preparations have been subjected to treatment with celite (Bovarnick and Snyder, 1949), bovine serum albumin (Bovarnick and Miller, 1950), cation exchange resin (Kawamura, 1962; Shishido, 1962a; Yamamoto *et al*., 1958) and/or sucrose (Thompson *et al*., 1971), or Renografin density gradient centrifugation (Dasch and Weiss, 1977; Weiss *et al*., 1975) to eliminate contaminants.

Renografin density gradient centrifugation in particular, is excellent for the purification of typhus and spotted fever group rickettsiae, but, as noted by Weiss *et al.* (1975), the method is not useful for the purification of *R. tsutsugamushi* because of the instability and fragility of the organisms.

However, Tamura *et al.* (1982) found that *R. tsutsugamushi* could be purified by Percoll density gradient centrifugation from infected L cells, and the rickettsiae thus purified retained their infectivity and intracellular morphology (Fig. 12). *R. tsutsugamushi* organisms are easily disrupted by mechanical treatment, such as strong homogenization and osmotic shock. Further, rickettsiae are sticky, and once they are pelleted, it is difficult to prepare homogeneous suspensions without strong agitation. With Percoll these problems are avoided since this material has no osmotic effect, and the purification procedure does not involve the pelleting of rickettsiae except at the final stage.

Procedure for Percoll density gradient purification

1. L cells in suspension culture are infected with *R. tsutsugamushi*, and, after 4 to 5 days, the massive growth of rickettsiae in many cells is confirmed by microscopic observation of cell smears stained with Giemsa. The preparation of 1–3 liters of culture,

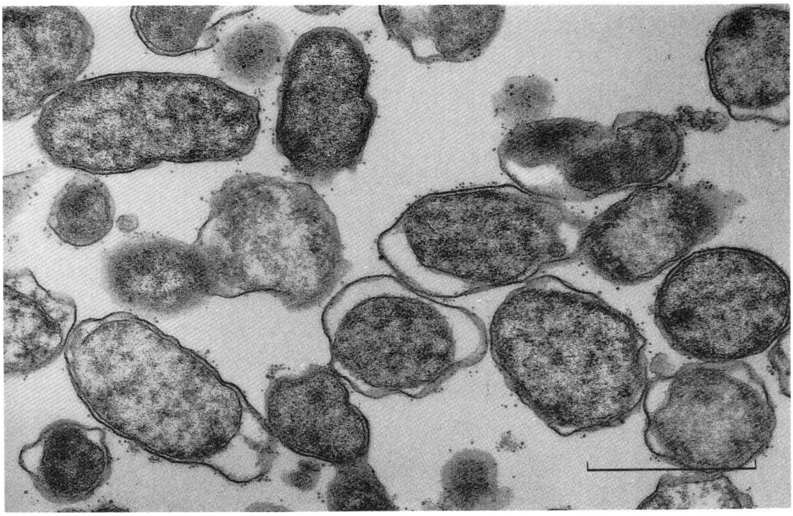

Fig. 12. Electron micrograph of a thin section of *R. tsutsugamushi* purified by Percoll density gradient centrifugation. Percoll particles are seen on the rickettsial surface.

containing 10^6 cells per ml, is desirable for purification.

2. Cells are harvested from the culture by centrifugation at $300 \times g$ for 10 min and are resuspended in 0.033 M Tris hydrochloride, pH 7.4, containing 0.25 M sucrose (TS-buffer) at a cell concentration of 10^8 or more (about 1/100 of the original culture volume).

3. Cells are homogenized with a Dounce stainless steel homogenizer (Kontes Glass Co., Vineland, N.J.) at 20–30 strokes or with a Polytron homogenizer (Wheaton, Inc, Millville, N.J.) at moderate speed for 1–2 min.

4. The homogenate is centrifuged at $200 \times g$ for 10 min and the supernatant is mixed with Percoll (Pharmacia Fine Chemicals, Uppsala, Sweden) suspended in TS-buffer at a final Percoll concentration of 40%. (The original Percoll suspension is taken to be 100%, but the results differ a little in each batch; a preliminary test is, therefore required.)

5. The mixture is divided into several 10 ml centrifuge tubes (polycarbonate tube with screw cap) and centrifuged at $25{,}000 \times g$ for 60 min in a Hitachi RP-55 angle rotor (Hitachi Koki, Tokyo Japan).

6. After centrifugation, two bands are observed. The upper band near the top consists of cell debris, and the rickettsiae are accumulated in the lower band near the bottom. The upper band is removed by suction, and portions of the lower band are harvested with a capillary pipette and pooled in a new centrifuge tube.

7. The pooled rickettsial suspension is centrifuged again, without dilution, at 77,000 × *g* for 30 min. (If the amount of suspension does not fill the tube, the suspension may be diluted with 40% Percoll in TS-buffer.)

8. Rickettsiae collected again in the same band by centrifugation are harvested and diluted several-fold with TS-buffer; the purified rickettsiae are recovered in the pellet after centrifugation at 6,000 × *g* for 20 min.

9. To eliminate Percoll from the preparation, the rickettsiae in the pellet are resuspended in TS-buffer with light agitation and centrifuged, and the procedure is repeated once or twice more.

b. Purification of rickettsial envelope

For the basic studies of a microorganism, purification of the microbial envelope is required. However, as noted above, *R. tsutsugamushi* has a very fragile and sticky cell envelope, and purification of the envelope has, therefore, been very difficult.

To purify the rickettsial envelope, Takahashi *et al.* (1985) examined methods for disrupting the rickettsiae, such as sonication, osmotic shock, and vigorous shaking with glass beads. They also compared various methods for separating the envelope from contaminants in the homogenate, such as treatment with RNase, DNase, and/or proteolytic enzyms; treatment with detergents and chemicals such as sodium dodecyl sulfate (SDS), sodium deoxycholate, Nonidet P40, Triton X-100, high concentrations of urea, and/or NaCl; and sucrose and potassium tartrate density gradient centrifugation.

From these preliminary trials, the following procedure was found to be the best for the purification of the cell envelope of this rickettsia. The final preparation obtained by the procedure consists of rickettsial cell walls and cell membranes (Fig. 13).

Procedure for purification of rickettsial envelope

1. Purified and concentrated rickettsiae suspended in 1.0 ml NET-buffer (0.14 M NaCl-0.001 M EDTA-0.033 M Tris-HCl buffer,

pH 7.4) are mixed with 2 g of glass beads (0.1 mm in diameter) and shaken vigorously in a cell mill shaker (Edmund Bühler, Tübingen, Germany) for 3 min at room temperature.

2. The disrupted rickettsial suspension is separated from the glass beads by decanting and the glass beads are washed several times with a small amount of NET-buffer.

3. Crystalline NaCl is added, at a final concentration of 2 M, to the combined mixture of the homogenate and washing fluid, and the mixture is incubated for 1 h in an ice bath.

4. One ml of the mixture is then layered on 4 ml of a 20–50% continuous sucrose density gradient column containing 2 M NaCl-0.033 M Tris-HCl buffer, pH 7.4, prepared in a 5 ml nitrocellulose centrifuge tube, and centrifuged at 33,000 × *g* for 60 min in a Hitachi RSP 50 swing bucket rotor.

5. Two bands are seen in the centrifuge tube after centrifugation. The upper band formed in the 34% sucrose region consists mainly of well-dispersed rickettsial envelopes. The lower band in the 39% sucrose region contains aggregates of the rickettsial envelopes with small granular materials; the homogeneity is not as good as in the upper band.

6. The upper band is harvested, diluted with NT-buffer (0.14 M

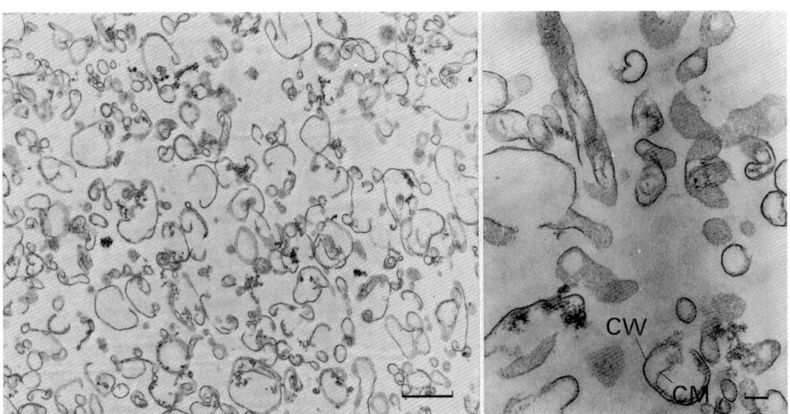

Fig. 13. Electron micrograph of a thin section of purified rickettsial envelopes at lower (left) and higher (right) magnification. CW: cell walls; CM: cytoplasmic membranes. Bars indicate 1.0 μm (in the left panel) and 0.1 μm (in the right panel).

NaCl-0.033 M Tris-HCl buffer, pH 7.4), and centrifuged at 33,000 × *g* for 30 min.

7. The pellet obtained is resuspended in NT buffer containing 0.02 M $MgCl_2$ and treated with bovine pancreatic RNase and DNase (each 100 μg/ml final concentration) for 2 h at 37°C.

8. The suspension is fractionated again by 20–50% sucrose density gradient centrifugation, and the band formed is recovered as described above.

5. Antigenic Variants of *Rickettsia tsutsugamushi*

a. Analysis of antigenic variation among strains

Antigenic heterogeneity among strains of *R. tsutsugamushi* has been recognized by cross-complement fixation (CF), cross-neutralization, and cross-protection tests (Bell *et al*., 1946; Bengston, 1945, 1946; Bennett *et al*., 1949; Fox, 1949; Rights and Smadel, 1948; Shishido *et al*., 1959). In early studies, the Karp strain, isolated in New Guinea; the Seerangayee strain, in Malaysia; and the Gilliam strain in Burma were at first distinguished serologically in cross-CF tests by using ether-treated antigens prepared from the infected yolk sacs of embryonated chicken eggs (Bengston, 1945, 1946; Craigie, 1945). By a similar technique, patient sera collected in Japan were classified into two groups, those that were reactive with either Gilliam or Karp antigen (Philip, 1947).

Kawamura and associates (Kawamura, 1962; Yamamoto *et al*., 1958) developed a procedure for the partial purification of intact rickettsiae from infected yolk sacs, using differential centrifugation and treatment with a cation exchange resin, Amberlite XE64 (Rohm & Haas Co., Philadelphia, Pa.).

Using antigens prepared by a similar purification method, Shishido (1962a, 1964) found that the Gilliam, Karp, and Kato types isolated in Japan were distinguishable from each other by the CF test, and also that many isolates from patients, field rodents, and chiggers in Japan could be classified as these three types.

Bozeman and Elisberg (1963) introduced indirect immunofluorescence (IF) to detect antibodies against *R. tsutsugamushi* in the sera of patients with Tsutsugamushi disease. Kawamura and associates (Iida *et al*., 1966a; Kawamura, 1969; Murata and Kawamura, 1980) succeeded in establishing highly specific direct and indirect IF for *R. tsutsugamushi*. Using direct IF, Iida *et al*. (1966a, 1966b) classified many isolates obtained in Japan from patients, rodents, and chiggers as Gilliam, Karp, and Kato types, while they also found evidence suggestive of the presence of mixed types among the isolates.

New antigenic types different from the three prototypes, Gilliam, Karp, and Kato, were found in Thailand (Elisberg *et al.*, 1967, 1968, 1978; Shirai *et al.*, 1981d), in Peninsular Malaysia (Shirai *et al.*, 1979b, 1981b), in the Pescadores Islands of Taiwan, in the Philippines (Shirai *et al.*, 1982c), and in North Queensland, Australia (Shirai *et al.*, 1982a). Elisberg *et al.* (1978) reported that five strains (TA678, TA686, TA716, TA763, and TH1817) isolated in Thailand were antigenically different from the prototype strains determined by cross reactivity in indirect IF with several polyclonal hyperimmune sera. Studies of 114 isolates from patients in Malaysia, using direct IF with antisera against each prototype and the five types in Thailand, led to the classification of 29 types (Shirai *et al.*, 1979b).

In Japan, the Shimokoshi strain, isolated from a patient in Niigata Prefecture, was identified as a new type that showed low cross reactivity with hyperimmune sera against the Gilliam, Karp, and Kato strains (Table 3) (Tamura *et al.*, 1984). The Kawasaki and Kuroki strains, isolated from patients in Miyazaki Prefecture, showed low cross reactivity with antisera against the prototype strains, but were highly reactive to the respective homologous antiserum (Table 4) (Yamamoto, 1984; Yamamoto *et al.*, 1989). These two strains were also shown to be distinct from the prototype strains by the more detailed characterization carried out by Yamamoto *et al.* (1986) and Ohashi *et al.* (1990b). Moreover, these rickettsial strains were isolated from patients using cyclophosphamide-treated mice, as some strains of *R. tsutsugamushi* have been confirmed to have low pathogenicity in mice.

Prior to the these findings, Kobayashi and coworkers had isolated the Irie (Kobayashi *et al.*, 1978) and Hirano (Tachibana *et al.*, 1982b) strains from patients in Miyazaki Prefecture, the same area in which the Kawasaki and Kuroki strains were isolated, employing cyclophosphamide-treated mice; however, the identity of the former two types with the latter types has not yet been confirmed, although it has been demonstrated that the Irie and Hirano strains are antigenically distinct from the Gilliam, Karp, Kato, and Shimokoshi strains (Tange *et al.*, 1991, 1992).

Table 3. Cross Reactivities of Gilliam, Karp, Kato and Shimokoshi Strains with Guinea Pig Antisera against Each Strain by Complement Fixation Test

Antigens	Antiserum			
	Gilliam	Karp	Kato	Shimokoshi
Gilliam	512	16	32	< 8
Karp	8	256	16	< 8
Kato	16	32	256	8
Shimokoshi	< 8	8	< 8	128

Table 4. Cross Reactivities of Gilliam, Karp, Kato, Kawasaki and Kuroki Strains with Guinea Pig Immune Sera against Each Strain by Indirect Immunofluorescence*

Antigens	Antiserum				
	Gilliam	Karp	Kato	Kawasaki	Kuroki
Gilliam	640	80	40	80	80
Karp	40	640	80	20	160
Kato	40	160	640	20	160
Kawasaki	20	40	80	640	40
Kuroki	40	160	80	20	640

* From Yamamoto *et al.*, 1989.

Analysis of these antigenic variations of this rickettsia proceeded in more depth with the use of monoclonal antibodies. Many investigators independently prepared various kinds of monoclonal antibodies for the typing of newly isolated strains (Chang *et al.*, 1990; Murata *et al.*, 1986; Tange *et al.*, 1991, 1992; Yamashita *et al.*, 1992). Some of these monoclonal antibodies were strain- or type-specific, and the others group- or subgroup-specific. Almost all strain-specific antibodies recognized the 56-kDa strain-specific antigen located on the rickettsial surface (Eisemann and Osterman, 1985; Hanson,1985; Kanemitsu, 1987; Murata *et al.*, 1986; Tange *et al.*, 1991).

Typing of the newly isolated strains was first performed by using three strain-specific monoclonal antibodies, 4B-6 (anti-Gilliam), I-19 (anti-Karp), and 2C-6 (anti-Kato). Consequently many isolates from patients, chiggers, and wild rodents in Japan were classified into three groups: reactive with 4B-6 (Gilliam type), reactive with I-19 (Karp type), and non-reactive with either of these antibodies (Murata *et al.*, 1986; Yamamoto *et al.*, 1986). This method of classification was very clear, since no isolate showed cross reactivity with multiple antibodies. Kato type rickettsia was not found among the isolates tested in these studies. Shimokoshi and Kawasaki strains were included in the non-reactive group.

The Kuroki strain was not identified well at that time, but it was recognized with the I-19 and 2C-6 antibodies by reacting slightly at 1:320 dilution or lower, whereas these antibodies reacted with the corresponding Karp and Kato type antigens at a dilution of 1:10,000 or higher (Yamamoto *et al.*, 1989). As shown in Table 5, the use of such alternative antibodies is now no longer necessary, since monoclonal antibodies specific against each of the Kawasaki, Kuroki, and Shimokoshi strains have been prepared (Furuya *et al.*, 1991b; Tange *et al.*, 1992).

In Korea, the presence of another antigenic type of *R. tsutsugamushi* (Boryong strain) was demonstrated in isolates from patient by reaction patterns with murine polyclonal and monoclonal antibodies (Chang and Kang, 1991; Chang *et al.*, 1990). It is interesting that recent analysis of the type-specific antigen, a 56-kDa protein, of this strain indicates that only five amino acids differ from those of the Kuroki strain (Kim *et al.*,1993a).

The entire base sequence of the gene coding for the 56-kDa type-specific antigen in the Gilliam, Karp, Kato, Kawasaki, Kuroki, Shimokoshi, and Boryong strains has recently been clarified (Kim *et al.*, 1993a; Ohashi *et al.*, 1990a, 1992a; Stover *et al.*, 1990a). Based on the sequence, polymerase chain reaction (PCR) and nested PCR methods have been introduced for the diagnosis of Tsutsugamushi disease and for the typing of *R. tsutsugamushi* (Furuya and Yoshida,

Table 5. Reactivities of Antigenic Types of *R. tsutsugamushi* with Strain-Specific Monoclonal Antibodies in Immunofluorescence*

Rickettsial strains	Monoclonal antibody				
	anti-Gilliam (4B–6)	anti-Karp (I-19)	anti-Kato (2C–6)	anti-Kawasaki (87)	anti-Kuroki (55–12)
Gilliam	10240	< 40	< 40	< 40	< 40
Karp	< 40	40960	< 40	< 40	< 40
Kato	< 40	< 40	20460	< 40	< 40
Shimokoshi	< 40	< 40	< 40	< 40	< 40
Kawasaki	< 40	< 40	< 40	20480	< 40
Kuroki	< 40	320	320	< 40	10240

* Yamamoto, S. (unpublished data).

1992; Furuya *et al.*, 1991b, 1993; Kawamori *et al.*, 1993; Murai *et al.*, 1992; Takahashi *et al.*, 1994c). Ohashi *et al.* (1992b), using several restriction enzymes, analyzed the restriction patterns of PCR-amplified whole genes of the 56-kDa antigen from different strains and found two groups with different reaction patterns in Gilliam type, three in Karp type, and two in Kuroki type. Recently, Ohashi *et al.* (1994) also succeeded in isolating ten rickettsial strains (nine Karp and one Gilliam types) from rodents captured in Taiwan and classified the nine Karp-type rickettsia into six subtypes; all these Karp and Gilliam types were different from prototype Karp and Gilliam strains and also from isolates in Japan, based on restriction fragment length polymorphism analysis.

Thus, antigenic analysis with monoclonal antibodies has revealed the existence of many antigenic variants in new isolates of *R. tsutsugamushi*, and DNA fragment analysis has shown that there are some variants in the same type confirmed with monoclonal antibody.

b. Distribution of rickettsial types

As noted above, various antigenic variants are recognized in *R. tsutsugamushi*. In Southeast Asia, different antigenic types of isolates (TA678, TA686, TA716, TA763, and TH1817), besides Gilliam, Karp, and Kato prototypes, have been identified in Thailand (Elisberg *et al.*, 1968, 1978; Shirai *et al.*, 1981d), and the distribution of these types was also recognized in Malaysia (Shirai *et al.*, 1979b, 1981b), in the Pescadores in Taiwan (Shirai *et al.*, 1982c), in the Philippines (Shirai *et al.*, 1982c), and in North Queensland, Australia (Shirai *et al.*, 1982a).

Rickettsia cross-reactive with multiple antisera by IF was also recognized in isolates from patients and chiggers in the above areas (Shirai *et al.*, 1979b, 1981b, 1981d, 1982a, 1982c, 1982d). As noted by these authors, it is not clear whether these are new antigenic types that contain a mosaic of antigenic determinants reactive with multiple antisera, or whether the rickettsiae in the specimens are a mixture of different antigenic types.

In Korea, Boryong-type rickettsia, which has been distinguished immunologically, has been isolated, and is distributed widely (Chang and Kang, 1991; Chang *et al.*, 1990). In Taiwan, ten isolates were classified by IF, which showed one Gilliam type and nine Karp types; however, the gene structures of these isolates were different from the authentic Gilliam and Karp strains (Ohashi *et al.*, 1994). In Jiangsu, China, the prevalent infection was due to Gilliam type (Guo *et al.*, 1993).

In Japan, in addition to the Gilliam, Karp, and Kato types, the Kawasaki, Kuroki, and Shimokoshi types have been found (Ohashi *et al.*, 1990; Tamura *et al.*, 1984; Yamamoto, 1984; Yamamoto *et al.*, 1986). The Irie and Hirano strains have also been isolated (Kobayashi *et al.*, 1978; Tachibana *et al.*, 1982b). The distribution of rickettsial types in each endemic area in Japan has been re-examined in recent years. In Niigata Prefecture, in the northern part of Honshu Island (the main island of Japan) facing the Sea of Japan, Gilliam and Karp types were predominantly isolated from patients (Murata *et al.*, 1986). In Akita Prefecture, also in the northern part of Honshu Island, most sera from patients showed high antibody titers against Karp antigen (Suto *et al.*, 1991a). These results suggest that Gilliam and Karp types are the predominant types in these areas.

In contrast, in Miyazaki Prefecture, in the southern part of the island of Kyushu, only Kawasaki or Kuroki types were isolated from patients in 1985 (Yamamoto *et al.*, 1989). The typical Gilliam and Karp types were rare in this area. These Kawasaki and Kuroki types were also recognized in Shizuoka, Kanagawa, and Chiba Prefectures, which are located along the coast of the Pacific Ocean in Honshu Island, although some Karp types and, occasionally, Gilliam types were also isolated in these areas (Furuya *et al.*, 1993; Kaiho *et al.*, 1993; Kawamori *et al.*, 1992). Thus, the distribution of rickettsial types differs greatly in each endemic area.

Kato type *R. tsutsugamushi*, which was frequently isolated in Niigata and Akita Prefectures in earlier years, is now rarely isolated in these areas, although a few patients showing a high titer of anti-Kato antibody have been detected in Akita Prefecture by serological tests performed during epidemiological surveys (Suto, 1991a). However, it should be noted that the rickettsial type indicated by serological examinations, even if there is a high titer of anti-rickettsial type antibody, does not always coincide with the rickettsial types isolated from patients in the same endemic area (Kaiho *et al.*, 1993). Recently, several isolates in Ehime Prefecture, Shikoku Island, were identified as Kato type by IF with monoclonal antibodies (Tange *et al.*, 1992). This may be the first case of that type in that area.

On one occasion, in 1984, the Shimokoshi strain was isolated from a patient in Niigata Prefecture (Tamura *et al.*, 1984), but it has not been isolated there since. In immunological tests carried out during epidemiological surveys, however, a few patients whose sera showed high antibody titers against the Shimokoshi strain were recognized in Niigata (Shibata *et al.*, 1984) and in others in Japan (Tamura *et al.*, unpublished data).

In Hokkaido, only the Gilliam type has been isolated from wild rodents and chiggers; no patient has ever been found (Kitaoka *et al.*, 1973).

Direct isolation of rickettsia from chiggers and identification of the rickettsial type have been reported by several investigators. In Japan, Shishido (1964) isolated both Gilliam and Karp types from *Leptotrombidium pallidum*. Iida *et al.* (1966b) also succeeded in isolating Gilliam type from the same species of chiggers. The authors of a recent study in which type-specific monoclonal antibodies were used reported that Karp type was recovered from *L. pallidum*, and Kawasaki type from *L. scutellare* in the same area (Kawamori *et al.*, 1992). Karp type was also isolated from an infected laboratory colony of *L. pallidum* (Takahashi *et al.*, 1988b).

In Niigata Prefecture, five isolates from *L. akamushi* were identified as Kato type (Shishido, 1964); and of 12 isolates from *L. akamushi* in Akita Prefecture, three were typed as Gilliam, one as Karp, and eight as Kato (Iida *et al.*, 1966b).

In Hokkaido, Gilliam type was isolated from *L. kawamuraii* (Kitaoka *et al.*, 1973). This finding agreed with the findings that almost all isolates from rodents in this area were Gilliam type (Shishido, 1962a), although no patient has ever been found (Kitaoka *et al.*, 1973).

In Southeast Asia, *L. arenicola*, *L. fletcheri*, and *L. deliense* were considered to be the main vectors of *R. tsutsugamushi*. Robinson *et al.* (1977) detected a mixture of Karp and TA763 types in *L. arenicola* maintained for seven generations in the laboratory. Shirai *et al.* (1982d) found a mixed infection of TA716, TA763, TA686, Karp, and Kato types in *L. arenicola,* and also a mixed infection of TA716, TA763, TA686, Karp, Kato, and Gilliam in *L. fletcheri*, both of which species had been maintained for succeeding generations in the laboratory. Unfortunately, as these analyses of rickettsial types were performed with polyclonal antibodies, it is anticipated that in-depth studies will be performed using modern techniques, such as type-specific monoclonal antibodies and genetic analysis by the PCR method.

Gotoh (1968) passaged three pairs of mixed infections with three prototype strains in mice once a week for either 25 or 50 weeks, and typed the series weekly by direct IF. Of the three strains injected, the infectivity of two strains was aligned. In a series involving Gilliam strain, the three types were always detected together with another type which was not added and always appeared beginning with the early passages. On the other hand, in a series involving Karp and Kato strains, only two types were detected, and no Gilliam type appeared at all. These results suggest that strain selectivity or mutation occurred during passage in mice.

Recently, Takahashi *et al.* (1994d) reported that only the Karp type was recovered from an infected laboratory colony of *L. pallidum* by passage in mice, whereas *R. tsutsugamushi* DNA obtained from the same mites detected directly by nested PCR included the Kawasaki, Kuroki, and unidentified types, in addition to the Karp type. These results should be kept in mind for future studies in typing rickettsia in chiggers.

6. Analysis of Antigens in *Rickettsia tsutsugamushi*

a. *Preparation of antisera in animals*

For immunological studies of *R. tsutsugamushi*, antisera to this rickettsia are commonly prepared by immunizing guinea pigs, rabbits, or mice. The procedures used for antibody preparation in these animals are briefly outlined in this section.

In guinea pigs : Antigens used for immunization are prepared from the spleens and livers of infected mice, or from the infected yolk sacs of embryonated chicken eggs as 10–20% suspensions of homogenates of these organs or tissues in sucrose phosphate-buffered glutamic acid (SPG) (Bovarnick *et al.*, 1950; Iida *et al.*, 1966a, 1966b; Shishido, 1962a, 1964). Rickettsiae prepared in cultured cells are also used as antigens. Each guinea pig is injected with 0.1 ml antigen intracerebrally, and the rectal temperature is measured every day for 2 weeks.

Infection is confirmed when the rectal temperature exceeds 40°C; this elevation begins 3–10 days after injection and continues for 2–7 days. The blood is harvested by cardiac puncture 4 weeks after infection, and the sera are pooled and stored after the antibody titer and its specificity have been examined by immunological tests.

In rabbits : Iida *et al.* (1966b) prepared antisera against *R. tsutsugamushi* as follows; rickettsiae were introduced to a primary renal cell culture prepared from the extirpated kidney of a rabbit, and, after massive rickettsial growth, a concentrated rickettsial suspension was prepared by centrifugation. This suspension was injected intravenously several times, at weekly intervals, into the rabbit whose one kidney had been extirpated. The antiserum obtained usually showed relatively high antibody titers and specificity, similar to the antisera obtained from guinea pigs.

Shirai and coworkers (Shirai and Wisseman, 1975; Shirai *et al.*, 1979b, 1980, 1981b) prepared antisera in rabbits by the intravenous injection of 20% liver and spleen homogenate of infected mice or infected yolk sac homogenate. In all cases, the rabbits do not show any symptoms after injection. Therefore, the antibody titer should be examined by indirect immunofluorescence (IF) or by any other test at appropriate intervals after injection by collecting a small amount of blood from an ear vein; if necessary, a booster injection is given. Satisfactory immunization results in elevated antibody titers, of 1:128 to 1:256 by indirect IF, or 1:8 to 1:64 by the CF test.

In mice : *R. tsutsugamushi* strains that are virulent and avirulent in mice have been found. Intraperitoneal injection of a virulent strain to mice results in the death of the animal before there is significant elevation of antibody titers. Therefore, subcutaneous injection should be used, since, with infection via this route, the appearance of symptoms is delayed and the survival of the animal is prolonged. With this method, if there are striking signs of infection, it is advisable to give antibiotic treatment, for example, 100 μl of doxycycline, at a concentration of 1 mg/ml, injected intraperitoneally once a day for 3 consecutive days.

Although blood can be harvested from the heart or vena cava caudalis for checking antibody titers during the immunization process, small amounts of blood (0.05–0.1 ml) can be obtained several times from the orbital sinus or plexus using a capillary tube, without killing the animal.

b. Preparation of monoclonal antibody

Monoclonal antibodies against *R. tsutsugamushi* are also useful for the serological and antigenic analysis of this rickettsia. The preparation procedures are described in this section (Murata *et al.*, 1986; Pontecorvo, 1975).

Immunization and preparation of spleen cells : A preparation of antigen, such as infected cells, purified rickettsial preparation, or fractionated component(s) of the rickettsia, is emulsified with Freund's adjuvant in phosphate-buffered saline without Ca^{2+} and Mg^{2+} (PBS(−), consisting of 140 mM NaCl, 2.6 mM KCl, 1.47 mM KH_2PO_4, and 9.10 mM Na_2HPO_4, pH 7.1) and injected intraperitoneally into 4- to 6-week-old male BALB/c mice. After 3–8 weeks, the mice receive a booster injection of the same antigen preparation, and 3 days later the spleen is harvested under sterile conditions.

The spleen is cut into several pieces with scissors, and the cells are dispersed into PRMI 1640 medium without fetal bovine serum (FBS) by pressing the cut pieces of spleen with the flat tip of forceps. The cell suspension obtained is passed through a stainless steel strainer (No. 200), and the cells, after being counted in the filtrate, are washed twice with FBS-free RPMI 1640 medium by centrifugation at 1,000 rpm for 5 min at room temperature.

Cell fusion : Myeloma cells such as P3X63Ag8U1 (P3U1), which are cultured in RPMI 1640 medium containing 10% FBS or in GIT medium (Nihon Pharmaceutical Company Ltd., Tokyo) without FBS, are washed twice with FBS-free RPMI medium by repeated centrifugation, and mixed with the spleen cells suspension in the same FBS-free RPMI medium at a ratio of myeloma to spleen cells of 1:3 to 1:10. The mixture is centrifuged at 1,000 rpm for 5 min and the supernatant is discarded. For cell fusion, 1 ml of sterilized 50% w/v polyethylene glycol (PEG) 4000 in FBS-free RPMI medium kept at 37°C is added dropwise to the cells in the centrifuge tube for 1 min while the tube is vigorously shaken. After 1-min incubation, FBS-free RPMI medium is added to the tube (at a speed of 2 ml in 2 min); then another 7 ml is added in 2 min in order to suspend the cell fusion reaction. The cells are recovered in a pellet after centrifugation at 1,000 rpm for 5 min, and are re-suspended, at a concentration of 10^6 spleen cells per ml, in RPMI 1640 supplemented with 10% FBS or GIT without FBS, which contains 10^{-4}M hypoxanthine, 4×10^{-7}M aminopterin and 1.6×10^{-5}M thymidine (HAT medium). One hundred-μl aliquots of the cell suspension are then added to each well of a 96-well culture multiplate, and incubated at 37°C in a

5% CO_2 atmosphere. Colonies of the spleen hybridoma and myeloma cells are observed after about 7 days. At this time, half of the culture medium is exchanged for new medium, 10% FBS-containing RPMI 1640 or FBS-free GIT medium supplemented with 10^{-4}M hypoxanthine and 1.6×10^{-5}M thymidine (HT medium). The culture is continued by repeating medium changes at 2- to 3-day intervals until the hybridoma colony is a suitable size, and antibody production in the culture fluid is examined by an indirect IF method or enzyme-linked immunosorbent assay (ELISA) method. *Cloning of hybridoma* : First, thymus or spleen is harvested from a BALB/c mouse and a cell suspension of the tissue used for feeder cells is prepared as outlined above. The cell number is adjusted to 10^6–10^7 cells/ml in 10% FBS-containing RPMI 1640 or FBS-free GIT medium. Hybridoma cells in each well in which antibody production is recognized in the culture fluid are suspended in the same medium, and the cell number is determined. Then a mixture of hybridoma and feeder cells is prepared, at a concentration of 5 hybridoma cells/ml and 10^6–10^7 feeder cells/ml. Aliquots of 100 μl are distributed to each well of a 96-well plate and incubated at 37°C in a 5% CO_2 atmosphere, for 7 to 10 days. Antibody production in each well is examined by an indirect IF or ELISA with the respective antigen, and this cloning procedure is repeated again for the cells in antibody-positive wells. The cloned cells obtained are cultured in 10% FBS-RPMI or FBS-free GIT medium.
Preparation of high-titer antibody : Hybridoma cells (10^6–10^7) are injected into 5- to 6-week-old BALB/c mice that have been intraperitoneally injected with 0.5 ml Pristan (2, 6, 10, 14-tetramethylpentadecane; Aldrich Chemical, Milwaukee, Wisconsin) 1–2 weeks prior to the injection of hybridoma cells. After 1–2 weeks, the peritoneal fluid is harvested, centrifuged and stored at –30°C or lower.

The antibody titer is determined by an indirect IF, and the antibody subclass is determined with antibodies against each subclass, using an indirect IF or the Ouchterlony's test.

c. Antigenic structure of R. tsutsugamushi

Eisemann and Osterman (1981) were the first to demonstrate that several components on the rickettsial surface showed antigenicity reactive with antibodies against homologous or heterologous strains of *R. tsutsugamushi*, this was shown in gel slices obtained after polyacrylamide gel electrophoresis (PAGE) by ELISA. More precise analysis of rickettsial antigenic components was performed by immunoprecipitation and PAGE autoradiography (Hanson, 1985) and by an immunoblotting technique (Tamura *et al.*, 1985). The reactivity of individual polypeptides on PAGE with the guinea pig hyperimmune polyclonal antibodies against each antigenic type of rickettsia is summarized below (Tamura *et al.*, 1985):

(i) The 56-kDa polypeptide, which polypeptide is present in the largest amount on the rickettsial surface, reacts strongly with homologous antiserum, but faintly or moderately with heterologous antisera, indicating that this polypeptide has strain- or type-specific antigenicity.

(ii) The 46–47-kDa and 70-kDa polypeptides react not only with homologous antiserum but also with heterologous antisera, suggesting that these polypeptides have the characteristics of group- or species-specific antigenicity.

(iii) Many guinea pig hyperimmune sera, prepared by the intracerebral injection of intact rickettsial suspension, showed a clear reaction with the 56-kDa, the 46–47-kDa, and the 70-kDa polypeptides, but not such a clear reaction with the other polypeptides on immunoblotting tests, as shown in Fig. 14.

However, on the immunoblotting test, sera from patients varied (Ohashi *et al.*, 1988). Most sera reacted with the 56-kDa polypeptide, suggesting that this polypeptide is the dominant antigen in the course of the infection. The other polypeptides, *i.e.*, the 60-, the 50–52-, the 46–47-, the 35- and the 21–25-kDa polypeptides were reactive with some sera, but not all. The 60 kDa is group- and 46–47 and 21–25 kDa are subgroup-specific antigens.

The antigenic components in *R. tsutsugamushi* have also been examined with monoclonal antibodies by various investigators (Eisemann and Osterman, 1985; Hanson, 1985; Murata *et al.*, 1986). Many strain-specific monoclonal antibodies show a reaction with the 56-kDa polypeptide (Hanson, 1985; Murata *et al.*, 1986). These strain-specific monoclonal antibodies react only with the homologous strain and do not react at all with the heterologous strains, as shown in Fig. 15. Therefore, these antibodies are useful for typing of isolated rickettsia (Furuya *et al.*, 1991b; Kawamori *et al.*, 1992; Murata *et al.*, 1986). However, some of the monoclonal antibodies reactive with the 56-kDa polypeptide show cross-reaction with some

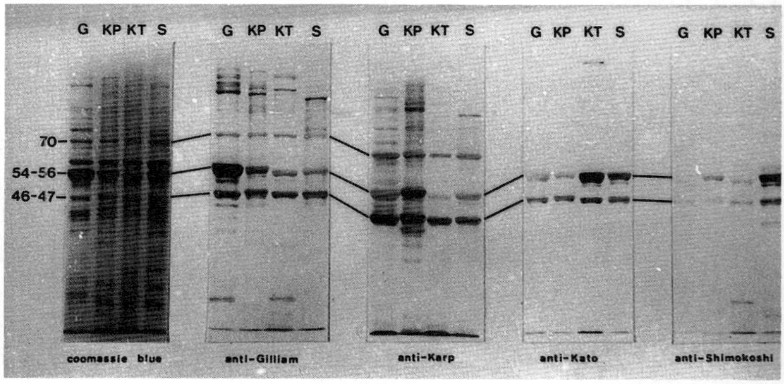

Fig. 14. Immunoblotting profiles of rickettsial polypeptides separated by PAGE. Rickettsial antigens were purified from L cell cultures, and antisera were prepared in guinea pigs immunized with rickettsiae also derived from L cell cultures. Characters at the top indicate the rickettsial strain of each column: G : Gilliam; KP: Karp; KT: Kato; S: Shimokoshi. Each of the four columns in each group was stained with Coomassie blue or reacted with antisera as indicated at the bottom of the columns. The numbers on the left side indicate the molecular sizes (in kDa) of the bands which were determined in comparison with migrations of standard proteins.

heterologous types (Eisemann and Osterman, 1985; Hanson, 1985), indicating that the 56-kDa polypeptide has epitopes that are both strain-specific and common among several strains.

On the other hand, the monoclonal antibodies against the 46–47- and 60-kDa polypeptides show, in many cases, cross-reactivity with several strains (Hanson, 1985; Furuya *et al.*, 1991b), indicating that these polypeptides have a group- or subgroup-specific antigenic nature. A monoclonal antibody against the 21–25-kDa polypeptide showed subgroup-specific properties.

d. Type-specific antigen

As noted above, the antigenic type of *R. tsutsugamushi* depends on the 56-kDa polypeptide, which is the major polypeptide located on the rickettsial surface. When the rickettsia is solubilized at 80°C or lower in SDS-containing buffer without 2-mercaptoethanol (2-ME), this antigenic polypeptide forms a band at 110 kDa or higher positions on PAGE analysis, suggesting that it is present as a dimer or oligomer in this rickettsia (Urakami *et al.*, 1986).

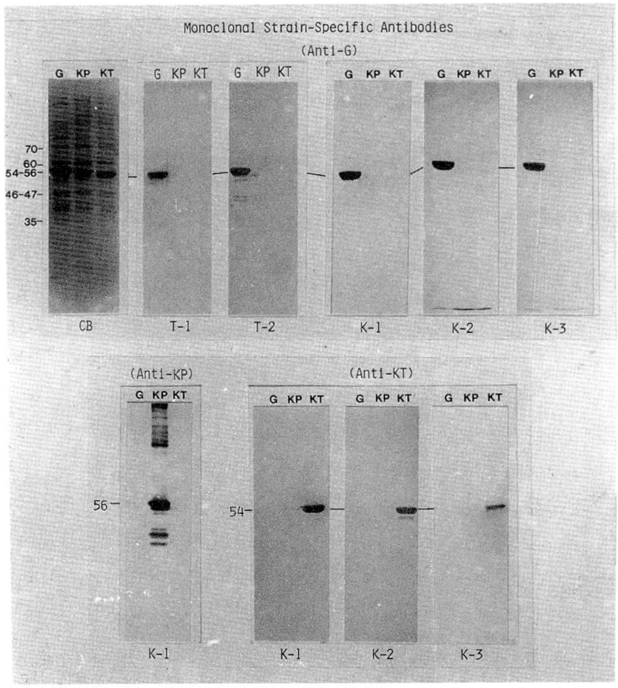

Fig. 15. Immunoblotting profiles of rickettsial polypeptides separated by PAGE with monoclonal antibodies which show strain-specificity to each prototype strain of *R. tsutsugamushi*. Rickettsial antigens were purified from L cell cultures. Letters at the top indicate the rickettsial strain of each column: G: Gilliam; KP: Karp; KT: Kato. Three columns in each group were stained with Coomassie blue or allowed to react with monoclonal antibodies as indicated at the bottom of the columns. The numbers on the left side are the same as in Fig. 14.

When the sample is treated with 2-ME, this oligomeric polypeptide is split into monomers of 43 kDa, suggesting intermolecular disulfide bonds. The 43-kDa polypeptide changes to the 56-kDa position on PAGE analysis when the solubilized sample is heated at more than 80°C for 10 min, indicating that this is a heat-modifiable polypeptide.

The 56-kDa polypeptide can be purified from the rickettsia by the method outlined below, and the N-terminal amino acid sequence has been determined (Ohashi *et al.*, 1989). Comparison of 35 amino acid sequences at the N-terminal side of the polypeptides in the Gilliam,

Karp, and Kato strains revealed that isoleucine was an N-terminal amino acid in all cases, replacements were observed at several amino acids, and there was about 70% homology among strains.

This finding indicates that the 56-kDa polypeptide may have a characteristic sequence in each strain. To determine in greater depth the differences in molecular structure among strains, the genes of the polypeptide were cloned and sequenced (see the following section on gene analysis).

e. Purification of the 56-kDa polypeptide

The purification procedure consists of three steps (Ohashi *et al.*, 1989): (1) The outer membranous proteins are separated from the others by treating the purified rickettsia with a mild nonionic detergent, Sarkosyl (Nakarai Chemicals, Kyoto, Japan). (2) The insoluble fraction obtained is solubilized with a strong anionic detergent, sodium dodecyl sulfate (SDS), and the proteins in the sample are fractionated by gel-filtration chromatography. By this procedure, a partially purified 56-kDa fraction is obtained. (3) This fraction is further fractionated by reverse-phase chromatography. The 56-kDa polypeptide is recovered in a sharp peak, and the purity is estimated to be more than 90%.

This procedure can be applied without any changes to the purification of 56-kDa polypeptides from the Gilliam, Karp, and Kato strains. The yield of these polypeptides from 2.2 to 3.0 mg of the outer membrane protein fraction (Sarkosyl-insoluble fraction) is approximately 0.12 to 0.18 mg. The purified polypeptide retains antigenicity in a dot blot immunoassay with strain-specific monoclonal antibodies.

The procedure (Ohashi *et al.*, 1989) is described in detail below:

(i) Purified rickettsiae are suspended in 10 mM sodium phosphate buffer, pH7.4, containing 0.1% Sarkosyl. After incubation at 37°C for 30 min, the suspension is centrifuged at 10,000 × *g* for 1 h.

Note : Sarkosyl at the concentration of 0.05–0.1% gives a satisfactory result. A concentration of 0.5% Sarkosyl results in the solubilization of almost all membranous proteins into the soluble fraction.

(ii) The insoluble pellet is solubilized with 10 mM sodium phosphate buffer, pH7.4, containing 2% SDS, 5% 2-ME, and 5 mM ethylenediaminetetraacetic acid (EDTA) by heating at 100°C for 10 min, followed by centrifugation at 15,000 × *g* for 10 min.

(iii) The supernatant fluid is loaded onto a TSK G3000SW glass column (8 by 300 mm; Tosoh, Tokyo, Japan) for high-performance liquid chromatography (HPLC; Ultrochrom GTi system; Pharmacia, Uppsala, Sweden), and the proteins are eluted, at a flow rate of 0.5 ml/min, with 0.05 M sodium phosphate buffer, pH7.0, containing 0.1% SDS and 0.1 M sodium chloride, monitoring absorbance at 280 nm. The fractions of each peak observed are analyzed by SDS-PAGE.

Note : Several peaks are observed during the retention times of 11 to 21 min. The 56-kDa polypeptide peak is the largest peak, seen at a retention time of about 14 min. The SDS-PAGE pattern of this fraction, shown by Coomassie blue staining, reveals one band of the 56-kDa polypeptide, but several bands are revealed on the column by silver staining.

(iv) The 56-kDa polypeptide fraction obtained is applied to the TSK Phenyl-5PW RP column (4.6 by 75mm; Tosoh) of an HPLC equipped with an automated gradient controller. The proteins are eluted with linear gradients of 0–20% acetonitrile in 0.05% trifluoroacetic acid for 5 min and then with 20–60% acetonitrile in 0.05% trifluoroacetic acid for 32 min, at a flow rate of 0.8 ml/min, monitoring absorbance at 215 nm. The fractions of each peak are pooled, and analyzed by SDS-PAGE.

Note : Although a gradual increase of absorbance at 215 nm is observed after a retention time of 10 min, a sharp peak is seen at the retention time of 27–28 min. The SDS-PAGE of this fraction reveals a single band of the 56-kDa polypeptide by silver staining.

7. Genetic Analysis

a. Genetic analysis of rickettsial proteins

Genes of rickettsial proteins that have been cloned are for the 150-, 110-, 72-, and 60-kDa proteins (the last of which has been described as a 58-kDa proteins by such investigators as Oaks *et al.*, 1987), and the 56-, 49-, 47-, and 22-kDa proteins (Hickman *et al.*, 1991; Kim *et al.*, 1993a; Oaks *et al.*, 1987, 1989; Ohashi *et al.*, 1990a, 1992a; Stover *et al.*, 1987, 1990a, 1990b). These eight proteins are all antigenic and react with hyperimmune sera against *Rickettsia tsutsugamushi*. Some of them also react with patient sera, indicating that B cell epitope(s) may exist in the protein molecules.

The nucleotide sequences of genes encoding the 60-, 56-, and 22-kDa proteins and their amino acid sequences have been determined (Hickman *et al.*, 1991; Kim *et al.*, 1993a; Ohashi *et al.*, 1990a, 1992a; Stover *et al.*, 1990a,b). The 56-kDa protein is the major type-specific antigen that determines the antigenic type of rickettsia, and the recombinant 56-kDa protein is used as an antigen for the serodiagnosis of Tsutsugamushi disease by ELISA and hemagglutination assay (Kim *et al.*, 1993a,b).

The 110-kDa protein also shows strain-specific antigenicity (Oaks *et al.*, 1989). On the other hand, the 72-, 60-, and 47-kDa proteins show cross-reactive antigenicity among strains (Oaks *et al.*, 1989). The antigenic specificity of the 150-, 49-, and 22-kDa gene products has not yet been reported in depth.

The role played by these proteins, except for the 60 kDa, in rickettsial cells is not known at present. The 60-kDa protein is considered to be a stress protein from its amino acid sequence homology with heat shock protein (HSP) 60 in other bacteria (Stover *et al.*, 1990b). The 47- and 22-kDa proteins have a T cell epitope, suggesting that they may activate cellular immunity, and some investigators consider that these proteins will be the first candidate for the development of a component vaccine for Tsutsugamushi disease (Hickman *et al.*, 1991, 1993).

b. Gene structure

Table 6 shows the nucleotide sequence of the promoter regions, ribosome-binding sites (RBS), and stop codons, summarized from the published sequences of various genes of *R. tsutsugamushi*. Two genes from *R. rickettsii* and *R. prowazekii* and the consensus sequence of *E. coli* are also shown in the table for comparison. Ohashi *et al.* (1992a) found recently that the gene for the 56-kDa protein of *R. tsutsugamushi* Kato strain is regulated by four main tandem promoters designated P1, P2, P3, and P4, which are located 100–500 bp upstream of the start codon; −10 and −35 regions for each locus were assumed. The same nucleotide sequences of the −10 and −35 regions were also found in other types of *R. tsutsugamushi*, *i.e.*, in the Gilliam, Karp, and Kawasaki strains. In the Shimokoshi and Kuroki strains, some nucleotide replacement was seen in the corresponding areas, but the sequences were similar. In the Boryong strain, P3 and P4 regions have not been identified (Kim *et al.*, 1993a).

Table 6. Comparison of Promoter Regions, Ribosome-Binding Sites (RBS) and Stop Codons of Several Rickettsial Genes

Bacteria	Strain	Product	Promoter No.	–35	–10	RBS	Stop codon	References
E. coli consensus				TTGACA	TATAAT	AGGAGGU	—	McClure, 1985
R. tsutsugamushi								
	Kato	56-kDa antigen	P1[a]	TATACT	TATAAA	AGGAG	UAG	Ohashi *et al.*, 1992a
	Kawasaki			******	******	******	***	〃
	Kuroki			******	******	******	***	〃
	Shimokoshi			*G****	******	******	***	〃
	Gilliam			******	******	******	***	〃
	Karp			******	******	******	***	Stover *et al.*, 1990a
	Boryong			******	******	******	***	Kim *et al.*, 1993a
	Kato		P2	TTTACA	TATACT			
	Kawasaki			******	******			
	Kuroki			******	******			
	Shimokoshi			****TG	*G****			
	Gilliam			******	******			
	Karp			******	******			
	Boryong			******	******			
	Kato		P3	TTGCGT	TATCTA			
	Kawasaki			******	******			
	Kuroki			******	******			
	Shimokoshi			****A*	******			

	Gilliam			******	******			
	Karp			******	******			
	Boryong			NI[b]	NI			
	Kato		P4	TTGATT	TATAAT			
	Kawasaki			******	******			
	Kuroki			******	**AT*A			
	Shimokoshi			******	******			
	Gilliam			******	******			
	Karp			******	******			
	Boryong			NI	NI			
	Karp	22-kDa antigen	—	TTGATA	TATATT	AGGA	UAA	Hickman *et al.*, 1991
	Karp	11-kDa protein	—	TTGAAA	TATGAT	GGAGGA	UAA	Stover *et al.*, 1990
				TTCACACTTGAA[c]				
		60-kDa antigen		cotranscribed with *stp 11*		AGGAG	UAA	Stover *et al.*, 1990
R. rickettsii		17-kDa antigen	—	TTTACA	TATACT	AGAGAGA	UAG	Anderson *et al.*, 1987
R. prowazekii		Citrate synthase	—	TTCTAA	TATACT	AUGAGGU	UGA	Wood *et al.*, 1987

[a] P1, P2, P3, and P4 indicate tandem promoters for 56-kDa antigen gene.
[b] Not identified.
[c] Heat shock promoter.

The putative promoter of the 22-kDa protein gene is similar to the consensus sequence of *E. coli*, with one nucleotide replacement in each of the −10 and −35 regions (Hickman *et al.*, 1991). Both the *stp11* and *sta58* genes, which encode the heat shock protein of *R. tsutsugamushi*, are regulated by a common promoter, suggesting that these genes are cotranscribed or coregulated (Stover *et al.*, 1990b). The presumed promoter sequence of the −10 region is TATGAT, but the −35 region consists of the overlapping promoter sequence of TTGAAA and heat shock promoter TTCACACTTGAA.

For comparison, the putative promoter sequences of the 17-kDa protein gene in *R. rickettsii* (Anderson *et al.*, 1987) and the citrate synthase gene (*gltA*) in *R. prowazekii* (Wood *et al.*, 1987) are also shown in Table 6. All these promoter sequences, including all types of *R. tsutsugamushi*, are similar to the consensus sequence of *E. coli* (McClure, 1985), suggesting that these rickettsiae have transcription mechanisms similar to those of *E. coli*.

In general, the nucleotide sequences of the ribosome-binding site (RBS) located a few bases upstream of the start codon are purine-rich. All the RBS of the rickettsial genes shown in Table 6 are also adenine- and guanine-rich sequences, which are similar to the Shine-Dalgarno RBS sequence of *E. coli* (Shine and Dalgarno, 1974). All the RBS of the 56-kDa protein genes from the seven strains shown in Table 6 had an identical sequence, AGGAG (Kim *et al.*, 1993a; Ohashi *et al.*,1990a, 1992a; Stover *et al.*, 1990a), and the other genes also had the AGGAG or AGGA sequence at the RBS (Hickman *et al.*, 1991; Stover *et al.*, 1990b). Thus, similarity of the nucleotide sequence at RBS has been recognized among the various genes reported to date.

The stop codons in the genes of *R. tsutsugamushi* are UAA (ocher) and UAG (amber), as shown in Table 6. The stop codon of UGA (opal) has not yet been found in *R. tsutsugamushi*. However, in the *R. prowazekii gltA* gene, UGA is effective as its stop codon (Wood *et al.*, 1987).

A hairpin loop structure was recognized approximately 20 bp downstream of the stop codons in the 56-kDa protein genes in five of the seven *R. tsutsugamushi* strains; but was not observed in the Kawasaki strain and not identified in the Boryong strain (Table 7) (Ohashi *et al.*, 1992a; Stover *et al.*, 1990a).

Table 7. Hairpin Loop Structures Which Are Seen in the 3′-side Flanking Regions of 56-kDa Protein Genes, and Comparison of the Structure among the Antigenic Variants of *R. tsutsugamushi*

Rickettsial strains	Hairpin loop structure* (spacing)
Gilliam	AAAAAGCAGCTAAAA—(14)—TTTTAGCTGCTTTTT
Karp**	AAAAAGCAGCTAAAA—(14)—TTTTAGCTGCTTTTT
Kato	AAAAAGCAGCTAAAA—(14)—TTTTAGCTGCTTTTT
Kawasaki	ATAAGGTAGCTAAAA—(14)—TTTTAGCCGCTTTCG
Kuroki	AAAAAGCAGCTAAAA—(14)—TTTTAGCTACTTTTT
Shimokoshi	AAAAAGCAGCTGAAA—(16)—TTTTAGCTGCTTTTG

* Unpaired bases are underlined.
** Referred from the report by Stover *et al.*, 1990a.

c. *Properties of individual rickettsial genes and their products*

56-kDa protein gene (type-specific antigen gene)

The 56-kDa protein, the predominant constitutional protein in *R. tsutsugamushi*, is located on the rickettsial surface and shows type-specific antigenicity. Genes of the type-specific protein from the Gilliam (Ohashi *et al.*, 1990a), Karp (Stover *et al.*, 1990a), Kato, Kawasaki, Kuroki, Shimokoshi (Ohashi *et al.*, 1992a), and Boryong (Kim *et al.*, 1993a) strains have been cloned and sequenced, each of which strains shows distinct antigenicity.

The length of the nucleotide sequences determined except in the Boryong strain, was 2260–2303 bp, which involved 555–592 bp of the 5′- noncoding region, 1563–1596 bp of the open reading frame (ORF), and 129–148 bp of the 3′-noncoding region. In the Boryong strain, the total length was 1874 bp, which involved 272 bp of the 5′-noncoding region and 1602 bp of the ORF, including the stop codon, without a description of the 3′-noncoding region.

As noted above, it has been shown that the transcription of these 56-kDa protein genes is regulated by at least four multiple tandem promoters. This suggests that mRNAs of different sizes are synthesized from each promoter locus by transcription, and that this predominant protein in the rickettsia is produced abundantly during rickettsial multiplication.

In the 3′-noncoding regions of the Gilliam, Karp, and Kato strains, a potential hairpin-like loop structure consisting of 15 paired bases is recognized. This demonstrates the characteristics of a rho-independent transcriptional terminator. The corresponding structure in the genes of the Kuroki and Shimokoshi strains is the sequence with an incomplete inverted repeat including one or two unpaired bases. In the gene of Kawasaki strain, however, five mismatched bases are included in the corresponding area, as shown in Table 7, showing that a hairpin-like structure may not be fabricated.

All the genes described above encode proteins consisting of 521–533 amino acids. The sequence of 22 amino acids at the NH_2-terminal was predicted to be a signal peptide, since the NH_2-terminal sequence of the mature 56-kDa protein, which was determined by chemical analysis of purified protein obtained from rickettsiae (Ohashi *et al.*, 1989), was recognized downstream of the putative signal peptide.

The amino acid sequence of signal peptides was identical in the six strains, Gilliam, Karp, Kato, Kawasaki, Kuroki, and Boryong, while purine-to-purine replacements of nucleotides were recognized at some positions in the corresponding region of the gene. In the signal peptide of the Shimokoshi strain, two amino acids differed from those of the other strains. All the signal peptides of *R. tsutsugamushi* strains consist of a basic region and a hydrophobic core, as seen in those characteristic of other prokaryotic cells (Oliver, 1985).

The three COOH-terminal amino acids of the signal peptide are Ala-Ser-Ala or Ala-Asn-Ala. This Ala-X-Ala sequence is included in the preferred amino acid sequences of signal peptides at the processing site proposed by Oliver (1985).

In the comparative analysis of amino acid sequence alignments of the 56-kDa proteins in antigenic variants of the Gilliam, Karp, Kato, Kawasaki, Kuroki, and Shimokoshi strains, substitutions or deletions of one or several contiguous amino acid residues are recognized throughout the molecules, but the significant difference in sequences among strains is in the variable domain (VD) regions I-IV, as shown in Fig. 16.

In the variable domains, there are both diversity and similarity among strains, and the relationships are complicated. For example, the Kuroki strain seems to be a chimera of the Gilliam and Karp strains, since the sequence of Kuroki strain is similar to that of Gilliam at VD I, to Karp at VD III, and to both Gilliam and Karp at VD IV. The sequences of Gilliam at VD II and VDIII resemble those

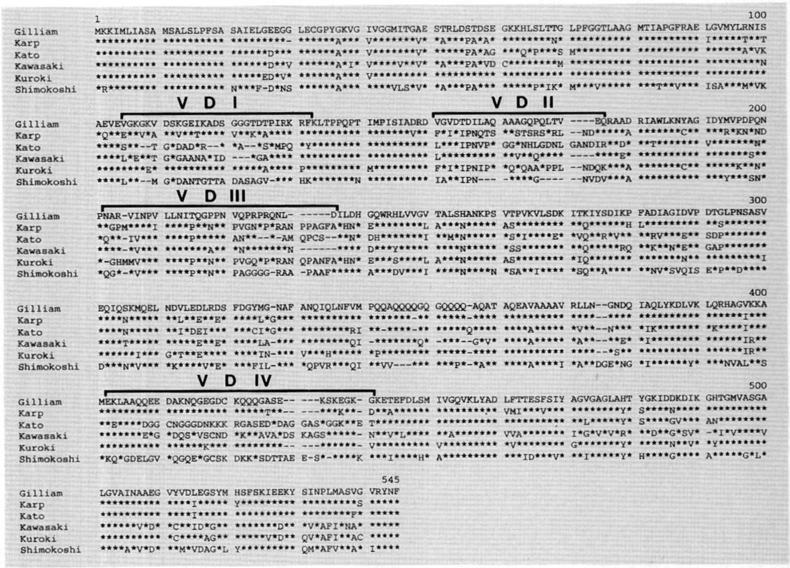

Fig. 16. Alignment of deduced amino acid sequences of 56-kDa protein homologues from six antigenic variants of *R. tsutsugamushi*. Aligned position of identical amino acids with the molecule of Gilliam strain are shown with asterisks. The sequence from Karp strain is from the report of Stover *et al.* (1990a). Gaps indicated by dashes were introduced for optimal alignment of all six homologues. Brackets indicate four variable domains (VDI, II, III, IV). Twenty-two amino acid sequences at the NH_2-terminal side are the signal peptide regions.

of Kawasaki, but the sequences at VD I and IV of both these strains differ greatly. It is not yet known how the polymorphism in the variable domains evolved, but this diversity appears to be due to a combination of point mutation and a recombinational process.

Hydropathy analysis shows that these 56-kDa proteins of all antigenic variants have an alternative succession of hydrophilic and hydrophobic motifs which is characteristic of transmembrane proteins (Fig. 17). All the variable domains noted above are located mostly in hydrophilic regions. This suggests that all or some of the domains are located on the rickettsial surface and may serve as antigenic determinant(s) of rickettsial types. Indeed, a type-specific B cell determinant for Karp was demonstrated at the VD I region (Stover *et al.*, 1990a).

Based on the homology of the amino acid sequence of these proteins in the six antigenic variants, the relationship among variants is

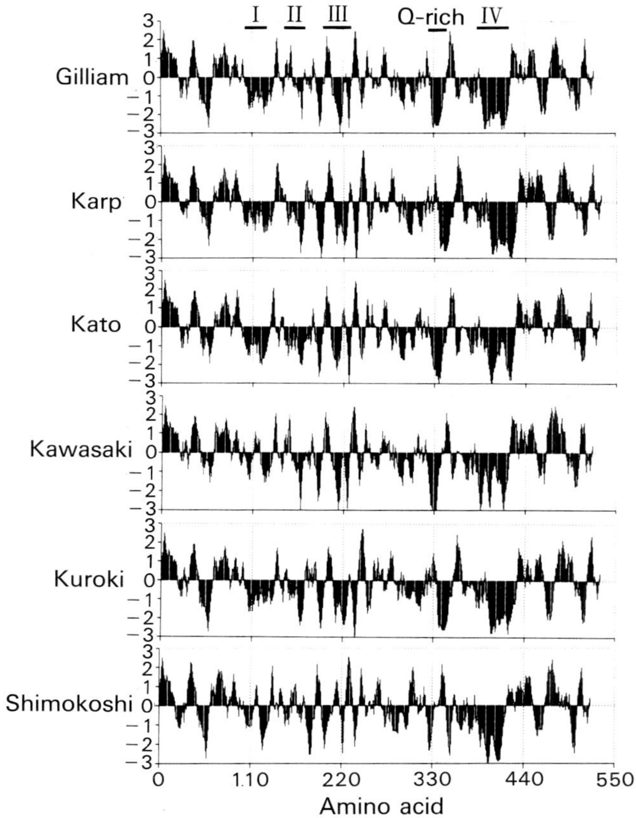

Fig. 17. Comparison of hydropathy profiles of 56-kDa protein homologues. Positive and negative values at the left indicate hydrophobicity and hydrophilicity, respectively, which were analyzed by the method of Kyte and Doolittle (1982) using a seven amino acid window. Variable domains and Gln-rich regions are barred with numbers and symbols at the top, respectively.

illustrated in a phylogenetic tree (Fig. 18). This tree was constructed by computer analysis using the unweighed pair-group method (Nei, 1987) in the program Gene Works. The Gilliam, Karp, and Kuroki strains form a closely related cluster, whereas the Shimokoshi strain is located far from the others.

The amino acid sequence of the 56-kDa protein of the Boryong strain presumed from the gene analysis performed by Kim *et al.* (1993a) is very similar to that of the Kuroki strain, with only five

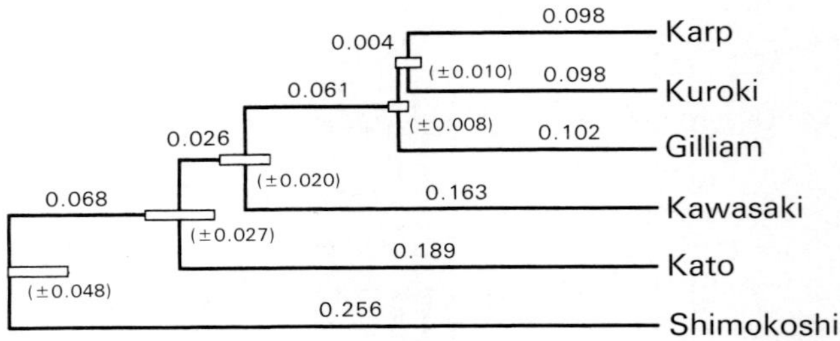

Fig. 18. Phylogenetic tree of *R. tsutsugamushi* antigenic variants based on the amino acid sequences of 56-kDa protein homologues. The graph was constructed with the unweighted pair-group method of analysis (Nei, 1987) in the program Gene Works. The numbers and those in parenthesis indicate genetic distance and standard errors at the branching points, respectively.

amino acid replacements in the whole molecule, one being located at VD II and the others at separate loci; the Boryong strain is therefore very closely related to the Kuroki strain.

60-kDa protein gene

In 1990, the gene for the 60 kDa of the Karp strain of *R. tsutsugamushi* was cloned and sequenced by Stover *et al.* (1990b); these investigators also found a gene encoding the 11-kDa protein upstream of the 60-kDa protein gene. The genes for the 60-kDa and 11-kDa proteins were designated *sta58* and *stp11*, respectively. The amino acid sequence of the products of the *sta58* and *stp11* genes was similar to those of GroEL and GroES in *E. coli* (Hemmingsen *et al.*, 1988), respectively, suggesting that these two products belong to the heat shock protein family, HSP 60 and HSP 10. Furthermore, the *sta58* and *stp11* genes are cotranscribed by a single common heat shock promoter, *i.e.*, the structure of these two genes is polycistronic, as in the case of GroEL and GroES.

In general, it is known that heat shock proteins in heterologous species show great similarity in their amino acid sequences (Vodkin and Williams, 1988) and also cross-reaction in their antigenicity. However, immunoblotting has revealed that anti-*R. tsutsugamushi* antibody reacted specifically with the 60-kDa protein of *R. tsutsugamushi*, but reacted only slightly with the corresponding proteins from other bacteria (Stover *et al.*, 1990b). This suggests that the 60-kDa protein of *R. tsutsugamushi* possesses species-specific B cell epitope(s). The B cell epitope(s) of the 60-kDa protein in *R. tsutsugamushi* was analyzed with synthetic oligopeptides (Lachumanan *et al.*, 1993).

Among 160 synthesized overlapping octapeptides, corresponding to the amino acid sequence of the 60-kDa protein, 15 peptides reacted with nine kinds of patient sera. By this examination, the amino acid sequence of the 15 immunoreactive peptides were found to be widely distributed within the hydrophilic regions of the 60-kDa protein. Additionally, it was found that IgM antibody in patient sera reacted with these peptides, but that IgG did not.

47-kDa protein gene

The gene encoding the 47-kDa protein, which is a group-specific antigen, was cloned from the Karp strain of *R. tsutsugamushi* by Oaks *et al.* (1987). However, its nucleotide sequence has not yet been published. Hickman, a colleague of Oaks (Hickman *et al.*, 1993), found in a [^{3}H] thymidine incorporation test that a recombinant 47-kDa protein induced proliferation in a polyclonal helper T cell line derived from *R. tsutsugamushi* immune mice, indicating that the 47-kDa protein possesses potential T cell epitope(s). To identify the T cell epitope(s), eight kinds of synthetic peptides corresponding to the 20–28 amino acid sequences of the 47-kDa protein were tested for capacity to induce proliferation in the T cell line. The peptide corresponding to the 81–100 amino acid sequence, Asp-Gly-Lys-Arg-Val-Ile-Val-Asn-Ala-Phe-Ala-Lys-Phe-Lys-Ile-Ile-Asp-Pro-Ile-Thr, elicited a proliferative response ten times greater than that of a control malarial peptide of similar length. The results suggested that this 20-amino acid residue peptide contained a stimulatory T cell epitope of the 47-kDa *R. tsutsugamushi* antigen. Hickman *et al.* (1993) have stated that this 47-kDa protein is a candidate for the development of a component vaccine for Tsutsugamushi disease.

22-kDa protein gene

The gene encoding the immunoreactive 22-kDa protein of the Karp strain has been cloned and sequenced by Hickman *et al.* (1991). The recombinant 22-kDa antigen was also found to elicit a proliferative response in a helper T cell line, suggesting the presence of a stimulatory T cell epitope(s) in the 22-kDa protein as well as in the 47-kDa protein. Consequently, Hickman *et al.* (1991) stated that this 22-kDa protein would be usable for a vaccine for Tsutsugamushi disease.

Phylogenetic analysis by 16S rRNA gene sequences

The 16S rRNA analysis has often been used for taxonomic studies of microbial organisms. Ohashi *et al.* (1995) determined the 16S rRNA gene sequences of *R. tsutsugamushi* six antigenic variants, Gilliam, Karp, Kato, Kawasaki, Kuroki, and Shimokoshi strains, and the phylogenetic positions of their variants in the 40 microbes of the Proteobacteria and two species of the order Chlamydiales. The phylogenetic tree illustrated in Fig. 19 indicates that almost all members of the order Rickettsiales are clustered in the α group of the Proteobacteria composed of 36 microbes in the figure, except *Coxiella bunetii* and *Wolbachia persica* located in the γ group consisting of 4 species. The 10 microbes of the genus *Rickettsia* are further clustered together with 11 species of the genera *Ehrlichia, Wolbachia, Cowdria,* and *Anaplasma*. Consequently, this taxonomic study reveals that a subcluster of *R. tsutsugamushi* six variants is located apart from that of the other species in the genus *Rickettsia* with a similarity value of 90.2–90.6%. The phylogenetic relatedness among the six antigenic variants in *R. tsutsugamushi* moderately reflects their antigenic relationship as known in closely and distantly related strains.

Recently, Tamura *et al.* (1995) proposed that *R. tsutsugamushi* should be taxonomically transferred from the genus *Rickettsia* to the newly established *Orientia,* as *Orientia tsutsugamushi*, because of the existence of several different characteristics from other species in genus *Rickettsia*: its lack of peptidoglycan and lipopolysaccharide; the differences in protein-constitution in the ultrastructure of the cell wall, and in the resistance to penicillin and quinolone chemotherapeutic agents; and the remote relationship among their phylogenetic positions in the 16S rRNA analysis.

8. Susceptibility to Chemotherapeutic Agents

In clinical practice, it is well known that some antibiotics — chloramphenicol, rifampicin, the tetracyclines, and the macrolides — have a clear therapeutic effect on Tsutsugamushi disease, whereas beta-lactam and related antibiotics do not. The *in vitro* evaluation of these antibiotics against the typhus and spotted fever

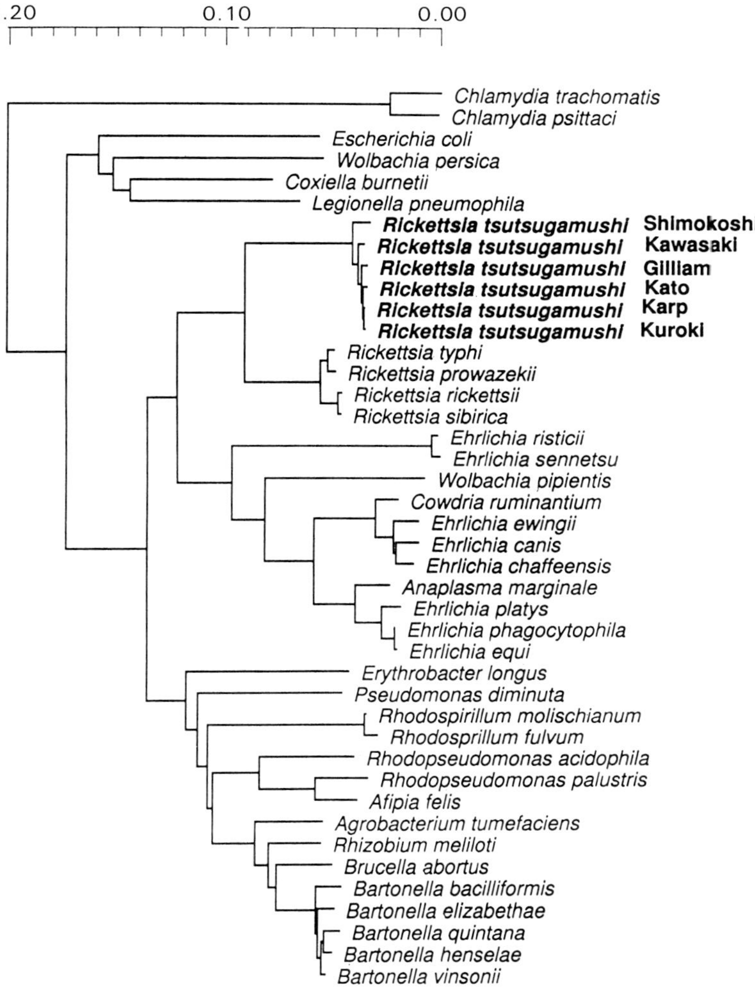

Fig. 19. Phylogenetic positions of *R. tsutsugamushi* Gilliam, Karp, Kato, Kawasaki, Kuroki, and Shimokoshi strains in members of the order Rickettsiales and Chlamydiales, and other species of α and γ groups of the Proteobacteria. The tree was constructed by the neighbor-joining method (Saito and Nei, 1987) based on the evolutionary distances estimated using the six-parameter method (Gojobori *et al.*, 1982) in the SINCA program of the BIORESEARCH software package (Fujitsu, Tokyo).

group of rickettsiae has been reported by many investigators (Raoult *et al.*, 1986, 1987b, 1987a, 1988; Wisseman and Ordonez, 1986; Wisseman and Waddell, 1982; Wisseman *et al.*, 1974), but there have been few *in vitro* studies of the effect of these antibiotics on *Rickettsia tsutsugamushi* (Brown *et al.*, 1978; Hopps *et al.*, 1959; Yamaguchi *et al.*, 1984).

The minimum inhibitory concentrations (MIC) of various chemotherapeutic agents, including a series of quinolone agents, against *R. tsutsugamushi* was reported in comparison with those against *R. prowazekii* in the typhus group, and *R. rickettsii* and *R. sibirica* in the spotted fever group (Miyamura and Ohta, 1991; Miyamura *et al.*, 1985, 1989; Urakami *et al.*, 1988a). The results, shown in Table 8, indicate that the tetracycline antibiotics (tetracycline, demethylchlortetracycline, doxycycline, and minocycline), chloramphenicol, kitasamycin (leucomycin, a macrolide antibiotic), and rifampicin all have strong inhibitory effects against all rickettsiae, with no significant difference among antibiotics.

R. tsutsugamushi strains showed a higher resistance to a series of quinolone agents (norfloxacin, ciprofloxacin, and ofloxacin) than typhus and spotted fever group rickettsiae.

R. tsutsugamushi was completely resistant to the beta-lactam antibiotics (benzylpenicillin, ampicillin, carbenicillin, cephaloridine, cefmetazole, and cefotaxime), whereas the growth of *R. prowazekii* and two species of the spotted fever group rickettsiae was inhibited by a high concentration of penicillin antibiotics (benzylpenicillin, ampicillin, and carbenicillin).

The susceptibility of newly isolated strains of *R. tsutsugamushi* to several antibiotics was found to be similar to the results shown in Table 8 (Urakami *et al.*, 1988a), and none of these strains were resistant to tetracycline, chloramphenicol, or leucomycin.

The addition of tetracycline, chloramphenicol, or erythromycin (a macrolide antibiotic) to cultured cells infected with *R. tsutsugamushi* results in the immediate cessation of rickettsial growth (Yamaguchi *et al.*, 1984). On days 1 and 2 after the addition of the antibiotic, the stainability of rickettsiae with Giemsa staining decreases gradually, and the number of rickettsiae in cells is greatly reduced on the third day. After the addition of antibiotics, enlargement of the rickettsia and disruption of the inner structure are observed under electron microscopy.

Table 8. *In Vitro* Activities of Various Antimicrobial Agents against Four Rickettsial Species

Antimicrobial agents	MIC (μg/ml)								
	R. tsutsugamushi						*R. prowazekii*	*R. rickettsii*	*R. sibirica*
	Gilliam	Karp	Kato	Shimokoshi	Kawasaki	Kuroki			
Tetracycline	0.02	0.02	0.09	0.04	0.04	0.09	0.09	0.005	0.78
Demethylchlortetracycline	0.01	0.01	0.04	0.04	0.01	0.04	0.02	0.01	0.39
Doxycycline	0.02	0.01	0.01	0.09	0.04	0.04	0.02	0.01	0.04
Minocycline	0.02	0.01	0.01	0.02	0.19	0.09	0.04	0.04	0.39
Chloramphenicol	0.39	0.19	0.19	0.39	0.39	0.39	0.19	0.04	0.78
Kitasamycin	0.02	0.04	0.02	0.04	0.04	0.04	0.09	0.09	0.09
Rifampicin	0.04	0.005	0.01	0.09	0.04	0.04	0.01	0.005	0.04
Norfloxacin	50	100	50	100	100	50	3.12	1.56	1.56
Ciprofloxacin	25	12.5	6.25	12.5	25	12.5	0.78	0.19	1.56
Ofloxacin	25	6.25	3.12	6.25	6.25	6.25	0.39	0.09	0.78
Benzylpenicillin	>1000	>1000	>1000	>1000	>1000	>1000	25	25	50
Ampicillin	>1000	>1000	>1000	>1000	>1000	>1000	100	100	100
Carbenicillin	>1000	>1000	>1000	>1000	>1000	>1000	1000	1000	>1000
Cephaloridine	>1000	>1000	>1000	>1000	>1000	>1000	>1000	>1000	>1000
Cefmetazole	>1000	>1000	>1000	>1000	>1000	>1000	>1000	>1000	>1000
Cefotaxime	>1000	>1000	>1000	>1000	>1000	>1000	>1000	>1000	>1000

MIC: minimum inhibitory concentration.

Assay procedure for determining MIC

The MIC of various chemotherapeutic agents for *R. tsutsugamushi* was determined by the following method (Urakami *et al*., 1988a):

(1) Rickettsia is inoculated to an L cell monolayer culture and, after the rickettsia has become adsorbed to the cells by incubation for 1.5–2 h, the cells are detached by trypsin treatment.

(2) The infected cells are suspended in Eagle's minimum essential medium (MEM) containing 2% calf serum, at a concentration of 7.5×10^4 cells/ml, and 400 μl of this suspension is inoculated into each well of a 24-well plastic multiplate (Corning Inc. Corning, N.Y.) in which a sterile glass cover slip has been placed at the bottom.

(3) The sample drug is dissolved in Eagle's MEM containing 2% calf serum, and 400-μl aliquots of two-fold serially diluted samples, diluted in the same medium, are added to the wells of the multiplate which have been inoculated with infected cells.

(4) After four-day incubation of the prepared multiplate in a 5% CO_2 atmosphere at 37°C, the cells on the cover slip are fixed with methanol and stained with Giemsa. Each cover slip is observed under a light microscope at 1,000 × magnification from the cover slip incubated in medium containing a higher dilution of the drug. The rickettsial multiplication profile in cells is seen at the lower concentration of the drug, but not at the higher concentration. The MIC of a drug is determined as the lowest drug concentration at which the rickettsial growth profile diminishes.

9. Pathogenicity

Many strains of *Rickettsia tsutsugamushi* have been isolated from patients and from wild animals. All the strains were isolated from patients who showed clinical symptoms; thus these isolates are mostly pathogenic to humans. However, when the isolates were injected to hairy mice, some strains showed different degrees of virulence.

Using mice treated with cyclophosphamide (an immunosuppressive agent), Kobayashi *et al.* (1978) first identified such a strain (Irie), obtained from a patient, which was avirulent in hairy mice. Similar avirulent strains were isolated by Kawamura *et al.* (1980) from a field rodent in an area endemic for Tsutsugamushi disease on

Miyake Island, one of the Shichito Islands, using athymic nude mice; by Tamura *et al.* (1984) from a patient (Shimokoshi) in Niigata Prefecture; and by Yamamoto *et al.* (1986, 1989) from patients (Kawasaki, Kuroki, and others) in Miyazaki Prefecture, using cyclophosphamide-treated mice.

Most isolates of Gilliam and Karp types in Japan are highly virulent in ddY mice, although some are of low virulence. Almost all isolates of Kawasaki and Kuroki types are avirulent in hairy mice. The laboratory strain of Kato is highly virulent in mice, but the Shimokoshi strain is avirulent. However, there are no reports on any relationships between antigenic types or genotypes and the symptomatic severity of human illness.

Of laboratory animals tested, rabbits show no symptoms after injection with rickettsiae. Guinea pigs exhibit elevated rectal temperature when they are inoculated with live rickettsiae, but there are no other significant symptoms.

The mouse is generally susceptible to rickettsial infection, but susceptibility depends on the mouse strain (Groves and Osterman, 1978; Groves *et al.*, 1980) and on the rickettsial strains, as mentioned above. Mice injected intraperitoneally with a strain that is highly virulent in mice became ill after a latent period of 3–10 days, depending on the amount of rickettsiae inoculated, and died after 2–5 days.

When an avirulent strain is injected to hairy mice, they survive the infection without manifestation of symptoms, or they may exhibit ruffled fur for a short period after the injection.

However, if the mice are treated with the immunosuppressant cyclophosphamide, they show clinical manifestations, such as ruffled fur and weakness, on rickettsial infection.

10. Immunity to Rickettsial Infection

a. Humoral and cellular responses to Tsutsugamushi disease

There are very few thorough reports suitable for evaluation of the immune response in patients with Tsutsugamushi disease. Bourgeois *et al.* (1982), at US Naval Medical Research Unit (NAMRU) 2, reported 103 Tsutsugamushi disease cases (all males) in members of the Chinese military garrisoned on the Pescadores Islands, Taiwan, during 1976–1977. This is the most comprehensive report among recent publications. The patients in the report exhibited typical symptoms of eschar, headache, fever, rash, conjunctivitis, and general lymphadenopathy, and were diagnosed definitively by indirect immunofluorescence (IF), and *Rickettsia tsutsugamushi* was isolated from all of them. Based on their IgM and IgG responses, 78 of the patients showed an elevated IgM level from day 8 and an elevated IgG level from day 12 (Type I). The remaining 25 patients showed an increased IgG level beginning on day 6, with the concomitant appearance of IgM in 16 of the 25 patients, but both the appearance and duration of immune response were variable (Type II). The IgA response occurred only transiently in six of the Type I cases. Only the IgG levels remained elevated for one year after day 40 in both types. Serological typing into three prototype (Gilliam, Karp, Kato) strains was performed using IgM, but this yielded ambiguous results. These results were not unexpected in view of the report of Shirai *et al.* (1982) on the typing by direct IF of 49 *R. tsutsugamushi* isolates, including some from patients in the island, using the three prototype strains and five Southeast Asian local types, which resulted in approximately 47% TH716 type and approximately 35% TH716 + Karp type. Bourgeois *et al.* (1982) confirmed reinfection (both types) in 14 patients during the course of the study; all of the patients were virtually asymptomatic and an IgG increase was observed. On the other hand, with respect to cellular immunity, the activated T cell response decreased during the acute phase (days 0–7) in both types; and in the early recovery phase (days 8–15), the Type I cases still showed a depression in T cell response. In contrast, the T cell response increased during the latter recovery phase in both types. These results imply that Type I represents an initial infection and Type II, a reinfection. A comparison of the Type II cases to the 14 reinfected cases showed that reinfection due to *R. tsutsugamushi* heterogeneity was common in highly endemic areas, and that cellular immunity played an important role, but was not a final decisive factor. This probably represents the same phenomenon as that reported in a highly endemic area (Niigata, Japan) where approximately 30% of 104 patients were infected twice and as many as 5% were infected three times or more (Tamiya, 1962), and the reports of Shishido (1962b), Kawamura *et al.* (1980), and Fan *et al.* (1987) that the presence of weakly pathogenic *R. tsutsugamushi* and inapparent infection due to *R. tsutsugamushi* heterogeneity were widespread throughout many localities. As described below, in the host defense in a mouse model, there was negligible involvement of antibodies in the elimination of *R. tsutsugamushi*, and T cells and macrophages played a major role in the presence of *R. tsutsugamushi*. However, in the cultured cells of patients, T3 (+) and T8 (+) lymphokine-activated killer cells (LAK) were found to be significantly inolved in the lysis of cells infected with a typhus group rickettsia in both an autologous system and a heterologous HLA system, whereas *R. tsutsugamushi*-infected cells could not be lysed (Carl *et al.*, 1988). In a nude mouse system, *Rickettsia* species other than *R. tsutsugamushi* produced IgM antibodies, whereas *R. tsutsugamushi* did so only following the transfer of *R. tsutsugamushi*-specific helper T cells. This phenomenon may be related to the finding that an ether-soluble protein-carbonydrate complex is present on the surface of the cell wall of *Rickettsia* species other than *R. tsutsugamushi*, but is absent in *R. tsutsugamushi* (Jerrells and Eisemann, 1983).

b. Immune responses to experimental rickettsial infections in monkeys

Prior to the identification of the causative agent of Tsutsugamushi disease in 1930, a small number of anthropoid apes (orang-utans) and several hundred domestic and imported macaques were used in Japan as sentinel animals to search for endemic areas or as experimental animals for pathogen detection, because they exhibited symptoms and a disease course, similar to that in humans (Kawamura, 1926). The majority of the animals were Japanese monkeys; since most of the monkeys did not die, those surviving a course of infection were also used for reinfection studies and to confirm immunity. Among such large numbers of animals, the reinfections reported ranged from those exhibiting no symptoms to slight symptoms. However, immunological investigation, other than by the Weil-Felix reaction, the standard at that time, was not performed.

MacMillan *et al.* (1985) infected cynomolgus monkeys (*Macaca fascicularis*) with *R. tsutsugamushi* (Karp strain), observed the symptoms (fever, eschar, lymphadenopathy, rickettsemia), and analyzed *R. tsutsugamushi*-specific antibodies and cell-mediated immune (CMI) responses. They found that the IgM level, measured by ELISA, increased initially, followed by IgG antibodies; lymphocyte proliferation and γ-interferon production due to peripheral blood mononuclear leukocytes were also found.

These monkeys were repeatedly challenged with either homologous or heterologous *R. tsutsugamushi* strains at various times. Eight months after the initial infection, they exhibited complete resistance to the challenge; after one year, only a localized cutaneous lesion resulting from the *R. tsutsugamushi* inoculation and enlarged lymph nodes were found; after eight years, the symptoms and the cell-mediated immune response were virtually the same as those exhibited during the initial infection, with the exception that only the IgG level was elevated. These results imply that immunity to Tsutsugamushi disease is not sustained for a prolonged period.

c. *Mouse model of host resistance to experimental* rickettsial infection

Host resistance to *R. tsutsugamushi* infection has been studied for decades in mouse strains. Kuwata (1952) reported that when he infected mice with an avirulent *R. tsutsugamushi* strain and subsequently challenged them with a heterologous virulent *R. tsutsugamushi* strain, *R. tsutsugamushi* invaded the tissue, causing a superinfection. When the mice were intraperitoneally challenged, they eventually died from the infection. However, the mice survived when a subcutaneous route of infection was used. Shishido *et al.* (1958, 1959) inoculated mice subcutaneously with *R. tsutsugamushi* and reported that all the animals tolerated an intraperitoneal challenge with homologous *R. tsutsugamushi* after 7–21 days. They also reported inter-strain cross-protection differences when the animals were rechallenged with heterologous strains after a 7-day interval, the animals tolerating the challenge after 14 days. They found virtually no neutralizing tests to perform with antibodies.

Shirai *et al.* (1976) in Osterman's group were the first to analyze mouse resistance to *R. tsutsugamushi* infection using modern immunological criteria. They used weakly virulent Gilliam and virulent Karp strains in BALB/c mice and demonstrated that protection against intraperitoneal challenge with the Karp strain occurred 7 days after an intraperitoneal inoculation of the Gilliam strain. As for humoral antibodies, they showed that anti-Karp antibodies were protective against certain levels of challenge, whereas anti-Gilliam antibodies were not protective. Passive protection against a Karp-strain challenge at days 7–28 occurred in mice receiving 3×10^7 spleen cells from Gilliam-immune mice, but the protective response decreased after day 42. T cells were involved in all of these phenomena. In 1979, Nacy and Osterman demonstrated using a macrophage tissue culture and an *in vivo* system that the final clearance of infected *R. tsutsugamushi* in cells was effected by macrophages, and that humoral antibody and the lymphokines released from T cells activated the macrophages. They also showed that macrophage populations activated *in vitro* or *in vivo* contained a small percentage of cells that supported the unrestrained growth of *R. tsutsugamushi*, and that an early immunological event in experimental Tsutsugamushi disease infection may be the development of activated macrophages capable of suppressing rickettsial proliferation prior to the appearance of antibodies.

Important advances in the mouse model system were reported by Groves and Osterman (1978), Groves *et al.* (1980), and Nacy and Groves (1981) with genetic analyses of natural resistance among inbred mouse strains to the *R. tsutsugamushi* Gilliam strain. This resistance is unrelated to the H-2 gene; it is controlled by a single autosomal dominant gene, the *Ric* gene, which has *r* and *s* (resistant and susceptible) alleles against *R. tsutsugamushi* infection. Analyses using a recombinant inbred mouse strain confirmed that the *Ric* locus was located on chromosome 5, closely linked to the retinal degeneration (*rd*) locus. Genetic analyses of cross-bred mouse strains showed that the resistant allele was dominant. The genetic dominance of the natural resistance of mouse strains against intraperitoneal infection by the Gilliam strain is transmitted by macrophages. Among *R. tsutsugamushi*-resistant and -susceptible mouse strains, macrophages were not activated in some of the susceptible strains because the lymphokines produced under normal conditions were not reactive. Subsequently, Osterman's group (Jerrells and Osterman, 1982b) performed extensive analyses of host defense mechanisms against *R. tsutsugamushi*, using *R. tsutsugamushi*-resistant and -susceptible mouse strains. They showed that a differential response for the expression of *Ric* gene occurred as a consequence of the route of challenge. With an intravenous challenge, mice from both strains were resistant, and *R. tsutsugamushi* replication occurred in the spleen [probably the same phenomenon reported by Kuwata (1952) as superinfection]. With an intravenous challenge following treatment performed to decrease macrophage activity by the administration of silica and carrageenan in the susceptible mice, these mice were still susceptible. When resistant mice were intravenously challenged following either irradiation or silica treatment, they were still resistant. However, when these treatments were concurrently administered, the mice became susceptible. When resistant mice were challenged intraperitoneally following sublethal irradiation, they showed susceptibility, but when they were administered silica or carrageenan, they remained resistant. Based on these findings, Jerrells and Osterman (1982b) concluded that both mouse strains were intrinsically resistant as a consequence of a fixed macrophage response to intravenous challenge. In addition, they reported that an irradiation-sensitive process was involved in resistant mouse strains challenged by intraperitoneal inoculation.

In 1983, Nacy *et al.* activated macrophages and elucidated the characteristics of the lymphokines and also purified them. Then, in 1984, Nacy and Meltzer pretreated susceptible mice with the purified lymphokines and demonstrated that the mice were able to tolerate the *R. tsutsugamushi* challange. This phenomenon was not observed in macrophages activated by sterile inflammatory agents. Therefore, it can be concluded that the main mechanism of protective immunity in the *R. tsutsugamushi* mouse model involves cell-mediated immunity. This was demonstrated by lymphocyte transfer, lymphokine or γ-interferon production by T lymphocytes, the activation of macrophages by lymphokines, the demonstration of a delayed-type hypersensitivity response following exposure to these organisms, and an *in vitro* lymphocyte proliferation assay, and so on. Lymphocyte transfer was reported by Shirai *et al.* (1976) as noted above. Catanzaro *et al.* (1977) transferred 3×10^7 spleen and ascites lymphocytes, respectively, of Gilliam strain-infected mice to mice and challenged them with the Karp strain at various time intervals. Comparing the efficiency of the two cell types, they found that ascites lymphocytes were more efficient than spleen lymphocytes although the spleen lymphocytes involved population inhibiting *R. tsutsugamushi* infection.

In 1982, Jerrells and Osterman (1982a) presented a detailed report regarding delayed-type hypersensitivity responses. They inoculated intraperitoneally with the Gilliam strain into *R. tsutsugamushi*-resistant and -susceptible mouse strains and traced delayed-type hypersensitivity responses. The responses appeared in the early stage by days 5–7 in both mouse strains, declined before death in the susceptible mice, but continued for 9–15 days in resistant mice. In addition, when the Gilliam strain was inoculated subcutaneously to susceptible mice, causing a chronic infection, delayed-type hypersensitivity peaked on day 21, a result which correlated with resistance to the intraperitoneal challenge. T cells were responsible for transferring the delayed-type hypersensitivity.

In order to determine the role played by lymphocyte proliferation, Jerrells and Osterman (1983a) subcutaneously inoculated mice with three live *R. tsutsugamushi* prototype strains, respectively, causing chronic infections; they then performed *in vitro* lymphocyte proliferation assays of the lymphocyte responses of these mice cross-reactively at various time intervals with the respective rickettsiae grown in irradiated tissue culture, and found lymphocyte proliferation in all cases. The lymphocyte proliferation appeared on day 14, and was manifested in all combinations, as in the delayed-type hypersensitivity study. However, the time of appearance of the peak was markedly strain-dependent. This is probably a consequence of differences in responding T cells.

Of the lymphokines produced as a result of the interaction between an *R. tsutsugamushi*-specific antigen and T-lymphocytes, γ-interferon was responsible for macrophage activation. However, when Palmer *et al.* (1984) inoculated the Gilliam strain subcutaneously into *R. tsutsugamushi* susceptible mice, causing chronic infection, and intravenously challenged them with irradiated Gilliam strain, interferon production peaked 4 h later. Similarly, interferon production peaked at 48–72 h in an *in vitro* system, and no interferon was produced in nude mice. Consequently, these investigators concluded that the interferon produced was *R. tsutsugamushi*-specific and did not react with other rickettsiae.

The role of antibodies is to help macrophages eliminate *R. tsutsugamushi,* thus facilitating *R. tsutsugamushi* clearance from the bloodstream. The interaction between *R. tsutsugamushi* and the antibodies rapidly eliminates *R. tsutsugamushi* from the bloodstream in concert with reticuloendothelial cells, and delivers the antigen to cells with antigen-processing ability. Hanson (1983) stated that antibodies in a tissue culture system functioned in a complement-independent manner to inhibit *R. tsutsugamushi* adsorption and invasion, but that they could not inhibit the growth of *R. tsutsugamushi* once the cells had been invaded since the phenomenon was antibody concentration-dependent and strain-specific.

Kobayashi *et al.* (1985) reported that in nude mice, where *R. tsutsugamushi* infection is always fatal, the transfer of homologous antibody had little effect, and the transfer of T cells from non-immune normal mice was also ineffective. However, mice receiving T cell transfers from immune normal mice survived the challenge. The protective capacity of the T cells was still low on the 10th immune day; it was sustained for 1–12 months. In addition, Kodama *et al.* (1987, 1988) showed that a T cell line, obtained following the long-term culture of *R. tsutsugamushi* Gilliam strain-immune splenocytes in the presence of *R. tsutsugamushi* antigen and syngeneic filler cells exhibited *R. tsutsugamushi*-specific helper T-cell characteristics, was Gilliam strain-specific in a lymphocyte proliferation assay, and produced Gilliam strain-specific γ-interferon; mice receiving these T cells survived a Gilliam strain-specific challenge. These findings demonstrate that antigen-specific helper T cells are required for defense against the infection. Furthermore, this T cell line (Kodama *et al.*, 1987, 1988) produced a cytotoxic factor that, selectively, acted on *R. tsutsugamushi*-infected macrophages.

Rollwagen *et al.* (1986) also showed that there was very little involvement of antibodies in the elimination of *R. tsutsugamushi* at the time of *R. tsutsugamushi* infection. However, they found that lymphocytes and macrophages played a major role when *R. tsutsugamushi* antigen was present, and immune splenocytes lysed *R. tsutsugamushi*-infected tissue culture cells. This activity is indicative of H-2-restricted killing, and the activity is lost when T cells are destroyed.

Jerrells and Osterman (1981) compared the inflammatory responses of susceptible and resistant mouse strains infected intraperitoneally with Gilliam strain; Jerrells (1983) studied the role of Ia antigen-positive macrophages in both susceptible and resistant mouse strains and found a correlation between Ia antigen-positive macrophages and resistance. Jerrells and Osterman (1983b) elucidated the complexity of T cell responses *in vivo* in delayed-type hypersensitivity responses by demonstrating that delayed-type hypersensitivity and lymphocyte proliferation occurred concomitantly in cell-mediated immunity against *R. tsutsugamushi* infection. Initially, these responses occurred at about the same level. However, after day 28, delayed-type hypersensitivity declined, and lymphocyte proliferation increased until day 45 and was sustained until day 90.

In addition, Jerrells *et al.* (1983) showed that when mice were immunized three times with γ-irradiated Karp strain antigen, the levels of cell-mediated immunity (both delayed-type hypersensitivity and lymphocyte proliferation) and lymphokine and antibody production increased. These animals were also completely tolerant of a viable Karp strain challenge. However, antibody levels were lower in mice immunized with irradiated rickettsia than in mice immunized with viable rickettsia. Jerrells (1985) inoculated BALB/c mice subcutaneously with *R. tsutsugamushi* and evaluated both the antibody and cellular immune responses during chronic infection, finding that transient immunosuppression appeared, irrespective of the *R. tsutsugamushi* strain used, and that splenomegaly occurred due to the inflow of inflammatory macrophages, accompanied by immunosupression. Consequently, he showed that the chronic infection was due to an interaction between immunosuppressive T cells and the activated macrophages involved in *R. tsutsugamushi* clearance. On the other hand, Lim *et al.* (1986) reported that, in an acute *R. tsutsugamushi* infection in BALB/c mice, the lymphocyte response was suppressed for 11–28 days, but humoral immunity increased during that time.

3

Epidemiology and Clinical Aspects

1 Geographical Distribution

Tsutsugamushi disease is an apparent or inapparent *Rickettsia tsutsugamushi* infection caused by the bite of larval trombiculid mites which harbor *R. tsutsugamushi* and which bite humans. The occurrence of the disease thus requires a point of contact between humans and the mites. In other words, contact between trombiculid mites and humans is restricted by the frequency and length of time that humans remain in areas infested by larval trombiculid mites that harbor *R. tsutsugamushi* during the epidemic season, and by the number of *R. tsutsugamushi*-positive individuals in a mite population and the density of micro spots containing *R. tsutsugamushi*-positive trombiculid mites, called mite islands.

Since mild or inapparent *R. tsutsugamushi* infections are confirmed, the mere tracking of patients is inadequate to comprehend the geographical distribution of *R. tsutsugamushi*. Consequently, it is necessary to study the enzootic cycle of *R. tsutsugamushi* in vertebrate animals centered around its main hosts, field rodents, to elucidate the distribution of *R. tsutsugamushi*.

As shown in Fig. 1, the distribution of *R. tsutsugamushi* today extends north to northern Japan, Russia, and the Primorski Karai region in the Russian Far East; south to northern Australia and the western Pacific islands; and west to Afghanistan, Pakistan, and areas neighboring the former USSR (WHO Working Group on Rickettsial Diseases, 1982). Naturally, human *R. tsutsugamushi* infections occur widely in these regions, but not everywhere.

After trombiculid mites, which had been proven to be *R. tsutsugamushi* vectors in Asia, were collected in eastern Africa, the

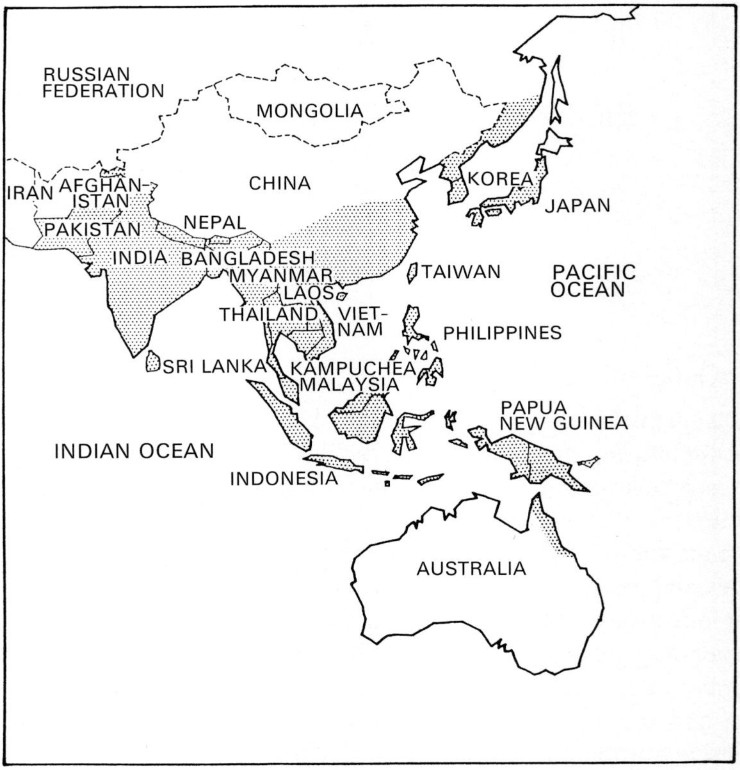

Fig. 1. Geographical distribution of *R. tsutsugamushi*

presence of Tsutsugamushi disease in Africa was also considered to be possible. Indeed, a Japanese man (53 years old) who traveled in the areas of Brazzaville, Gamboma, Okoyo, Owando, and Makoua in the People's Republic of the Congo on a business trip as a construction consultant from October 11 to November 2, 1989, returned to Japan on November 4, became ill on November 10, and was diagnosed as having typical Tsutsugamushi disease.

Although the isolation of *R. tsutsugamushi* was not attempted, the diagnosis was confirmed by the indirect immunoperoxidase method. Among the *R. tsutsugamushi* strains used for the tests, significantly elevated IgM and IgG antibody titers were found with paired sera particularly against Kato and Malaysian USAMUR 6989 strains, and a primary infection by *R. tsutsugamushi* was confirmed. Infection by spotted fever group rickettsia was completely negative (Osuga *et al.*, 1991). This result suggests that *R. tsutsugamushi* may be widely distributed in Africa.

Not all geographical regions in which *R. tsutsugamushi* is found are sites of human outbreaks. For example, even in Japan, a small island nation, no Tsutsugamushi disease patients have been identified in either Hokkaido or Okinawa. Although *R. tsutsugamushi* reservoirs are abundant in Hokkaido, and *R. tsutsugamushi* infection by *Leptotrombidium kawamurai*, which does not bite humans, was found among field rodents (Kitaoka *et al.*, 1973) and distribution of *L. pallidum*, the principal vector species in Japan for non-*L. akamushi* type Tsutsugamushi disease, has been confirmed (Tamiya, 1962), not a single clinical case has been reported to date.

As for Okinawa Prefecture, despite the fact that cases continue to occur in mainland Kagoshima Prefecture to the north and in Taiwan to the south, with more than 100 infections reported in each of these regions in recent years, *R. tsutsugamushi* has not yet been found even though very rigorous studies have been made (Otsuru, 1992). One exception is a report of Tsutsugamushi disease in two patients in October 1961 in the US Army in Okinawa Prefecture. In both patients, elevated antibody titer was found against Gilliam type, using the complement fixation test with paired sera. However, even though these patients were affiliated with the military troops in Okinawa Prefecture, there was no description as to where they had become infected, and the question thus remains (406th Med. Gen. Lab. Prof. Rept., 1962).

On the other hand, it has been known for many years that in Honshu (the main island of Japan), areas in which there were frequent human infections (called mite islands, infective spots, or hot spots) containing *R. tsutsugamushi*-positive mites were found as micro spots, some of which shifted yearly, even within regions endemic for classical Tsutsugamushi disease transmitted by *L. akamushi* (Kawamura and Tanaka, 1988). The existence of these mite islands has also been confirmed in non-*L. akamushi*-transmitted Tsutsugamushi disease (Takahashi *et al.*, 1990b).

Such occurrences of *R. tsutsugamushi*-positive trombiculid mites in a limited locale within a broader region were elucidated in a report by Tsutsugamushi disease specialist teams of the US and British armed forces organized during World War II (Audy, 1949, 1961;

Philip, 1948a; Philip *et al.*, 1949). Audy, who participated in the war as a British military physician, reported a sudden outbreak of Tsutsugamushi disease in 756 British soldiers (1.5% fatality) during maneuvers in grassy fields near Embilipitiya, in the south of Ceylon, in 1943, although there had been absolutely no occurrence of the disease among the soldiers participating in maneuvers at various other locations on the island. He confirmed that the vector was *L. deliense*, which infested field rodents captured in the grassy fields, and he called such areas of concentrated outbreaks with vector mites "hot spots" or "infective spots."

Philip (1948a) reported an outbreak of Tsutsugamushi disease in 1,469 patients in only a 2-month period among US troops who landed in 1944 on Biak and Owi Islands, north of western New Guinea. The disease afflicted 90% of the troops garrisoned on the coast of Cape Samsapor; the fatality rate (0.6%), however, was extremely low.

The US Army established a laboratory in Kuala Lumpur, Malaysia, after the war, where Philip *et al.* (1949) confirmed the existence of several concentrated outbreak regions with *R. tsutsugamushi*-positive trombiculid mites in the vicinity, using volunteers and sentinel animals (rats, mice), calling such outbreak regions "hyperendemic areas." Additionally, Philip *et al.* reported that the vector trombiculid mites of *R. tsutsugamushi* in these regions were *L. deliense* and Malaysian *L. akamushi* (= *L. fletcheri*).

Evidently, although Tsutsugamushi disease exhibits typical symptoms in newcomers to the enzootic areas and in some natives, the more important finding was the result of an indirect immunofluorescence study of acute fevers among the natives in the enzootic foci which showed that the majority of the unknown fevers were Tsutsugamushi disease (WHO Working Group on Rickettsial Diseases, 1982). Moreover, their clinical picture was atypical, lacking eschar, rash, and lymphadenopathy, and *Proteus* OXK agglutination tests were negative (WHO Working Group on Rickettsial Diseases, 1982). In addition, as described previously, mild cases were also observed, which included people who had contracted Tsutsugamushi disease one or more times in the past. Such repeated reinfections indicate that the heterogeneity among *R. tsutsugamushi* strains is so broad that all the various strains cannot be responded by cellular immunity. On the other hand, there are, among *R.*

tsutsugamushi strains, those that exhibit milder pathogenicity to humans, causing only abortive or inapparent infections. Unless the specific *R. tsutsugamushi* antibody is detected serologically, the true nature of these cases cannot be understood. In addition, as noted in Chapter 1, there are *R. tsutsugamushi* strains that are only mildly pathogenic to mice while causing typical Tsutsugamushi disease in humans. Consequently, it has become necessary to devise an ingenious method for isolating *R. tsutsugamushi* strains. The above finding also implies the possible existence of *R. tsutsugamushi* strains that are mere symbionts to trombiculid mites exhibiting absolutely no pathogenicity to humans or to mice.

In order to clarify this subject, it is necessary to either isolate *R. tsutsugamushi* directly from trombiculid mites, using tissue culture cells, or to detect *R. tsutsugamushi* DNA in the trombiculid mites by polymerase chain reaction (PCR) or nested PCR (Furuya and Yoshida, 1992).

At any rate, it appears that Tsutsugamushi disease is implicated in the patients with acute fever requiring hospital care who live in enzootic foci. Local medical professionals and health administrators should be aware of this problem.

2 Seasonal Occurrence

The seasonal occurrence of Tsutsugamushi disease parallels the time of emergence of the vector, larval trombiculid mites, and this is determined by the natural environment (temperature, humidity, rainy season, dry season, vegetation, etc.), which controls larval life in the region of emergence. As noted by Kawamura and Tanaka (1988), the seasonal prevalence of the principal vector species for Tsutsugamushi disease in Japan is as follows:

Leptotrombidium akamushi larvae emerge from the end of July to early September when the temperature exceeds 25°C, at river terraces on the northern coast of the Sea of Japan (Niigata, Yamagata, and Akita Prefectures).

L. pallidum larvae emerge in the vicinity of their habitat during the period when the temperature is 18–20°C, *i.e.*, from autumn to winter and from late spring to early summer. Regarding the emergence of these trombiculid mites, Takahashi (1988a) and Takahashi *et al.* (1993a) confirmed that the same colony of larvae occurs twice annually and that this is not a bimodal occurrence of two colonies with different emerging times in the same area.

L. scutellare larvae also emerge when the outside temperature is 18–20°C. However, these trombiculid mites emerge only once a year, from autumn to winter, because of their habitat, and the time of emergence is slightly later than that of *L. pallidum* (Tamiya, 1962).

The seasonal prevalence of Tsutsugamushi disease transmitted by *L. pallidum* and *L. scutellare* is also controlled by these external factors in areas other than Japan, such as Korea, the People's Republic of China, Taiwan, and the Primorye region in Russia. In addition, *L. pavlovskyi* in Primorye also emerges under virtually the same conditions as *L. pallidum* and *L. scutellare*.

In contrast, *L. deliense*, *L. fletcheri*, and *L. arenicola* (Traub and Wisseman, 1974b), which are the principal Tsutsugamushi disease vectors in Southeast Asia and the southwest Pacific are distributed in tropical to subtropical regions. Consequently, these larvae are present throughout the year, independent of the season. Furthermore, it has been confirmed by studies of volunteers in hyperendemic areas and by sentinel animal experiments that the larvae occur in relatively dry periods; their primary active time is the morning, and they become less active as the temperature rises during the daytime (Philip *et al.*, 1949).

3 Isolated *Rickettsia tsutsugamushi* Strains

a. Heterogeneity of R. tsutsugamushi *strains*

Rickettsia tsutsugamushi strains are isolated from human patients, field rodents, trombiculid mites, and other sources mainly by using mice. For antigenic analysis, *R. tsutsugamushi* grown in the yolk sacs of embryonated eggs were used in the post-World War II period; currently, *R. tsutsugamushi* is grown in tissue culture cells for this use. Cox-Craigie type antigens (Craigie, 1945) obtained by the ether treatment of yolk sac suspensions were used as complement fixation (CF) test antigens. However, as early as 1945, it had already been shown that, unlike other similar antigens of the typhus group of rickettsiae or spotted fever group rickettsiae, there were scarcely any *R. tsutsugamushi* group-specific soluble antigens. However, strain specificity due to species-specific particulate antigens was strongly expressed. Consequently, it has been proposed (Bengtson, 1945, 1946; Philip, 1947) that Karp strains (New Guinea) and Gilliam strains (Burma) be used in combination as prototype strains in order to allow for the heterogeneity. In 1969, the above-mentioned soluble antigens were fractionated with difficulty, using sucrose density gradient centrifugation of tissue culture-derived material (Shishido *et al.*, 1969), but no practical applications ensued. However, there was no progress in analysis due both to the low titers of yolk sac-derived CF test antigens and to the presence of anti-complementary reactions. The Kawamura group (Kawamura, 1962; Yamamoto *et al.*, 1958) succeeded in the partial purification of *R. tsutsugamushi* using a cation exchange resin (Amberlite XE 64) and 8% KCl treatment. Modifying this method, Shishido *et al.* (1962a, 1964) produced CF test antigens, added the Kato strain (Niigata, Japan) to the Karp and Gilliam prototype strains, and performed serological typing of many strains isolated in Japan. The serological typing of *R. tsutsugamushi* was also performed widely in Thailand, by Elisberg *et al.* (1967, 1968), using the above three prototype strains. However, neither research group was able to account for all the antigenic diversity.

In 1963, indirect immunofluorescence (IF), which had a higher sensitivity than the CF test, was first introduced by Bozeman *et al.* (1963) for typing. However, there were non-specific fluorescence problems with this method, and Kawamura *et al.* (Iida *et al.*, 1966a; Kawamura, 1977; Murata and Kawamura, 1980) improved the labeling method, purified the labeled antibodies, and established highly accurate direct IF and indirect IF. *R. tsutsugamushi* derived from patients, field rodents, and trombiculid mites were typed by IF in Japan (Iida *et al.*, 1966b; Shishido *et al.*, 1967), Thailand (Elisberg *et al.*, 1978), and Malaysia (Shirai *et al.*, 1979b). Subsequently, in addition to *R. tsutsugamushi* strains that reacted singly with the three prototype strains, mixed types of the three prototypes were also found in Japan. Strains that were believed to be different from the three prototype strains also appeared (Kobayashi *et al.*, 1978). Meanwhile, there were strains that appeared in Thailand and Malaysia also that could not be classified into the three prototype strains, and five additional strains (TA678, TA686, TA716, TA763, and TH1817) were selected from the strains isolated in Thailand. Analyses were performed in Southeast Asia with the eight strains, and as many as 29 new types, including single strains and mixtures, were identified. Typing with the eight strains produced virtually the same results in other regions also (Shirai *et al.*, 1982a, 1982b). In particular, the results obtained in Malaysia (Shirai *et al.*, 1981b) and Thailand (Shirai *et al.*, 1981d) by direct IF typing of *R. tsutsugamushi* directly from trombiculid mites showed marked heterogeneity of *R. tsutsugamushi*; although the Karp type was dominant, many composite strains were identified. *Leptotrombidium arenicola* and *L. fletcheri*, which were maintained as naturally *R. tsutsugamushi*-infected laboratory-reared trombiculid mite colonies, were confirmed to be mixtures of 5 or 6 types, at all times throughout all generations (Shirai *et al.*, 1982c).

Subsequently, with the introduction of monoclonal antibodies (Eiseman and Osterman, 1985; Murata *et al.*, 1986; Tange *et al.*, 1991, 1992; Yamashita *et al.*, 1992) and the addition of an indirect immunoperoxidase technique (IP) (Suto, 1982; Yamamoto and Minamishima, 1982) with better sensitivity than IF, the analysis of the antigenic diversity of *R. tsutsugamushi* progressed further. In Japan, the Shimokoshi strain (Niigata, Japan) (Tamura *et al.*, 1984), the Kawasaki strain (Miyazaki, Japan) (Yamamoto *et al.*, 1986), and the Kuroki strain (Miyazaki) (Ohashi *et al.*, 1990b; Yamamoto *et al.*, 1989) were identified in succession as different types from the three prototype strains. They were added to the prototype strain group for *R. tsutsugamushi* typing and are currently in use. A background to this work was the development of type-specific antigens (TSA) for each strain, made possible by recent rapid advances in the molecular biological research on *R. tsutsugamushi* made by the Tamura group and others and by progress made in genetic analysis (Ohashi *et al.*, 1988, 1989, 1990a, 1992a; Stover *et al.*, 1990a; Tamura *et al.*, 1985). These activities made the elucidation of types possible by the chemical identification of TSA. In other words, proteins of 54,000–58,000 molecular weight (56-kDa proteins) which are present on the surfaces of *R. tsutsugamushi* cells are type determinants of TSA, and the respective TSA types are expressed based on the differences of the 56-kDa genes (*tsg 56*) that encode the TSAs. In Japan, in order to account for the various *R. tsutsugamushi* types, it is necessary to perform analysis that includes at least the Shimokoshi, Kawasaki, and Kuroki strains in addition to the previous three prototype strains. The Tamura group (Ohashi *et al.*, 1989, 1990a, 1992a) analyzed the genetic structures and total amino acid sequences of the 56-kDa proteins of the above six strains and compared the inter-strain homology of the open reading frames of these 56-kDa genes. The results showed that the Gilliam, Karp, and Kuroki strains were closely related; the Kawasaki strain was closely related to the Gilliam strain but different from the other strains, and the Shimokoshi strain was the least related to any of the strains. These differences in TSA which lead to type diversity and strongly influence both diagnosis and immune responses explain why the reinfection of patients is not at all rare, as well as explaining the difficulties that have been encountered in developing an *R. tsutsugamushi* vaccine.

Although it is troublesome to chemically determine the TSA of isolated *R. tsutsugamushi* strains each time, it has become possible to detect *R. tsutsugamushi* DNA by polymerase chain reaction (PCR) or nested PCR using, as primers, part of the sequence of the 56-kDa gene (*tsg 56*) encoding the TSAs of the six strains elucidated. In other words, *R. tsutsugamushi* DNA detection in patients' blood, in infected mice, or in the vector trombiculid mites, has become relatively simple by PCR (Furuya and Yoshida, 1992; Furuya *et al.*, 1991a, 1993). This has presented a useful means for the accurate diagnosis of Tsutsugamushi disease, the isolation of *R. tsutsugamushi*, and the elucidation of *R. tsutsugamushi* transmission. However, this is not to say that the methodology is without problems. For example, Takahashi *et al.* (1994d) reported that *R. tsutsugamushi* recovered with mice from a laboratory-reared colony of *L. pallidum* was consistently Karp type, showing no change throughout generations; whereas *R. tsutsugamushi* DNA detected directly from trombiculid mites by nested PCR also included Kawasaki and Kuroki types, in addition to Karp type. Further study is thus required to determine whether selection occurred through isolation with mice, or whether the difference occurred at the annealing region of the *R. tsutsugamushi* DNA of trombiculid mites with the primer used for PCR typing. In addition, regarding mouse passage, Gotoh (1967), from the Kawamura group, repeated passages in mice once a week (for 50 weeks and 25 weeks) with three series of mixed infection sets in which the infectivity of two strains of the previous three prototypes was aligned, and typing of the three series was performed with direct IF at each passage. Gotoh found that in the series involving the Gilliam strain, the one type which was not added always appeared from the early passages, and the three types were always found during the experiment; whereas in the series involving the Karp and Kato strain combinations, only two types were found, and the Gilliam type did not appear at all. These results suggest that strain selectivity or mutation occurred during passage in mice.

b. Distribution of R. tsutsugamushi *types*

This subject has already been described in detail in the preceding chapter. Here, we shall consider the significance of *R. tsutsugamushi* type distribution from the epidemiological point of view. *R. tsutsugamushi* is markedly heterogenic; could it be that some antigen-specific types are regionally distributed? In the case of post-World War II typing, results were, to some extent, influenced by methodology. However, in recent years, the true nature of TSA has been clarified by the analysis of TSA-encoding genes, and whether the previous results are usable as references is questionable. However, as we reviewed the studies prior to the introduction of monoclonal antibodies and the analysis of *tsg 56* genes, no obvious regularities were found in the distribution of the *R. tsutsugamushi* types based on complement fixation test or IF/IP.

In Japan, all *R. tsutsugamushi* isolates from field rodents and trombiculid mites (*L. kawamurai*, *L. pallidum*) in Hokkaido were of the Gilliam type (Kitaoka *et al.*, 1973; Shishido, 1962a), without a single exception. However, in Honshu, Japan, virtually no consistency was found in their distribution with respect to either origin or region (Iida *et al.*, 1966b; Shishido *et al.*, 1967). In Korea, the situation is similar to that in Japan, and Korean indigenous isolated strains are being studied centered around the Karp type strains (Chang *et al.*, 1990). Typing in Southeast Asia, on the other hand, shows a complex pattern, ranging from single type to mixtures involving eight strains (Elisberg *et al.*, 1978; Shirai *et al.*, 1979b, 1981b, 1981d, 1982a, 1982b, 1982c). For example, the 114 isolates recovered from Malaysian patients typed by direct IF were classified into 29 types, 86% of which were TA763, TA716, Karp, and TA686, either single or in mixtures (Shirai *et al.*, 1979b). In the strains recovered from Pescadores (Taiwan) patients (17 strains), field rodents (17 strains), and trombiculid mites (15 strains), 47% were of the TA716 type and 35% were of the Karp + TA716 type, showing polarization (Shirai *et al.*, 1982b). However, one may say that, as a trend, these strains were mainly Karp or Karp-analogue types. After monoclonal antibodies and analysis by TSA became available, *R. tsutsugamushi* isolates, and their distribution were analyzed in various regions of Japan, Miyazaki (Tange *et al.*, 1991; Yamamoto *et al.*,1986, 1989), Ehime (Tange *et al.*, 1992), Gifu Prefectures (Yamashita *et al.*, 1992), the slopes of Mt. Fuji (Kawamori *et al.*, 1992), Chiba Prefecture (Kaiho *et al.*, 1993), and elsewhere. The type in Ehime was different from that in Miyazaki; the Kawasaki and Kuroki types were distributed in Gifu, on the slopes of Mt. Fuji, in Kanagawa, and in Chiba, as they were in Miyazaki; and these isolates had low virulence in mice and overlapped with the *L. scutellare*-dominant district.

c. Relationship between vector and R. tsutsugamushi *types*
A relationship between *R. tsutsugamushi* type and the vector, trombiculid mites, was assumed earlier on. However, the results obtained thus far have confirmed only a relationship with the Gilliam type and *L. kawamurai* (which does not bite humans) in Hokkaido, and with the Gilliam type and *R. tsutsugamushi* isolates from field rodents (Kitaoka *et al.*, 1973; Shishido, 1962a). In Japan, *R. tsutsugamushi* isolates from the chief vectors of Tsutsugamushi disease, *L. akamushi*, mainly consisted of Kato and Gilliam types in Niigata and Akita Prefectures (Iida *et al.*, 1966b; Shishido, 1962a, 1964); *R. tsutsugamushi* isolates from *L. scutellare* were the Kawasaki and Kuroki types, intermixed with the Karp type (Asanuma *et al.*, 1974; Kaiho *et al.*, 1993; Tange *et al.*, 1991; Yamamoto *et al.*, 1986, 1989; Yamashita *et al.*, 1992); and those from *L. pallidum* were reported (Iida *et al.*, 1966b) as predominantly Gilliam type (in Akita, Niigata, and Kanagawa Prefectures), although some studies (Kawamori *et al.*, 1992; Shishido, 1964) reported that the Karp type was dominant.

On the other hand, in the serological typing of *R. tsutsugamushi* recovered directly from trombiculid mites in Southeast Asia, the *R. tsutsugamushi*-positive rate in Malaysia was 3.7%, with a single Karp type being dominant (63.7%); the majority of the remainder were mixtures (Shirai *et al.*, 1981b). In Thailand, the positive rate was 3.9%, with single Karp (50.7%), TA763 (11.6%), and TA716 (8.9%) types accounting for 76.7% and the remainder being mixed types (Shirai *et al.*, 1981d). In laboratory-reared chiggers, the mixture of 5 or 6 types did not deviate throughout the generations of two species colonies of rearing chiggers (Shirai *et al.*, 1982c).

However, an analysis of the relationship between *R.*

tsutsugamushi isolates and trombiculid mites in data gathered in the limited area of the slopes of Mt. Fuji (Kawamori *et al.*, 1992) is worth evaluating. In this area, the indirect IF typing of *R. tsutsugamushi* strains isolated from patients (24 strains), field rodents (30 strains), and trombiculid mites (5 strains; 4 to 125 mites pooled to form one series) by monoclonal antibodies resulted in the identification of 7 Karp strains, 13 Kawasaki strains, and 4 Kuroki strains among the isolates from patients, 25 Karp strains and 5 Kawasaki strains among the isolates from field rodents, 2 Kawasaki strains in the isolates from *L. scutellare*, and 3 Karp strains in the isolates from *L. pallidum*. Moreover, the Kawasaki type isolates from patients and field rodents overlapped with *L. scutellare,* and the Karp type overlapped with *L. pallidum*. However, when we consider that the isolates from trombiculid mites were all from a multiple number of pooled samples, that the above-mentioned *R. tsutsugamushi* isolates identified directly from trombiculid mites in Southeast Asia were not only single types but mixtures as well (Shirai *et al.*, 1981b, 1981d), and that the laboratory-reared trombiculid mite series were also mixtures (Shirai *et al.*, 1982c; Takahashi *et al.*, 1994d), it is evident that the relationship between *R. tsutsugamushi* types and trombiculid mites cannot be always so hastily resolved.

d. Pathogenicity of R. tsutsugamushi *strains*

R. tsutsugamushi strains are isolated from human patients, field rodents, and trombiculid mites predominantly by using mice, although tissue cultures are also used. At issue here is the differing pathogenicity of *R. tsutsugamushi* strains in mice. *R. tsutsugamushi* isolation with tissue culture cells is indifferent to such pathogenicity, but the isolation efficiency is not always good. Although there are mouse lines identified as having genetic resistance to *R. tsutsugamushi* infection or defense against such infection (Groves and Osterman, 1978; Groves *et al.*, 1980; Jerrells and Osterman, 1981), many rickettsia researchers have empirically acknowledged the existence of *R. tsutsugamushi* isolates that have low virulence in mice. Furthermore, it has been shown that inapparent infections occurred more often than would be expected in areas endemic for Tsutsugamushi disease, and these have been shown to be caused by *R. tsutsugamushi* strains with low virulence in humans (Fan *et al.*,

1987; Kawamura *et al.*, 1980; Shishido, 1962b). Because these *R. tsutsugamushi* strains with low virulence were isolated using mice, the development of a method (Kobayashi *et al.*, 1978; Tachibana and Kobayashi, 1975) in which cyclophosphamide was used as an immunosuppressive agent in mice led to the isolation of the abovementioned Shimokoshi, Kawasaki, and Kuroki strains, which are of different types, and the method also resulted in the isolation of the Irie and Hirano strains in Miyazaki Prefecture, which are also of different types. In addition, the use of nude mice was helpful in restoring *R. tsutsugamushi* pathogenicity weakened by yolk sac or mouse passage, and the usefulness of this method was confirmed (Kawamura *et al.*, 1980; Murata and Kawamura, 1977) for the isolation or passage of *R. tsutsugamushi* strains with low virulence in hairy mice.

4. Significance of Vector Mites as the Source of Infection

a. Trombiculid mites

Trombiculid mites belong to subfamilies of the families Trombiculidae and Leeuwenhoekiidae, which are included in the order Acarina, class Arachnida, phylum Arthropoda. More than 1,600 species of trombiculid mites are known worldwide, of which approximately 110 are found in Japan (Takada, 1990). These mites are noteworthy because some are vectors of Tsutsugamushi disease. The life history of trombiculid mites consists of four stages — egg, larva, nymph, and adult — as shown in Fig. 2. Nymphs and adults are totally independent of humans or other hosts and live a predatory life underground, whereas larvae have a parastic stage in which they generally suck the tissue fluids of their small vertebrate hosts (especially rodents).

Among the trombiculid mites are some which feed on humans in their larval stage, and if these larvae harbor *Rickettsia tsutsugamushi*, they infect the hosts including humans. Consequently, in order to elucidate various aspects of Tsutsugamushi disease, it is important to investigate the species of trombiculid mites that harbor *R. tsutsugamushi* and their seasonal prevalence. To this end, engorged trombiculid mites are collected from their hosts, such as field rodents; unfed mites are collected on black plates or sheets placed on the soil surface at target sites, or from the soil with a Tullgren funnel.

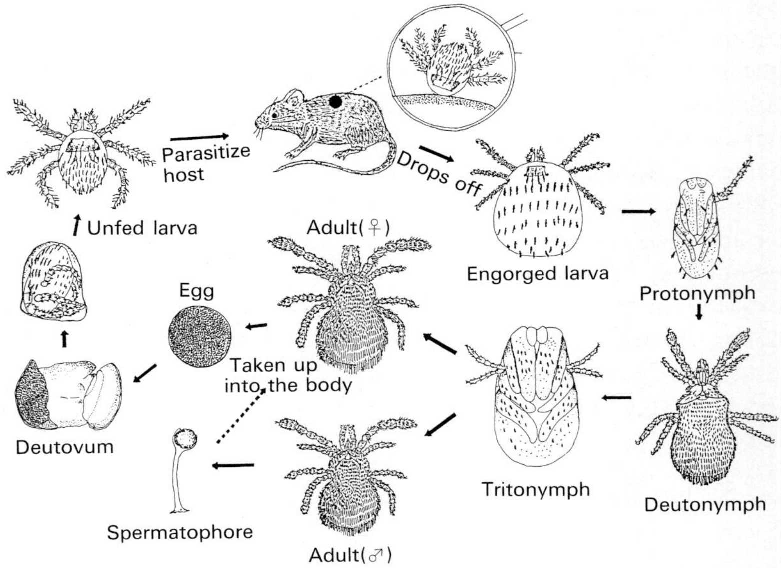

Fig. 2. Life cycle of *Leptotrombidium pallidum*

When humans or field rodents are bitten by *R. tsutsugamushi*-positive larval trombiculid mites and become infected, this indicates that *R. tsutsugamushi* has already been vertically transmitted from female adult mites to the unfed larvae by the transovarian route. This *R. tsutsugamushi* is a symbiotic organism and is not the *R. tsutsugamushi* that is transmitted to *R. tsutsugamushi*-negative mites up to the next generation.

The larvae have three pairs of legs; the body length of those hatched from eggs and unfed is approximately 0.2–0.3mm, a size barely visible to the naked eye. They parasitize their hosts and suck tissue fluids until they are engorged, at which time they drop off the host and burrow into the soil. The time of parasitization varies according to the trombiculid mite species and ranges from a minimum of approximately 2 days to as long as 7–10 days, but is generally 3–4 days. As a rule, larvae parasitize their host only once. A great many species of larval trombiculid mites have been found and classified using a synthesized classification formula (Vercammen-Grandjean and Langston, 1976).

The engorged larvae that return to the soil soon become dormant (protonymphs), after which they molt into deutonymphs, which have four pairs of legs. The deutonymphs prey on insect eggs in the soil or on the surface and again become dormant (tritonymphs), after which they molt into adults, which also have four pairs of legs. The adult's life is the same as the deutonymph's. Trombiculid mites do not propagate by direct copulation, but by indirect copulation, in which male adult mites drop off spermatophores and female adult mites are fertilized by taking in these spermatophores. The female mites produce eggs repeatedly. Larvae hatched from the eggs await the opportunity to parasitize hosts either under the soil or on the soil surface. Larvae sense the presence of a host by sensing its exhaled carbon dioxide in the air (Tanaka *et al.*, 1955).

b. Epidemiological association of vector trombiculid mites

In order to determine the vector trombiculid mite of Tsutsugamushi disease, the first step is to determine the larval trombiculid mite species present in the areas of activity of Tsutsugamushi disease patients at the time of onset, as well as to determine the seasonal prevalence and determine the epidemiological association of their relationship. For example, searches for vector trombiculid mites began with the epidemiological surveys carried out as part of the Tsutsugamushi disease research conducted in Japan. These studies were performed in the regions of classical Tsutsugamushi disease infection — Niigata, Yamagata, and Akita Prefectures; in the foothills of Mt. Fuji; and in the Izu Shichito Islands, where a new type of Tsutsugamushi disease, occurring from autumn to winter, was found after World War II. In Niigata and Akita Prefectures, the new type of Tsutsugamushi disease was found to occur from autumn to winter and from spring to early summer, the offseason for *Leptotrombidium akamushi*.

In particular, the conclusion that *L. akamushi* was the vector species of classical Tsutsugamushi disease during the period 1910–1925 was reached on the basis of data far more meager than today's, derived from a comparison with four other species of trombiculid mites found during the same period (Kawamura, 1926; Tamiya, 1962).

Similar epidemiological techniques allowed the inferences to be made that the culprits were *L. scutellare* in the new type of Tsutsugamushi disease, Shichito fever, found after the war in the Hachijo Islands of Izu Shichito, and *L. pallidum* for the

Tsutsugamushi disease occurring in the offseason of *L. akamushi* in Niigata Prefecture. However, in the foothills of Mt. Fuji, the seasonal prevalance of *L. scutellare*, *L. pallidum*, and *L. fuji* was similar; in Izu Oshima Island, both *L. scutellare* and *L. pallidum* were also present, and it was impossible to reach a conclusion based on the incidence of Tsutsugamushi disease patients and the seasonal prevalence of trombiculid mites alone. In order to derive more scientific conclusions from these speculations, a technique to detect *R. tsutsugamushi* in the larval stage had already been developed during approximately the same period, as discussed below.

Prior to 1920, larvae found on the bodies of humans who had entered endemic areas were identified at the sites of occurrence of classical Tsutsugamushi disease. Alternatively, monkeys were placed as sentinels in the endemic areas, larvae were recovered from the monkeys, and the clinical symptoms of the monkeys (fever and eschar) were observed to confirm the onset of the disease. These methods confirmed that *L. akamushi* was directly or indirectly involved with more than epidemiological factors (Kawamura, 1926; Tamiya, 1962).

In the Hachijo Islands, where Shichito fever occurred, *R. tsutsugamushi* was isolated from *L. scutellare* (Kitaoka, 1959), and to determine the vector species of autumn-to-winter Tsutsugamushi disease in Niigata Prefecture, field rodents were captured throughout the year, and the species composition of engorged trombiculid mites, their seasonal prevalence, and the *R. tsutsugamushi* harboring rate of the field rodents as well as attached trombiculid mites were studied. Concurrently, the use of sentinel animals, discussed below, was combined with *R. tsutsugamushi* isolation from rodents rather than from trombiculid mites (Asanuma *et al.*, 1964a, 1964b).

No human infection was found during the survey for the outbreak of Tsutsugamushi disease that was believed to have occurred in the summer in Kochi Prefecture, Shikoku, even though *R. tsutsugamushi* was isolated there from field rodents. Although, epidemiologically, *L. tosa* was considered the vector trombiculid mite, these mites are present throughout the year, and their infestation is not restricted to the summer, when infections occurred. However, the number of mites collected in June through September was four times greater than during other periods; *R. tsutsugamushi* was successfully isolated only once from *L. tosa* engorged on a field rodent.

Even in this case, as this was an engorged trombiculid mite, it is possible that the *R. tsutsugamushi* was acquired incidentally from *R. tsutsugamushi*-positive field rodents; further, this finding was not conclusive (Kawamura *et al.*, 1952; Nakaya, 1957).

In Kagawa Prefecture, which is also in Shikoku, Umayado disease, which occurs in the summer, was diagnosed as Tsutsugamushi disease, based on the clinical picture of the patients and on the *R. tsutsugamushi* isolated. However, as was the case in Kochi Prefecture, the vector species was not confirmed as *L. tosa*, although this was the most likely vector (Hamada, 1954; Nokihara, 1955; Ono, 1956). These findings indicate that the time of occurrence, the seasonal prevalence of the trombiculid mites, and the isolation of *R. tsutsugamushi* from attached trombiculid mites are by themselves not sufficient for the determination of the vector trombiculid mite.

c. *Confirming vector trombiculid mites and their predilection for humans*

As noted above, an epidemiological association is not sufficient for determining the vector trombiculid mite. To be certain, *R. tsutsugamushi* must be detected in unfed larvae. If *R. tsutsugamushi* is isolated from engorged larvae, one cannot discount the possibility that *R. tsutsugamushi*-negative larvae temporarily acquired *R. tsutsugamushi* from an *R. tsutsugamushi*-bearing host, as stated above. However, the collection of unfed larvae is often difficult, and not only is the *R. tsutsugamushi*-harboring rate of larvae low, but there are large variations according to trombiculid mite species.

Further, more than one type of *R. tsutsugamushi* is symbiotic to trombiculid mites, and multiple types frequently coexist. Consequently, the ideal method of identifying *R. tsutsugamushi* today would be to look for larvae that parasitize persons in areas endemic for *R. tsutsugamushi,* dig them out, confirm that the trombiculid mites have a predilection for humans, and determine the species, and then either wait to see if the person develops Tsutsugamushi disease or identify the DNA type of *R. tsutsugamushi* the larva is harboring, using either the polymerase chain reaction (PCR) or nested PCR (Furuya *et al.*, 1991a, 1993).

However, even in an endemic area, parasitized larvae on persons who have not developed Tsutsugamushi disease would be detected only in the course of a well planned study (Kitaoka *et al.*, 1974) or by chance. In 1956 and 1970, Kitaoka *et al.* (1974) carried out such studies, examining 386 local residents who had visited areas endemic for *R. tsutsugamushi*. They identified 87 of 93 trombiculid mite larvae parasitizing the subjects as *L. akamushi*, and they noted 45 of 386 cases of Tsutsugamushi disease (11.7%). These results provided valuable data. The *R. tsutsugamushi* harboring rate of *L. akamushi* calculated in this study was 2.5%.

The detection of *R. tsutsugamushi* by collecting larvae while they are biting humans is not always easy. The methods used to detect *R. tsutsugamushi* directly from unfed larvae collected in the natural environment include the mouse passage technique, electron microscopy, immunofluorescence (IF), biotin-avidin-IF, PCR, and nested PCR; these will be described in detail in Chapter 4.

The season of Tsutsugamushi disease occurrence, the *R. tsutsugamushi*-positive rate of field rodents, and the season of emergence of the vector trombiculid mite larvae coincide well; and field rodents are just as much victims of *R. tsutsugamushi*-harboring trombiculid mites as are other hosts (Fukuzumi, 1953; Kitaoka, 1959; Suzuki, 1959). Consequently, even though there are problems in the detection of *R. tsutsugamushi* in trombiculid mite larvae engorged on field rodents, such detection aids in the assessment of endemicity and has been frequently used in the past as a technique to facilitate drawing inferences regarding the vector trombiculid mites. The findings of *R. tsutsugamushi* detection assays in unfed and engorged larvae are discussed in detail in the next chapter.

As stated above, unfed larvae are not easily collected. Consequently, the technique used since the early phase of the research to identify the vector trombiculid mites and to determine *R. tsutsugamushi* endemicity is to place animals uninfected with *R. tsutsugamushi* in a target area (sentinel animals), recover and identify engorged larvae in these animals, and, at the same time, confirm *R. tsutsugamushi* infection of the animals themselves.

Nagayo *et al.* (1920) and Kawamura (1926) placed monkeys in areas endemic for classical Tsutsugamushi disease in Japan, and recovered and identified engorged *L. akamushi* as the vector trombiculid mites, confirming disease onset (fever and eschar) in the monkeys as well as providing epidemiological data. Ducks and chickens were also used as sentinel animals during this period, although without notable success (Hatori, 1919–20, 1920; Kawamura,

1926). However, the use of sentinel animals as a tool for identifying vector trombiculid mites and for locating endemic areas actually began after World War II. Phillip *et al.* (1949) and Traub and Frick (1950), using volunteer human subjects and rats, confirmed the transmissibility of *L. deliense* and Malaysian *L. akamushi* (= *L. fletcheri*), as well as the existence of endemic areas. Hubert and Baker (1963) used sentinel rabbits to confirm the transmissibility of *L. fletcheri*, which was classified as Malaysian *L. akamushi* at that time.

After *L. akamushi* was confirmed as the vector of classical Tsutsugamushi disease, widespread experiments with sentinel animals were conducted in Japan, proving that *L. scutellare* and *L. pallidum* were vectors for the new type of Tsutsugamushi disease. Asanuma *et al.* (1959b, 1959c) isolated *R. tsutsugamushi* from pooled material (a total of 14 engorged *L. pallidum*) obtained from nine rats placed in an endemic area in Nagaoka (Niigata Prefecture), and also from pooled material (four engorged *L. scutellare*) obtained from four mice in Shirahama, Chiba Prefecture.

Asanuma *et al.* (1962a) conducted 18 trials with a total of 785 rats and 419 mice in the Miura and Izu Peninsulas and isolated *R. tsutsugamushi* from two lines of rats which harbored *L. pallidum*. However, since sentinel mice and rats did not produce a satisfactory number of engorged mites, another study was conducted, in which Kitaoka and Asanuma (1968) placed 22 field voles, *Microtus montebelli*, as experimental animals in an area endemic for classical Tsutsugamushi disease, Oomagari in Akita Prefecture. This was done in two August trials, and 11 *R. tsutsugamushi* strains were successfully isolated from 36 pooled (100 individuals) *L. akamushi* lines. The *R. tsutsugamushi*-harboring rate of *L. akamushi* during the same period was 11.1–11.4%.

Similarly, Kitaoka *et al.* (1976) carried out a study with sentinel animals, using chickens. These birds, which do not fly, are potential carriers of the vector. Studies were carried out in Jyumonji, Akita Prefecture, three times (April 24–28 and October 6, 1970, and September 1, 1971), and the focus was on *L. pallidum*, the dominant vector along with *L. akamushi*. As shown in Table 1, *R. tsutsugamushi* was isolated only from the pooled group of 22 *L. pallidum* recovered in the third experiment, from 13 sentinel birds. *R. tsutsugamushi* was also isolated from the pooled spleens and liv-

Table 1. Isolation of *Rickettsia* from Sentinel Chickens Placed on the Tsutsugamushi Disease Endemic Area and Chigger Mites Collected from Host Chickens

Experiment	Date of placing chickens	No. of chickens attacked by chigger mites (No. of rickettsia-positive chickens)	Species and no. of chigger mites collected	No. of positive pools / no. of pools tested
I	April 24–28, 1970	5 (0) 12 (0)	*L. pallidum* 5 *L. palpale* 46	N. D. N. D.
II	October 6, 1970	1 (0)	*L. pallidum* 1	N. D.
III	September 1, 1971	4/13* 1 pool blood negative 1 pool spleen-liver positive	 *L. pallidum* 22 *L. pallidum* 4	 1 / 1 0 / 1

* Out of 13 chickens 4 were tested for rickettsia from their pooled blood and pooled spleen-liver.
N. D. : not done. (Modified from Kitaoka *et al.*, 1976)

ers of four chickens. Both of the above rickettsiae were the Kato strain.

To observe the trombiculid mites' predilection for humans, Arai (1955) used volunteer subjects in an area endemic for *L. scutellare*, on Hachijo Island where Shichito fever occurs, and confirmed that the mites were engorged on humans (no disease was observed). Similarly, Kitaoka *et al.* (1953a) examined schoolchildren from the island and also found engorged mites on them. Sasa *et al.* (1953a) and Kitaoka *et al.* (1953a) also confirmed that unfed *L. scutellare* from the island became engorged when placed on the skin of volunteers though they did not cause disease.

However, in a volunteer exposed to 50 trombiculid mites (a mixture of *L. fuji*, *L. kitasatoi*, and *L. pallidum*) collected from Izu Peninsula at about the same time, only eight mites were found to have become engorged. After they dropped off, the mite species was identified as *L. pallidum*. The volunteer developed typical Tsutsugamushi disease 15 days later (Asanuma *et al.*, 1958, 1962a; Kitaoka *et al.*, 1953a).

In recent studies, Takahashi *et al.* (1990b) used as sentinel animals the field vole, *Microtus montebelli*, for which trombiculid mites have a stronger predilection than for rats, mice, or rabbits. The animals were exposed six times during 1985–1986 in a limited area (350 × 35 m) of Chichibu City (Hitsujiyama Park), Saitama Prefecture, an area endemic for the new type of Tsutsugamushi disease, to study the distribution of the vector mites and their *R. tsutsugamushi*-harboring rate. Takahashi *et al.* (1990b), in the first two experiments, selected four spots where trombiculid mites occurred most frequently; in the subsequent four experiments, each selected spot was divided into 2 × 2 m quadrats, and one *M. montebelli* was placed in each quadrat. According to the literature, the trombiculid mite infestation rate on *M. montebelli* is, on average, approximately tenfold that on other sentinel animals.

The total number of engorged trombiculid mites found in the study was 331 *L. pallidum*, 175 *L. fuji*, and 16 *Gahrliepia saduski* (Takahashi *et al.*, 1990b). Each mite was assayed for *R. tsutsugamushi* by the BA-IF or by the mouse passage technique. In *L. pallidum*, 31/286 (10.8%) *R. tsutsugamushi* were of the Karp type; no *R. tsutsugamushi* was found in the other trombiculid mites. In particular, in *L. pallidum*, *R. tsutsugamushi* was detected in three *M. montebelli* at prevalence of 6/11, 2/5, and 3/5, respectively, and *R. tsutsugamushi* (Karp type) was isolated at a prevalence of 12/14 (85.7%) from a sentinel *M. montebelli*. These findings confirmed that *L. pallidum* was an *R. tsutsugamushi* vector and that the experimental sites were mite islands (hyperendemic areas) of *R. tsutsugamushi*-positive trombiculid mites.

Based on these results, it was confirmed that the majority of Tsutsugamushi disease in Japan was transmitted by three mite species, *L. akamushi*, *L. pallidum*, and *L. scutellare*, the detection of *R. tsutsugamushi* from unfed trombiculid mites showing approximately the same results as those assessed in engorged trombiculid mites. It was also found that *L. kawamurai*, which is not considered to parasitize humans, was a vector trombiculid mite in field rodents.

It has been confirmed that the species of mites infesting humans in Japan are *L. akamushi* (Asanuma, 1959; Ito and Obata, 1961; Kitaoka *et al.*, 1974, etc.), *L. pallidum* (Asanuma, 1959, 1962b; Kawamura, 1926; Kitaoka *et al.*, 1953a, etc.), *L. scutellare* (Arai, 1955; Asanuma 1959, 1962b; Kitaoka *et al.*, 1953a, etc.; Sasa *et al.*, 1953a), *L. palpale* (Asanuma, 1959; Kawamura, 1926), and *Eutrombicula wichmanni* (Asanuma, 1959; Kitahara, 1952; Sasa, 1956). Repeated attempts were made to isolate *R. tsutsugamushi* from one of these species, *L. palpale*, collected at numerous sites, with very limited success (it is possible that *R. tsutsugamushi* migrated from the infected animals to the trombiculid mites), and the isolation of *R. tsutsugamushi* from *Eutrombicula wichmanni* has not been successful (Asanuma, 1959, 1983; Sasa, 1956).

In other countries where Tsutsugamushi disease occurs, reports of the direct determination of the vector trombiculid mites in unfed mites or their determination by means of sentinel animals are relatively sparse. However, transmissibility by *L. deliense* and *L. fletcheri* has been confirmed through volunteers or sentinel animals, as stated previously (Hubert and Baker, 1963; Philip *et al.*, 1949; Traub and Frick, 1950). Although *R. tsutsugamushi* strains derived from other trombiculid mites have been isolated primarily from engorged ones, when the predilection for humans and the epidemiological data for Tsutsugamushi disease occurrence are taken into consideration, it is apparent that *L. deliense*, *L. fletcheri*, *L. arenicola*, *L. pallidum*, *L. pavlovskyi*, and *L. scutellare* are the six major vector species (Traub and Wisserman, 1974b).

d. Association of vector mite species with R. tsutsugamushi *type and pathogenicity*

As stated previously, *R. tsutsugamushi* is extremely heterogeneous, and this had led to problems in its typing. Consequently, its relationship to trombiculid mite vectors has become a subject of interest to researchers. However, until recently, no consistent relationship was shown. In recent years, molecular biological research on *R. tsutsugamushi* has made it possible to chemically confirm *R. tsutsugamushi* heterogeneity, using a type-specific antigen (TSA) for each *R. tsutsugamushi* strain, and to carry out genetic analysis. There is also a report demonstrating a relationship between the vector trombiculid mites and *R. tsutsugamushi* types (Kawamori *et al.*, 1992), based on the data obtained from the Gotemba-Oyama district at the foot of Mt. Fuji. Kawamori *et al.* (1992) conclude that *L. scutellare* transmits the Kawasaki type and *L. pallidum*, the Karp type of *R. tsutsugamushi*. However, the findings of Kawamori *et al.* (1992) appear to be controversial in the light of the findings, noted above, that *R. tsutsugamushi* identified in trombiculid mites in Southeast Asia were not only single types but also mixed types (Shirai *et al.*, 1981b, 1981d), and that the *R. tsutsugamushi* lines in the infected laboratory colonies were all mixed types (Shirai *et al.*, 1982c). Recent studies by Takahashi *et al.* (1994d) have resolved these questions, indicating that rickettsia type isolated from a mite species may have been due to the method used for isolation, *i.e.*, mouse passage, in which type selection could have occurred.

Takahashi *et al.* (1994d), using mice, reported that the *R. tsutsugamushi* types recovered from laboratory-reared *R. tsutsugamushi*-positive *L. pallidum* colonies were all Karp type throughout all generations, whereas probing of *R. tsutsugamushi* DNA from trombiculid mites by nested PCR showed the presence of Kawasaki and Kuroki strains as well. However, only the Karp type *R. tsutsugamushi* could be isolated, as before, from the mice on which the trombiculid mites were engorged.

Based on these results, one should consider two possibilities: (1) that *R. tsutsugamushi* type selection can occur in the isolation procedure in which mice are used , or (2) that a partial mutation may occur in the sequence of the *R. tsutsugamushi* DNA in a trombiculid mite to be annealed with the PCR typing primers. In any case, it is still premature to assert a consistent relationship between *R. tsutsugamushi* type and species of trombiculid mite.

The pathogenicity of *R. tsutsugamushi* in humans is as diverse as the heterogenicity of the strains, ranging from causation of typical Tsutsugamushi disease to inapparent infections. Similarly, the pathogenicity of *R. tsutsugamushi* in mice, exclusive of genetic resistance, also exhibits diversity. Moreover, the two cases do not necessarily take a parallel course; it has been confirmed that the *R. tsutsugamushi* causing typical Tsutsugamushi disease in humans is only mildly pathogenic to mice. Naturally, there could also be *R. tsutsugamushi* which show disease in mice and no pathogenicity in humans, or those showing only inapparent infections in both humans and mice. Perhaps these relationships among *R. tsutsugamushi* type, trombiculid mite species, and pathogenicity could be explained in terms of differences in TSA. However, no conclusion in this regard can be reached unless, first, all *R. tsutsugamushi* strains are established in tissue culture so that the strains with different pathogenicity in humans and mice can be analyzed.

5 Reservoir Hosts

As stated previously, the fact that humans and field rodents are infected with *Rickettsia tsutsugamushi* as a consequence of being infested by the same species of larval trombiculid mites which have been recovered and confirmed to be *R. tsutsugamushi*-positive in a sentinel animal experiment is indicative of transovarian transmission of *R. tsutsugamushi* from female adult to larva. The question is whether *R. tsutsugamushi* is a symbiont of trombiculid mites or is transferred from other *R. tsutsugamushi*-harboring animals during feeding. It has now been confirmed that *R. tsutsugamushi* is a symbiont of trombiculid mites, since no transovarian transmission occurs even when *R. tsutsugamushi* is transiently acquired by trombiculid mites from *R. tsutsugamushi*-infected animals.

Nevertheless, why do *R. tsutsugamushi*-positive larvae occur only in a subset of the population even within the same species? And why do *R. tsutsugamushi*-positive larvae form clusters like mite islands? There is still a great deal to be studied about the ecology of trombiculid mites in relation to *R. tsutsugamushi*. To make some progress toward solving this problem, it is necessary to use infected and uninfected laboratory colonies (laboratory-colonies of *R. tsutsugamushi*-positive and -negative trombiculid mites) and to analyze their interaction with *R. tsutsugamushi*-harboring animals.

The discussion here is based on rearing of trombiculid mites in the laboratory, the transovarian transmission of *R. tsutsugamushi* using infected colonies, and the experimental transfer of *R. tsutsugamushi* from *R. tsutsugamushi*-harboring animals to *R. tsutsugamushi*-negative trombiculid mites. (These methods are described in detail in Chapters 4 and 5.) When *R. tsutsugamushi* is transferred, even transiently, to larval trombiculid mites, from *R. tsutsugamushi*-harboring animals, it is necessary to determine how long the animals harbor *R. tsutsugamushi* and how long their antibodies are sustained. In this section, we also address the relationship between *R. tsutsugamushi* infection and pregnancy, including that in humans.

a. Laboratory-reared trombiculid mites and transovarian transmission of R. tsutsugamushi

Although the life cycle of trombiculid mites was elucidated relatively early in Tsutsugamushi disease research (Kawamura, 1926; Sasa, 1956), such details of the life history as propagation and life span were not understood until many years later, because of our inability to determine the food habits of free-living nymph and adult mites. After World War II, ecological studies of trombiculid mites began. In countries other than Japan, mosquito eggs (Wharton and Carver, 1946) and collembolan eggs (Lipovsky, 1951) were found to be useful for feeding trombiculid mites in the laboratory rearing. These eggs were also used successfully in Japan for the laboratory rearing of *Leptotrombidium akamushi* (Miura, 1960). A group at the US Army Medical Research Unit (Rapmund, 1984) in Kuala Lumpur succeeded in producing infected colonies of *L. deliense*, *L. fletcheri*, and *L. arenicola*, which are the principal vector species of Tsutsugamushi disease in Southeast Asia. This directly demonstrated that *R. tsutsugamushi* was vertically passed to the next generation of trombiculid mites by ovarian transmission.

In the meantime, laboratory colonies of *L. pallidum* were also established in Japan, and the same vertical transmission was observed (Takahashi *et al.*, 1988b). In order to verify the maintenance of the above-mentioned Kuala Lumpur colonies, the Kawamura group was requested to keep, and received laboratory colonies from the Kuala Lumpur group, and these are still being reared by Takahashi. Currently, infected and uninfected colonies have been established with *L. fletcheri*, *L. arenicola*, and *L. pallidum*; and uninfected colonies, with *L. deliense* and *L. akamushi*.

b. R. tsutsugamushi *transmission from* R. tsutsugamushi*-harboring animals to trombiculid mites*

As will be discussed in detail in Chapter 5, it has been shown that *R. tsutsugamushi* is actually transferred to larval trombiculid mites while infesting *R. tsutsugamushi*-harboring animals at a certain ratio. This was confirmed by the experiment in which the *R. tsutsugamushi*-infected animals were infested with larvae from the uninfected colonies, and *R. tsutsugamushi* was traced to the engorged larvae. The resulting ratios reported by various workers showed wide variations (ranging from 1.2% to 25.6%) depending on the trombiculid mite species and on the experimental conditions. However, since the laboratory conditions are usually not likely to be sustained in nature, the transfer ratios are not believed to be very high in the field condition. It is certain, however, that *R. tsutsugamushi* persists until mites reach the adult stage. As to whether secondarily acquired *R. tsutsugamushi* is transmitted to the next generation of trombiculid mites, results with experimental transmission to F_1 obtained by many researchers have been negative, with the exception of Traub *et al.* (1975), who found *R. tsutsugamushi* transmission to F_1 *L. deliense* in one out of 23 pools (one pool averaged 140 individuals). This observation is interpreted in Chapter 5, Section 2. The localization of *R. tsutsugamushi* living in trombiculid mite tissues after engorgement is unknown. However, it is inconceivable that rickettsiae invade ova in their bacteriostatic state.

c. Persistence of R. tsutsugamushi *in* R. tsutsugamushi*-harboring animals, and anti-*R. tsutsugamushi *antibody*

Numerous studies have attempted to predict *R. tsutsugamushi* infections of animals in nature by studying both the persistence of *R. tsutsugamushi* infection in experimental animals and anti-*R. tsutsugamushi* antibodies. However, because of variations in *R. tsutsugamushi* strain, dose, site of inoculation, and experimental animal lines and individual differences, neither the duration of the *R. tsutsugamushi* infection nor the duration of the antibody response has always been consistent.

Fox (1948) confirmed the presence of *R. tsutsugamushi* and its antibodies examined by complement fixation test for up to 610 days in mice after subcutaneous inoculation with the Karp strain, and for up to 269 days in cotton rats after subcutaneous inoculation with the Seerangayee strain. Suzuki (1959) traced *R. tsutsugamushi* for 94 days in rats following the subcutaneous inoculation of the human *R. tsutsugamushi* Kikuchi strain, recovering *R. tsutsugamushi* up to day 35. Meanwhile, rats receiving a subcutaneous inoculation with an *R. tsutsugamushi* field rodent strain were studied from days 79–417, and *R. tsutsugamushi* was recovered only on day 97.

In 1979, Shirai *et al.* (1979a) intraperitoneally inoculated mice with the *R. tsutsugamushi* TA678 strain, which is avirulent to mice, and found that *R. tsutsugamushi* persisted up to day 565.

Fukuzumi (1953), in a study of *R. tsutsugamushi* persistence in field voles, reported that, in *Microtus montebelli* which they trapped and reared, *R. tsutsugamushi* was positive on day 160 but negative on day 270. Suzuki (1959) subcutaneously inoculated *M. montebelli* and *Apodemus speciosus* captured in the field with the human *R. tsutsugamushi* Kikuchi strain, studying *R. tsutsugamushi* from days 79 to 131 in the former and days 79 to 190 in the latter animals; he was able to recover rickettsia up to day 79 in the former and up to day 190 in the latter. He also subcutaneously inoculated laboratory-reared *M. montebelli* with the Kikuchi strain of *R. tsutsugamushi*, traced rickettsia from days 30 to 190, and successfully recovered it up to day 190.

Van Peenen *et al.* (1977) used indirect immunofluorescence to determine the anti-*R. tsutsugamushi* antibody titer of field rodents captured in the Philippines and reported that all individuals in which *R. tsutsugamushi* was isolated were antibody-positive and the antibody response persisted for at least 11 months. And the antibody response persisted for up to 7 months in the individuals experimentaly inoculated with *R. tsutsugamushi*.

As can be seen from the references cited above, observations on the persistence of *R. tsutsugamushi* in infected animals and on the duration of anti-*R. tsutsugamushi* antibodies vary among researchers. Consequently, in order to determine the suitability of voles as *R. tsutsugamushi* reservoir hosts, Takahashi *et al.* (1990c) reared typical Japanese voles, *i.e.*, the Japanese grass vole, *Microtus montebelli*, large Japanese field mice, *Apodemus speciosus*, and small Japanese field mice, *A. argenteus*, as well as experimental animals such as the European grass vole, *M. arvalis*, in the laboratory. They confirmed in advance that none of the animals had anti-*R. tsutsugamushi* antibodies, and inoculated them subcutaneously at the base of the ear with the Karp strain of *R. tsutsugamushi*. Subsequently, every 30 days, they attempted to isolate *R. tsutsugamushi* by mouse passage and determine the presence of antibodies by indirect immunofluorescence. They found that the maximal periods of persistent infection with *R. tsutsugamushi* were 5 months for *M. montebelli*, 9 months for *M. arvalis*, 3 months for *A. speciosus*, and 3 months for *A. argenteus* (smaller numbers of animals). Antibody titers increased over 160-fold on day 150 in *M. montebelli*, over 320-fold on day 270 in *M. arvalis*, 80-fold on day 240 in *A. speciosus*, and 20-fold on day 90 in *A. argenteus*. These data highlight the differences among species of the experimental field rodents, as well as among individuals within the same species (Tables 2, 3, and 4).

In addition, on days 30 and 240 after the inoculation of *M. montebelli* and *M. arvalis* with *R. tsutsugamushi*, various organs were tested for *R. tsutsugamushi* by the mouse passage method.

Table 2. Persistence of Infection with *Rickettsia tsutsugamushi* in *Microtus montebelli* 30–300 Days after Subcutaneous Inoculation with *R. tsutsugamushi* at the Back of the Neck. Results in Terms of Ratios of Voles with Successful Isolation of *R. tsutsugamushi* and Detection of Anti-*R. tsutsugamushi* Antibody to the Infected Voles.

	Days after infection										
	30	41	60	90	120	150	180	210	240	270	300
Isolation of *R. tsutsugamushi*	2/4	1/2	3/4	0/4	1/4	1/4	0/2	0/3	0/3	0/4	0/4
Detection of antibody[a]	3/4	1/2	3/4	2/4	2/4	1/4	0/4	0/4	0/4	0/4	0/4
Sum of *R. tsutsugamushi* (+)	3/4	1/2	4/4	2/4	2/4	1/4	0/4	0/4	0/4	0/4	0/4

[a] Detection of antibody in mice for passage by indirect immunofluorescence using *R. tsutsugamushi* infected L cells as antigen. Antibody was regarded to be positive when reactions were positive at 1:10 serum dilution or more.

Table 3. Persistence of Infection with *Rickettsia tsutsugamushi* in *Microtus arvalis* 30–300 Days after Subcutaneous Inoculation with *R. tsutsugamushi* at the Back of the Neck. Results in Terms of Ratios of Voles with Successful Isolation of *R. tsutsugamushi* and Detection of Anti-*R. tsutsugamushi* Antibody to the Infected Voles.

	Days after infection									
	30	60	90	120	150	180	210	240	270	300
Isolation of *R. tsutsugamushi*	4/4	3/4	2/4	3/4	3/4	2/4	1/4	4/4	1/4	0/4
Detection of antibody[a]	4/4	2/3	2/4	2/3	3/4	3/4	2/4	4/4	1/4	0/4
Sum of *R. tsutsugamushi* (+)	4/4	3/4	2/4	3/4	3/4	3/4	2/4	4/4	1/4	0/4

[a] The same as Table 2.

Table 4. Persistence of Infection with *Rickettsia tsutsugamushi* in *Apodemus speciosus* 10–270 Days after Subcutaneous Inoculation with *R. tsutsugamushi* at the Back of the Neck. Results of Ratios of Rodents with Successful Isolation of *R. tsutsugamushi* and Detection of Anti-*R. tsutsugamushi* Antibody to the Infected Rodents.

	Days after infection				
	10	20	90	240	270
Isolation of *R. tsutsugamushi*	3/3	2/2	2/8	0/2	0/2
Detection of antibody[a]	3/3	2/2	2/8	1/2	0/2
Sum of R. tsutsugamushi (+)	3/3	2/2	2/8	1/2	0/2

[a] The same as Table 2.

These results, along with the anti-*R. tsutsugamushi* antibody measurements in these passaged mice, are shown in Tables 5 and 6.

The findings with *M. montebelli* on day 30 showed individual differences, but with *M. arvalis*, *R. tsutsugamushi* was detected in the organs of all individuals tested. On day 240, neither *R. tsutsugamushi* nor antibody was detected from *M. montebelli*, whereas with *M. arvalis*, *R. tsutsugamushi* was detected from the lungs, liver, spleen, and brain of some individuals tested, and the antibodies were also found in the passaged mice associated with these individuals.

On the other hand, the peritoneal smears of all individuals of *M.*

Table 5. Distribution of *R. tsutsugamushi* in Organs of 2 Species of *Microtus* 30 Days after Subcutaneous Inoculation with *R. tsutsugamushi* at the Back of the Neck

Organs	*M. montebelli*		*M. arvalis*	
	Isolation of *Rt*[a]	Ab[b]	Isolation of *Rt*[a]	Ab[b]
Lung	2/3	2/3	3/3	3/3
Liver	1/3	2/3	3/3	3/3
Spleen	2/3	1/3	3/3	3/3
Kidney	2/3	2/3	3/3	3/3
Blood	1/3	2/3	3/3	1/3
Lymph node	2/3	2/3	3/3	1/3
Brain	1/3	1/3	3/3	2/3

[a] Isolation of *R. tsutsugamushi* by mouse passage.
[b] Detection of anti-*R. tsutsugamushi* antibody from mice for passage.

Table 6. Distribution of *R. tsutsugamushi* in Organs of 2 Species of *Microtus* 240 Days after Subcutaneous Inoculation with *R. tsutsugamushi* at the Back of the Neck

Organs	*M. montebelli*		*M. arvalis*	
	Isolation of *Rt*[a]	Ab[b]	Isolation of *Rt*[a]	Ab[b]
Lung	0/3	0/3	3/4	3/4
Liver	0/3	0/3	3/4	3/4
Spleen	0/3	0/3	2/4	3/4
Kidney	0/3	0/3	0/4	0/4
Blood	0/3	0/3	0/4	0/4
Lymph node	0/3	0/3	0/4	0/4
Brain	0/3	0/3	1/4	1/4

[a, b] The same as Table 5.

montebelli and *M. arvalis* in which anti-*R. tsutsugamushi* antibodies (an increase of over 80-fold) were demonstrated on days 30 and 240 following *R. tsutsugamushi* inoculation were examined to detect *R. tsutsugamushi* by immunofluorescence and were all negative.

d. R. tsutsugamushi *infection and pregnancy*

A long time ago, at the areas endemic for classical Japanese Tsutsugamushi disease (Niigata Prefecture), the inhabitants believed that when a pregnant woman was infected by *R. tsutsugamushi*, she might miscarry, but would not die. To confirm in experimental animals whether this was true, Yamané (1955), raised male and female mice separately; these mice had received subcutaneous inoculation of *R. tsutsugamushi* Ozeki strain (Gilliam type) and survived the infection. After it was confirmed that the mice had harbored *R. tsutsugamushi* in the spleen for more than 7 months, the animals were paired so that the females would be impregnated. In the female mice, *R. tsutsugamushi* disappeared from the spleen toward the end of gestation. Although *R. tsutsugamushi* reappeared in the spleen after delivery, it was at a level far lower than that prior to the pregnancy; only those mice that had been pregnant did not survive a direct challenge with *R. tsutsugamushi*. Moreover, despite *R. tsutsugamushi* being isolated at a high rate from the placenta at the time of birth, all attempts at isolation from fetuses and offspring failed, and antibodies could not be detected after weaning.

Shirai *et al.* (1984a) found that mice did not conceive when inoculated with *R. tsutsugamushi*, and nearly half of the population died when the mice were inoculated with *R. tsutsugamushi* after they became pregnant, thus confirming that *R. tsutsugamushi* had an adverse effect on pregnant mice. They attempted to isolate *R. tsutsugamushi* from the placentas and fetuses on the day before the scheduled delivery in pregnant mice that had survived *R. tsutsugamushi* infections, as Yamané (1955) had done previously. *R. tsutsugamushi* was detected only in the placentas; furthermore, anti-*R. tsutsugamushi* antibodies in the offspring were undetectable after 1–2 days.

In a study of 111 postpartum women in areas endemic for *R. tsutsugamushi*, Shirai *et al.* (1981a) examined the mother's milk and the umbilical blood for anti-*R. tsutsugamushi* IgM and IgG antibodies. They found that, although IgG antibody was present, IgM antibodies could not be detected. Based on these findings, they reported that *R. tsutsugamushi* infection of fetuses was extremely rare.

Takahashi *et al.* (1992) investigated the relationship between *R. tsutsugamushi* infection and pregnancy in voles (*M. montebelli* and *M. arvalis*) and in the field mouse (*A. speciosus*). They found no difference in the pregnancy rate or in the rate of miscarriage between *R. tsutsugamushi* infected and uninfected groups, and concluded that *R. tsutsugamushi* infection had virtually no effect on pregnancy in these animals, that *R. tsutsugamushi* did not infect the fetuses, and that only IgG antibody migrated from dams to fetuses.

6 Transport of Mites by Birds

In Japan, as described above in Sections 1 and 2, the seasonal prevalence and distribution of trombiculid mites, the principal vectors of Tsutsugamushi disease have been elucidated, and it has been established that infected colonies are distributed in mite islands in limited locales, these islands shifting annually (Kawamura and Tanaka, 1988; Takahashi *et al.*, 1990b). These phenomena have also been observed in Southeast Asia and in those areas in the southwestern Pacific region that were World War II battlefields, where Tsutsugamushi disease is endemic, as the vector trombiculid mites occur year-around (Audy, 1949, 1961; Philip, 1948a; Philip *et al.*, 1949).

When the regions where Tsutsugamushi disease is endemic shift, as described above, it can be concluded that the trombiculid mite vectors must have migrated. However, their ability to migrate on their own is very limited, and their movement thus is mainly associated with the movement of hosts infested with larvae. However, the activity range of field rodents, the principal parasitized host of trombiculid mites, is also ecologically limited. Therefore, birds must also be considered as the phoretic hosts spreading trombiculid mites to distant locations or to other islands.

Hatori (1919–20, 1920), in Taiwan, was the first to describe trombiculid mites parasitizing birds (pheasant, quail, chicken, etc.). Subsequently, Hayashi *et al.* (1919) described *Leptotrombidium akamushi* parasitization of warblers and quails in Niigata Prefecture, Japan. At about the same time, Kawamura *et al.* (1921) captured and examined 412 birds of 31 species inhabiting an area in Niigata Prefecture where Tsutsugamushi disease was endemic. They found five species of trombiculid mites — *L. akamushi*, *L. scutellare*, *L. palpale*, *L. pallidum*, and *Neotrombicula tamiyai* (Kawamura's classification of types A, B, C, D, and E″, in use at the time, matched with the current classification) — in 18 species of terrestrial birds and reported that no parasitization occurred in aquatic or raptorial bird species. Both Hayashi *et al.* (1919) and Kawamura *et al.* (1921) proposed that measures to prevent Tsutsugamushi disease should include a consideration of birds in addition to field rodents.

In view of the fact that monkeys were used as sentinel animals in place of human volunteers in search of the pathogen for Tsutsugamushi disease (Kawamura, 1925, 1926; Nagayo *et al.*, 1920), it was a far-sighted concept of Hayashi *et al.* (1924, 1925) at that time to use chickens and ducks as sentinel animals in experiments by loose-housing them in an area where they anticipated Tsutsugamushi disease would occur, in an attempt to determine the sites and numbers of the vector trombiculid mites. However, there was a hiatus of some 20 years in which studies of the relationship between birds and trombiculid mites did not progress.

Following World War II, studies of this relationship were rekindled. Trombiculid mites that infested birds in the western Pacific region were studied, and bird-specific species in the genus *Neoschoengastia* and trombiculid mites that also infested other vertebrates as well as birds (*e.g.* the genus *Euschoengastia*) were investigated in pioneering studies in the field (Wharton and Hardcastle,

1946). It was later reported (Philip, 1948a; Philip *et al.*, 1949) that two *R. tsutsugamushi* strains were isolated in Malaysia from pools of trombiculid mites (250 *L. deliense* and 100 *L. fletcheri*) recovered from quails infested with Tsutsugamushi disease vector mites.

Meanwhile, at the time when the existence of Tsutsugamushi disease transmitted by non-*L. akamushi* vectors had been confirmed in Japan, trombiculid mites infesting birds were being studied extensively, and numerous new findings were made concerning trombiculid mites whose natural hosts were birds (Asanuma, 1959; Kamo, 1954, 1956; Kunitomo, 1956; Sasa, 1956; Tamiya, 1962). In Asamuma's study reported in 1959, a total of 1,985 birds of 125 species and 8,920 trombiculid mites of 31 species were recovered and examined. In addtion, they carried out periodic searches concentrated in the foothills of Mt. Fuji, and collected 1,052 birds of 78 species and 3,608 trombiculid mites of 10 species. In addition to species such as *N. asakawai* and *E. miyagawai*, and the above-mentioned genera of trombiculid mites, which may be considered to primarily infest birds, they recovered non-*L. akamushi*-transmitted Tsutsugamushi disease vectors (108 *L. scutellare* and 21 *L. pallidum*) from seven species of land-based birds at the foot of Mt. Fuji. A common characteristic of all these birds is that they are terrestrial winter birds inhabiting grassland. Uchikawa *et al.* (1985) studied the relationship between *L. pallidum* dispersion and pheasants, and confirmed that all six pheasants they captured were infested with *L. pallidum*. These results suggest that birds are involved in the transport of the Tsutsugamushi disease vector, trombiculid mites.

Studies of the susceptibility of birds to *R. tsutsugamushi* showed that when birds (chicken, pigeon, etc.) were experimentally inoculated with *R. tsutsugamushi*, transient rickettsemia occurred. Latent but transient *R. tsutsugamushi* was confirmed from the spleens of these birds, demonstrating that birds are also susceptible to *R. tsutsugamushi* (Kitaoka, 1959). However, Kitaoka and Okubo (1953) reported that, in six species of birds captured in Miyake Island of the Izu Shichito Islands, where Shichito fever (Tsutsugamushi disease) was epidemic, all attempts to isolate *R. tsutsugamushi* were negative.

In order to determine whether the Tsutsugamushi disease vector, trombiculid mites, which occur in Akita Prefecture after autumn, were *L. akamushi* or *L. pallidum*, Kitaoka *et al.* (1976) used chickens as non-flying sentinel birds in the area where Tsutsugamushi disease occurred. *R. tsutsugamushi* was isolated from *L. pallidum* (22 mites/pool) as well as from the spleens and livers of the chickens. The finding that the *R. tsutsugamushi* isolated were Kato type, common to both mites and chickens, suggests that Tsutsugamushi disease is transmitted by *L. pallidum* in autumn there.

7 Seroepidemiology

a Seroepidemiology of field rodents and humans on Miyake Island

As noted in Chapter 1, a survey of the resurgence of Shichito fever (the name for Tsutsugamushi disease in the Izu Shichito Islands) on Miyake Island in November 1976 identified only 12 patients (Kawamura *et al.*, 1980). And, in January 1977, all attempts to isolate *Rickettsia tsutsugamushi* in DDD mice from 25 captured field rodents failed, as did attempts at isolation from engorged and unfed trombiculid mites (*L. scutellare* and *L. pallidum*) collected from the soil (Kawamura *et al.*, 1980). In addition, a survey of rodents for anti-*R. tsutsugamushi* antibody, carried out by indirect immunofluorescence (IF) in the first survey was all negative (Kawamura *et al.*, 1980).

As shown in Fig. 3, additional surveys were conducted in November 1977, February 1978, November 1978, November 1979, February 1980, and November 1980. Each time, nude mice, BALB/c (*nu/nu*), were used to isolate *R. tsutsugamushi* from the captured wild rodents, and trombiculid mites, both engorged and unfed, were collected. Nevertheless, only one strain, Karp type *R. tsutsugamushi* (Miyake strain), to which only nude mice are susceptible, was isolated from one anti-*R. tsutsugamushi* seronegative *Rattus norvegicus* in the second survey; all others were negative.

Although the Miyake strain was not pathogenic in conventional mice, its anti-*R. tsutsugamushi* antibody response was positive in proportion to the quantity of *R. tsutsugamushi* inoculated. Seroepidemiological studies, using indirect IF of captured field rodents, showed increases in anti-*R. tsutsugamushi* seropositive rates, from 0% to 37.5%, 55.0%, and 83.3%, with a subsequent sustained level of about 50% in rodents sera of each survey, as shown in Fig. 3. The seropositive rate and the antibody titer were low for *R. rattus*, which is predominantly domiciliary, and high for *R. norvegicus* and

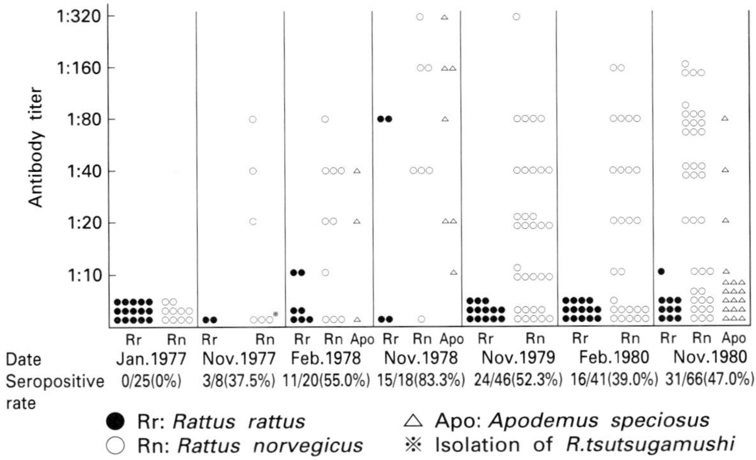

Fig. 3. Antibody titers against *R. tsutsugamushi* in sera from field rodents captured on Miyake Island (by indirect immunofluorescence)

Apodemus speciosus, which are sylvatic by nature (Kawamura and Tanaka, 1988; Kawamura *et al.*, 1980). Incidentally, the life span of these field rodents is approximately one year, and the duration of seropositivity to *R. tsutsugamushi* in these field rodents is also about one year (Van Peenen *et al.*, 1977). Studies of these field rodents showed that, during the 4-year period from 1977 to 1980, they were infected at a high rate with *R. tsutsugamushi* strains such as the Miyake strain, which is nonpathogenic to mice (Kawamura *et al.*, 1980).

From May to October 1978, a seroepidemiological study was conducted, using an indirect IF assay of anti-*R. tsutsugamushi* antibody, in the healthy general population of Miyake and Toshima Islands (Izu Shichito Islands). In particular, Tsutsugamushi disease had never been reported in Toshima Island. As shown in Table 7, approximately 25% of the inhabitants of both islands were antibody-positive, and no difference was found between men and women. Moreover, interviews with all antibody-positive persons failed to confirm a history of Tsutsugamushi disease in anyone, or any symptoms of the disease in the preceding 2 years. Since these results were obtained from sera collected for other purposes, no statistical correlations by sex and age were possible. However, there is no doubt that

Table 7. Age and Sex Distribution of Seropositive Rate among Inhabitants of Miyake and Toshima Islands

	Miyake Island			Toshima Island		
Age	male	female	total	male	female	total
10–19	2/10*	14/63	16/73	0/0	0/1	0/1
20–29	1/2	0/1	1/3	1/8	0/4	1/12
30–39	1/2	2/3	3/5	2/8	2/5	4/13
40–49	0/9	1/8	1/17	4/15	4/11	8/26
50–59	1/6	4/12	5/18	2/7	2/9	4/16
60–69	5/13	6/18	11/31	2/11	1/10	3/21
70–79	2/7	2/5	4/12	0/1	2/5	2/6
80–	1/1	0/1	1/2	1/1	0/2	1/3
Total	13/50	29/111	42/161	12/51	11/47	23/98
Positive rate	26.0%	26.1%	26.1%	23.5%	23.4%	23.5%

* Positive no. / no. examined.

there was a high rate of inapparent infection of *R. tsutsugamushi* in the residents of both islands (Kawamura *et al.*, 1980).

The findings obtained from *R. tsutsugamushi* isolates and the seroepidemiological findings from field rodents and residents indicated that the recent resurgence of Tsutsugamushi disease on Miyake Island, which began in 1976, has been a transient manifestation of trombiculid mites harboring *R. tsutsugamushi* pathogenic to humans. Alternatively, this resurgence may have been due to the presence of *R. tsutsugamushi* that is avirulent to hairy mice but pathogenic to some humans. At any rate, it is evident that a strain of *R. tsutsugamushi* which is nonpathogenic to mice, and which, therefore, cannot be isolated using hairy mice, played a major role in this resurgence of the disease.

In the performance of seroepidemioloical studies, the antigens used were prescreened against the three prototypes well known at that time; it was determined that the epidemic strain was a Karp type, and Karp antigens were used. However, in order to assess the seroepidemiological results described later (Kawamura *et al.*, 1980; Ujiiye, 1981), it would have been necessary to select antigens more precisely by taking the heterogeneity of *R. tsutsugamushi* into consideration. Further, because of the unexpectedly high seropositive rate found by indirect IF in that survey, control experiments that repudiated non-specific reactions were performed, and specificity was confirmed using these experiments (Kawamura *et al.*, 1980).

b. Evaluation of positive results in seroepidemiological studies

As noted in Chapter 1, *R. tsutsugamushi* strains are extremely heterogeneous, and reinfection of Tsutsugamushi disease or multiple infections in humans in endemic areas are not at all uncommon. The clinical picture in repeated reinfections often lacks typical characteristics (Bourgeois *et al.*, 1982; Tamiya, 1962) (see Section 8 below). On the other hand, as described previously, some *R. tsutsugamushi* strains are clearly mildly pathogenic to both humans and mice, and when a host is infected, no reaction other than an immune response occurs. Consequently, in some areas, seroepidemiology is the only proof of the actual state of endemicity. At times, it is difficult to distinguish whether inapparent endemicity is due to reinfection of humans or to avirulent rickettsia.

Shishido (1962b) first described the existence of such very mild or abortive Tsutsugamushi disease and inapparent *R. tsutsugamushi* infections in humans. In the autumn of 1959, seven cases of typical Tsutsugamushi disease occurred among Self-Defense Force soldiers during maneuvers at the food of Mt. Fuji, an area endemic for Tsutsugamushi disease. During the same period, 10 of 148 soldiers who visited the infirmary for a "common cold" were found to be *R. tsutsugamushi*-seropositive by the complement fixation (CF) reaction. In parallel with the above survey, Shishido confirmed that the majority of those who had been infected with Tsutsugamushi disease was seronegative, as determined by CF, within 5 years. Based on this result, Shishido conducted a seroepidemiological survey in May through Octorber 1960 determining the CF in healthy residents of Hachijo Island, Izu Shichito Islands, where the Shichito fever (Tsutsugamushi disease) epidemic had occurred in 1951–1952. Although anti-*R. tsutsugamushi* antibodies in parents with a history of Tsutsugamushi disease were assumed to have disappeared, the seropositivity rate among young cohorts was high, especially among schoolchildren, of whom 45% (45/100) were seropositive. Only four of the 45 seropositive subjects had a history of manifest Shishido fever.

Meanwhile, because of the existence of inapparent *R. tsutsugamushi* infection, as shown by the seroepidemiological testing of healthy inhabitants on Miyake and Toshima Islands, seroepidemiological testing using indirect IF was conducted in residents of various regions of Japan centered around areas endemic for Tsutsugamushi disease, which was beginning to become epidemic in its new type (Kawamura *et al.*, 1980; Ujiiye, 1981).

Seropositive rates were amazingly high: 56.3% on Hachijo Island in the Izu Shichito Islands; 30% at Akeno and 22% at Shirane in Yamanashi Prefecture, where Tsutsugamushi disease patients were found; in Toyama Perfecture, 43.9–60.7% at Urayamashin, an epidemic site where patients were found, and 37.9–45.6% in Nizayamashin, where no patients were found; 12.5–22.6% in an area where no *R. tsutsugamushi*-positive field rodents or trombiculid mites were found; 2.5% (12.0% in Uonuma where patients were found) in the northern part and 5.7% (6.1% in Itoigawa where patients were found) in the western part of Niigata Prefecture where both the classical and the new type of Tsutsugamushi disease exist. The rate was 9.0% in the region upstream of the Shinano river and 4.3% downstream, and 4.3% in the region around the Agano river, which areas are associated with classical Tsutsugamushi disease. Of 3,781 subjects tested in Niigata Prefecture as a whole, 171 (4.5%) were positive. The seropositivity rate was 24.5% in Nakanojo, Gumma Prefecture, where Tsutsugamushi disease occurred. These results suggest that the trombiculid mites in these areas retain strains of *R. tsutsugamushi* that are very mildly pathogenic to humans and field rodents. These findings are perhaps attributable to the occurrence of multiple infections due to the heterogeneity of *R. tsutsugamushi*.

In the People's Republic of China also, seropositivity for *R. tsutsugamushi* is being studied (Fan *et al.*, 1987). Outbreaks of Tsutsugamushi disease occurred during the period 1952–1954 in the southwestern region of China. Subsequently, the outbreaks decreased, but they began to occur again after 1981. In contrast, in Hainan Island, which is in the tropics, Tsutsugamushi disease continues to occur every year. Seroepidemiological testing for *R. tsutsugamushi* in healthy inhabitants of Hainan Island was conducted in 1983 and 1984, using the CF test, and seropositive rates were found to be 52.5% and 31.8%, respectively. This is a highly endemic site of *R. tsutsugamushi*; and, when the heterogeneity of *R. tsutsugamushi* is considered, it is conceivable that multiple infections occur.

However, the anti-*R. tsutsugamushi* seropositive rate in healthy residents of Sha Wan County in the Xinjian Uygur autonomous region, where no Tsutsugamushi disease occurred, was 36.1%, determined by indirect IF, which result suggests the possiblility of inapparent infection by mildly pathogenic *R. tsutsugamushi*, in addition to reinfection.

The new type of Tsutsugamushi disease, similar to that which occurred in Niigata Prefecture, also continues to occur in Akita Prefecture, an area endemic for classical Tsutsugamushi disease in Japan (see Chapter 1). Kamiya (1983) assayed anti-*R. tsutsugamushi* antibodies in captured dogs in Akita Prefecture using indirect IF. As a preliminary experiment, he infected seronegative dogs with three *R. tsutsugamushi* prototypes, and assayed IgM and IgG antibody levels to the respective antigens for one year, confirming that IgM antibodies were present from the first through the seventh week and that IgG antibodies were present for 5 months, from the first week. Of 627 pound dogs tested, 101 (16.1%) were seropositive. Since dogs display no symptoms of *R. tsutsugamushi* infection, the findings in dogs cannot be extrapolated to determine pathogenicity or non-pathogenicity in humans or mice. However, these results were useful for determining the endemicity of *R. tsutsugamushi*-positive trombiculid mites in Akita Prefecture as a whole.

The seroepidemiological results described in this section show that presence of *R. tsutsugamushi* strains pathogenic to humans (or mice), repeated *R. tsutsugamushi* infections due to heterogeneity, or inapparent infections with *R. tsutsugamushi* non-pathogenic to humans (or mice) characterized, solely or mingled, an area endemic for *R. tsutsugamushi*.

8 Clinical Aspects

a. Outlines

Until the advent of chemotherapy, the average annual fatality rate for classical Tsutsugamushi disease, which afflicts the inhabitants of river terrace regions on the northern coast of the Sea of Japan in Niigata, Yamagata, and Akita Prefectures, was as high as 30–40% (with the highest rate exceeding 60%) (Kawamura, 1926; Tamiya, 1962). However, the fatality rate for Tsutsugamushi disease in the Pescadores, Taiwan, was low, at approximately 3% (Kawamura, 1926; Yamamiya and Honda, 1933). Fatality due to Tsutsugamushi disease in military forces in the western Pacific region, where World War II battles were fought, was high in some places, such as Goodenough Island (27.5%) and Finchhaven of New Guinea (35.3%), but was generally low as in Embilipitiya, Ceylon (1.5%), and Owi and Biak Islands, north of western New Guinea (0.6%) (Audy, 1949; Audy *et al.*, 1947; Philip, 1948a). The mean fatality rate overall for Allied forces in World War II battlefields in Southeast Asia and the western Pacific regions was 3.85%, and marked regional differences were noted. Troops in wartime experienced varied fighting conditions, and regional differences in the fatality rate cannot be hastily ascribed to the severity or mildness of Tsutsugamushi disease.

However, the fatality rate due to classical Tsutsugamushi disease in northern Japan caused by *Leptotrombidium akamushi* has been consistently high, indicating that this type of the disease is extremely severe (Kawamura, 1925, 1926; Tamiya, 1962).

On the other hand, in Tsutsugamushi disease patients in various places during and after World War II — a group with a low fatality rate (new type Tsutsugamushi disease in Japan) — the clinical symptoms were not greatly different from those who contracted classical Tsutsugamushi disease (Arai and Komine, 1952; Bourgeois *et al.*, 1982; Misao *et al.*, 1967; Saito *et al.* 1981; Suto, 1986; Tachibana, 1985, 1987; Tamiya, 1962; Ueno, 1956). After the war, antibiotics exhibiting unique efficacy against *Rickettsia tsutsugamushi* were developed, and naturally, these antibiotics were administered to patients at relatively early stages in those areas where Tsutsugamushi disease occurred. Consequently, the disease was immediately curable, and clinical symptoms were mild. This factor makes it difficult to compare the clinical symptoms of the classical to those of the new type of Tsutsugamushi disease.

However, in areas where medical practitioners do not suspect Tsutsugamushi disease, patients are often subjected to useless treatment, due to the lack of a definitive diagnosis, and the outcome can thus be severe disease; there is even a report of a fatality (Suzuki and Sekikawa, 1981). Because of these occurrences, one cannot state decisively that the new type of Tsutsugamushi disease always has mild symptoms (Misao *et al.*, 1967; Saito *et al.*, 1981; Suto, 1986; Suzuki and Sekikawa, 1981; Tachibana, 1985, 1987). Patients in whom the disease is severe or fatal exhibit a hemorrhagic tendency and blood coagulation disorders during the course of the illness and are frequently complicated with disseminated intravascular coagulation (DIC) (Suzuki and Sekikawa, 1981; Tachibana, 1985). Regarding this issue, Baelz and Kawakami (1879), who first described the severe type, or classical Tsutsugamushi disease, by modern medical methods, reported very early on a marked decline in blood coagulability in the patients. Subsequently, Kawamura (1925, 1926), based on data in numerous severe and fatal cases, concluded that the inhibition of blood coagulation disorder and hemorrhagic tendency were the important characteristics of this disease, and that these characteristics were related to fatality. Allen and Spits (1945) performed autopsies on US military Tsutsugamushi disease fatalities (78 cases) during the war and found microvasculature thrombi at times in the kidneys, heart, lungs, or other organs in histopathological examinations. The seemingly contradictory phenomena of blood coagulation disorder and thrombus formation are now understood as the clinical entity DIC.

As noted above, there are regional differences in fatality due to Tsutsugamushi disease, and there are mild and severe clinical symptoms of the disease. However, in the actual areas endemic for Tsutsugamushi disease, heterogeneity in the causative *R. tsutsugamuahi* strains is marked. Consequently, cellular immunity to *R. tsutsugamushi* does not function adequately, resulting in reinfections and multiple infections. Thus, in such areas endemic for Tsutsugamushi disease, patients may exhibit typical symptoms at the time of initial infection, whereas they frequently show either mild or negligible symptoms at the time of reinfection and thereafter.

However, these phenomena are limited to native residents in these areas endemic for Tsutsugamushi disease, and newcomers exhibit typical symptoms. Further, the pathogenicity of *R. tsutsugamushi* varies by strain; there are *R. tsutsugamushi* strains that cause a range of clinical symptoms from typical to mild or abortive, even at the time of initial infection. The mildly pathogenic *R. tsutsugamushi* frequently results in a completely inapparent infection (Fan *et al.*, 1987; Kawamura *et al.*, 1980; Shishido, 1962b; Ujiiye, 1981). Moreover, *R. tsutsugamushi* pathogenicity varies in humans and mice. The *R. tsutsugamushi* strain transmitting Tsutsugamushi disease in Takahara-machi, Miyazaki Prefecture, causes fairly severe symptoms in humans, but shows almost no virulence in mice

(Kobayashi *et al.*, 1978; Misao *et al.*, 1967). Based on the differences in pathogenicity of these *R. tsutsugamushi* strains, a technique to isolate mildly pathogenic *R. tsutsugamushi* was devised, and an *R. tsutsugamushi* strain mildly pathogenic to mice was isolated from Tsutsugamushi disease patients. This led to the establishment of the Shimokoshi, Kawasaki, and Kuroki strains currently used as new *R. tsutsugamushi* types in Japan (Kobayashi *et al.*, 1978; Murata and Kawamura, 1977; Tamura *et al.*, 1984; Yamamoto *et al.*, 1986, 1989).

Naturally, it is possible that *R. tsutsugamushi* exists in a range of pathogenicities, from non-pathogenic in either humans or mice to non-pathogenic to humans but pathogenic to mice. The fact that Tsutsugamushi disease exhibits highly diverse clinical symptoms must be taken into consideration.

b. Typical clinical features and clinical course

Although, as stated above, there appears to be essentially no difference between the clinical symptoms of classical Tsutsugamushi disease and new type of the disease with lower rates of fatality, some studies have reported that, in the other type of the disease with low fatality, the fever tends to be intermittent rather than the continuous type seen in the non-classical type and symptoms such as rash and lymphadenopathy are somewhat milder or lacking in the non-classical type (Arai and Komine, 1952; Tamiya, 1962). Another study has reported finding no eschar in more than 40% of the patients with the non-classical type (Blake *et al.*, 1945).

However, it is necessary to consider the possibility that eschar may have been present at sites difficult to find, or that eschar, being a primary infection focus, did not appear due to the disease being a reinfection or one of multiple infections caused by the heterogeneity of *R. tsutsugamushi* strains. Consequently, the differences in clinical symptoms of patients with initial infection may be considered to be within the range of individual differences in patients (Arai and Komine, 1952; Saito *et al.*, 1981; Suto, 1986; Tachibana, 1985; Tamiya, 1962; Ueno, 1956).

With the clinical symptoms of classical Tsutsugamushi disease (Kawamura, 1925, 1926; Tamiya, 1962) as the basis, the clinical symptoms of Tsutsugamushi disease in other regions are summarized and listed below (Misao *et al.*, 1967; Saito *et al.*, 1981;

Tachibana, 1985, 1987; Tamiya, 1962):

1) Typical clinical features

a) Incubation period

The incubation period is 5–20 days, with the average being 10 days.

b) Symptoms

Symptoms always include headache, and other complaints include loss of appetite, general malaise, feverishness, and myalgia. The symptoms are exacerbated 7 days after onset.

c) Findings

Typical Tsutsugamushi disease is characterized by fever, rash, regional or generalized lymphadenopathy, and eschar.

(1) Eschar

The detection of eschar (which is found even at an early stage of illness) is essential for clinical differentiation from other febrile eruptive diseases. Even in cases of the spotted fever group (other than Rocky Mountain spotted fever) eschar is sometimes found at the sites where a tick was biting. Recurrent epidemics of a new type of Tsutsugamushi disease in Japan, Shichito fever, began in 1950. In December 1951, when surveying and research began in earnest, the eschar identification rate in patients was 54.3% (19/35), a result comparable to that of 51% in Tsutsugamushi disease patients among US Military Forces on the New Guinea Islands of Owi and Biak during World War II (Arai and Komine, 1952; Blake *et al.*, 1945). However, a local physician's follow-up study (Ueno, 1956) found eschar in virtually all Tsutsugamushi disease patients in the Hachijo Islands, where the epidemic was concentrated. These results suggest that eschar frequently occurs in difficult-to-find spots, and the reported differences are possibly due to differences in the thoroughness with which physicians investigate the eschar.

Tsutsugamushi disease in humans is caused by the infestation of human-preferring trombiculid mites harboring *R. tsutsugamushi*. The growth focus of *R. tsutsugamushi* in the initial infection caused by these trombiculid mites is the eschar. The predilection of *R. tsutsugamushi*-harboring trombiculid mites for humans, the sites and time of the mites' attachment, the number of eschars per individual, and the symptoms following attachment are described in detail in the following chapter. Here, we discuss the course of eschar changes in patients where observation was possible, and the dermatological changes that accompanied the experimental infestation of trombiculid larvae on volunteers. In the experimental infestation of trombiculid mites on the volunteers, it appeared that the larvae, with one exception noted below, did not carry *R. tsutsugamushi*; all subjects exhibited only dermatitis, none formed an eschar or developed the disease. Thus, differences in time of infestation and symptoms according to the species of trombiculid mite were clarified.

Dermatitis appeared as a redness around the sites of infestation beginning approximately 6–10 h after infestation; the area of dermatitis gradually enlarged, reaching maximum diameters ranging from 1 to 182 mm. However, there were marked individual differences. Further, the dermatitis caused by *L. akamushi* manifested only as redness, whereas *L. scutellare* caused pustules. In the abovementioned case in which the volunteer developed Tsutsugamushi disease, 8 unfed *L. pallidum* from the Izu Peninsula had been used 15 days earlier. However, the sites of infestation showed only dermatitis, and no eschar was formed. Since the isolation of *R. tsutsugamushi* from the engorged mite larvae was not performed, it was not confirmed that these larvae had caused the Tsutsugamushi disease (Arai, 1955; Kitaoka *et al.*, 1953a; Obata and Aoki, 1958; Takahashi *et al.*, 1991b; Tamiya 1962).

In regard to eschar in patients, the sites favored by trombiculid mites for infestation are frequently soft regions and are difficult to find unless the patient's body is thoroughly searched. There may occasionally be more than one site. Although there are variations in eschar characteristics according to the species of trombiculid mite causing the dermatitis, studies of eschar sites from the very early stage revealed bright red papules with induration around the site of attachment. The peripheral area of the papule is not always well demarcated. Subsequently, the blister developed in the center becomes pustular, the red circle around it is enlarged, and a small ulcer with a blackish-brown scab occurs in the center. The surrounding red circle becomes darker, the scab enlarges, and, with time, the red circle disappears, followed by the dropping off of the scab (Fig. 4). *R. tsutsugamushi* can be found in the eschar tissue (Arai and Komine, 1952; Takahashi *et al.*, 1991a; Tamiya, 1962; Ueno, 1956).

(2) Fever

The body temperature usually rises suddenly to 38°C or above 39°C, and this persists for about 10 days, exhibiting a remittent, or at

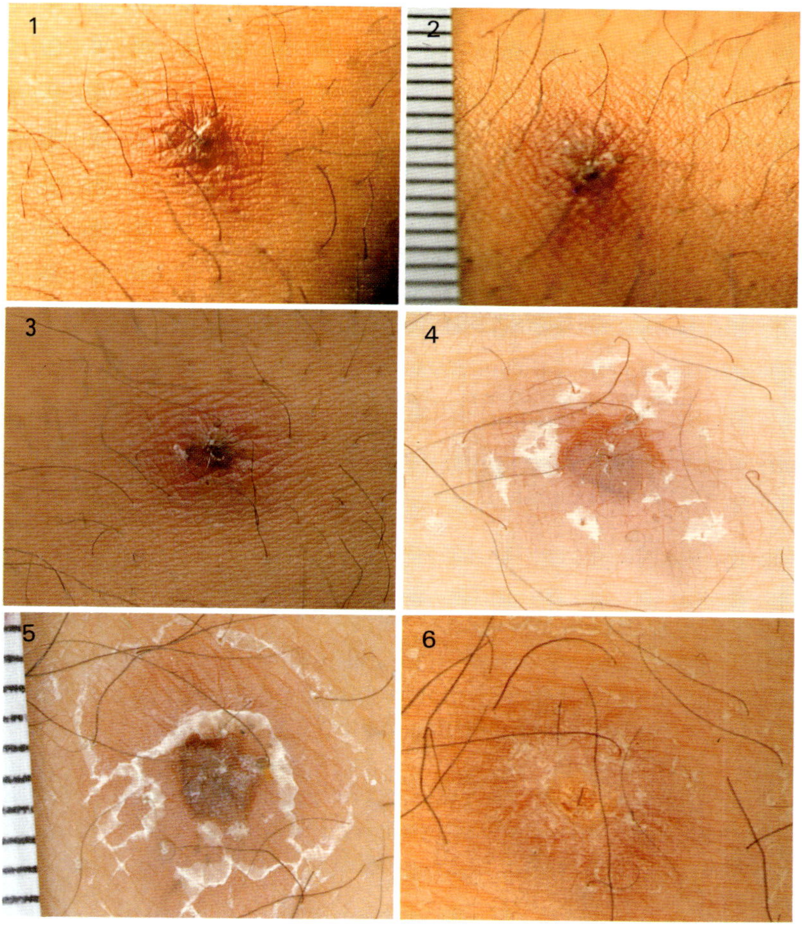

Fig. 4. Change of the eschar observed in a case of Tsutsugamushi disease (M.T., 36, male) (Takahashi *et al.*, 1991a)

1. 3rd day of illness, with pustule (4mm) and solar erythema (24mm).
2. 5th day of illness, with eschar and erythema (18mm).
3. 7th day of illness, with blister and reddish-black scab.
4. 10th day of illness, with tenderness and redness surrounding the lesion.
5. 12th day of illness, with a black crust over the eschar.
6. 15th day of illness, eschar has fallen off.

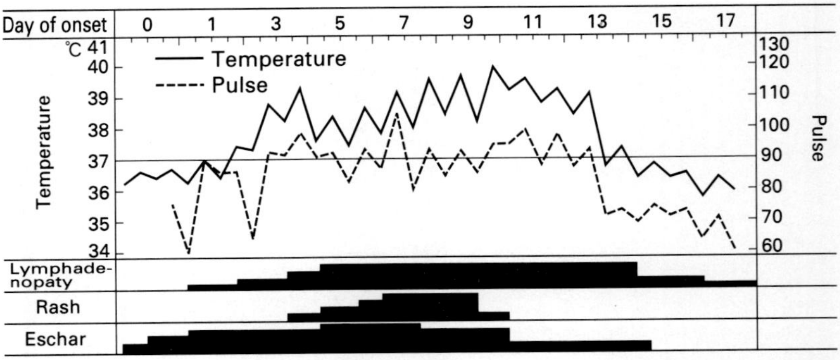

Fig. 5. The clinical course of Tsutsugamushi disease in one recovered patient, before the advent of chemotherapy

times continuous, fever type. This is frequently accompanied by headache, low-back pain, chills, and sweats (Fig. 5).

(3) Rash

A rash with round eruptions of approximately 5 mm dispersed on the trunk, face, and limbs. This usually lasts for 3–7 days (Fig. 5).

(4) Lymphadenopathy

Enlargement of the lymph nodes accompanied by tenderness is sometimes limited at local lymph nodes of the eschar site, but generally leads to systemic lymphadenopathy (Fig. 5).

(5) Other findings

The liver and spleen are enlarged by approximately 30%, and a hemorrhagic tendency becomes marked in serious cases. In more severe cases, disturbance of consciousness and circulatory insufficiency develop.

2) Laboratory findings

Generally, the white cell count of peripheral blood, especially the lymphocyte count, is decreased during the initial onset of the disease and increased during the latter half of the fever stage. Therefore, during this time, as discussed below, one should pay attention to the presence or absence of DIC findings. Further, 4–5% of lymphocytes are atypical.

The ratio of T4/T8 T lymphocyte subtypes decreases markedly at an acute stage. This trend continues in some patients even 7 days after onset; it is necessary to perform further functional studies to confirm an increase in lymphocytes towards the recovery stage.

In the liver function test, the elevation of lactic acid dehydrogenase (LDH) is prominent, with an increased LDH5 fraction. An elevated glutamic oxaloacetic transaminase (GOT) level was observed in 60% of patients, with GOT values being approximately 100 Karmen unit/ml. Abnormalities in glutamic pyruvic transaminase (GPT) levels are less marked than those in GOT. Values returned to normal relatively quickly after treatment in all patients. Additional findings included strongly positive C-reactive protein (CRP) (above 10.0 mg/dl), a moderate increase in the erythrocyte sedimentation rate, and decreased albumin in the serum protein fraction (Tachibana, 1985).

As stated at the beginning of this section, in severe cases of Tsutsugamushi disease, especially in those patients who do not receive appropriate treatment due to undetermined diagnosis, a hemorrhagic tendency and coagulation disorder are exhibited during the course of the disease; and when complicated with DIC, this at times is fatal. Consequently, it is necessary to pay attention to the test results and to evaluate them to provide a clinical diagnosis of DIC (Suzuki and Sekikawa, 1981). In other words, in addition to determining the bleeding time and clotting time of blood, one should look for laboratory results that include: (1) a decreased platelet count (below $10–15 \times 10^4/mm^3$), (2) elevated fibrin degradation product (FDP) level (above 10 μg/ml), (3) fibrinogen levels below 150 mg/dl, (4) extended prothrombin time (PT), and (5) extended partial thromboplastin (PTT) time. Other relevant laboratory test results include increases in β-thromboglobulin and LDH, and elevation of thrombin III, which promotes DIC.

The hemorrhagic tendency that occurs in severe Tsutsugamushi disease has long attracted attention, as thrombocytopenia, in the other rickettsiosis, Rocky Mountain spotted fever, and its cause had been studied. The causative rickettsiae, *R. tsutsugamushi* and *R. rickettsii*, described below, show such biological characteristics as acute toxicity and hemolytic activity due to the rickettsial toxins, which are harbored only by live rickettsiae. The components of the rickettsial toxins have not yet been identified, but they are related to vascular endothelial cell permeability factors.

Rickettsial toxins

When a large number (more than 10^8) of live rickettsiae are injected intravenously or intraperitoneally into rodents (mice, rats, rabbits), the animals die from acute toxicity within 1–8 h (Gildemeister and Haagen, 1940). Alive rickettsiae have the capacity to lyse mammalian (rabbit, sheep), and chicken red blood cells (hemolytic activity) both *in vitro* and *in vivo* (Clarke and Fox, 1948; Paterson *et al.*, 1954). These biological characteristics of rickettsiae appear to resemble those of bacterial endotoxins, exotoxins, and hemolysins; however, the most important difference is that the rickettsiae must be alive to display these characteristics.

The above-mentioned acute toxicity was first reported by Gildemeister and Haagen (1940) using mice and an *R. typhi* line. A similar phenomenon occurs with *R. prowazekii*, *R. rickettsii*, and *R. tsutsugamushi*; the effect was demonstrated with rats and rabbits in addition to mice (Paterson *et al.*, 1954; Price, 1953; Smadel *et al.*, 1946). Regarding *R. tsutsugamushi*, Smadel *et al.* (1946) reported that only the Gilliam strain possessed toxic activity. However, it so happened that the Gilliam strain had grown more actively than other strains in yolk sac culture; by modifying the growth and purification/concentration methods, we found all *R. tsutsugamushi* strains used in the quantified experiment to possess rickettsial toxins (Kawamura, 1962; Yamamoto *et al.*, 1958).

The *in vivo* mode of action of rickettsial toxins was analyzed by Neva and Snyder (1955), who demonstrated that animals injected with toxins first exhibited progressive pyknemia, and subsequently succumbed to terminal hypotension and died; adrenocorticotropic hormone (ACTH) and cortisone had no effect on the toxic symptoms. Wattenberg *et al.* (1955) showed that the permeability of peripheral vessels changed markedly when animals were injected with rickettsial toxins; and Greisman and Wisseman (1958), using the vascular bed of rat mesoappendix, showed that increased permeability of the capillary vessels was specific for rickettsial toxins.

From these results, it was evident that live rickettsiae evoked direct injury specific to the vascular system, probably to the epithelial cells. This finding agrees well with the finding that the sites or rickettsial growth in human rickettsiosis are the epithelial cells, and this results in the subsequent vascular changes. These rickettsial toxins are neutralized by antibodies, inhibited by an enzymatic inhibitor (KCN or CH_3ICOOH), and activated by an enzymatic accelerator (cysteine) (Suzuki, 1951).

Snyder *et al.* (1954) carried out an *in vitro* study of the mechanism of hemolytic activity, another biological characteristic of rickettsial toxins. They reported that this hemolytic activity required the presence of glutamate or Mg^{2+}, which serves as the basis for rickettsial respiration, and that metabolic inhibitors inhibited this reaction and antibodies neutralized it. Allen *et al.* (1954) irradiated purified rickettsiae with ultraviolet (UV) light to eliminate only the infectivity and succeeded in obtaining residual toxicity to mice. These investigators also observed that, as they increased the doses of UV light, the hemolytic activity weakened, followed by the respiratory system.

3) Clinical course and prognosis

We have discussed the clinical symptoms and laboratory findings primarily in patients in whom Tsutsugamushi disease ran its natural course without antibiotic treatment. Except in severe cases that exhibit a hemorrhagic tendency and coagulation disorder and complicated with DIC, patients recover 2 or, at most, 3 weeks after onset (Fig. 5).

In areas endemic for Tsutsugamushi disease, the majority of patients are properly treated with antibiotics following clinical diagnoses, without waiting for definitive serodiagnosis as discussed below, and symptoms immediately improve. Consequently, it is possible for patients to receive treatment as out-patients, without hospitalization. The clinical symptoms are either mild or abortive, as in the case of reinfection or multiple infections of *R. tsutsugamushi.*

On the other hand, in areas endemic for Tsutsugamushi disease, one should be aware that the residents can be infected several times, due to *R. tsutsugamushi* heterogeneity, with symptoms being abortive. These patients develop only a fever, which is known as a fever of unknown origin. Increasingly more cases are being identified as Tsutsugamushi disease after definitive serodiagnosis. In addition, in regions where Tsutsugamushi disease rarely occurs, the local physicians' lack of knowledge of the disease results in patients being given treatments ineffective for *R. tsutsugamushi*, such as the administration of beta-lactam antibiotics used for infectious diseases, which, at times, lead to severe or fatal cases. A system that provides accurate, definitive serodiagnosis of Tsutsugamushi disease is essential.

In short, if it is possible to verify the patient's activity regarding whether they have been in an area in which there are *R.*

tsutsugamushi-harboring trombiculid mite larvae about 10 days prior to the onset of the disease, and if the characteristic symptoms of Tsutsugamushi disease, especially eschars, are detected, proper treatment can be administered at once, in which case prognosis very favorable. However, if erroneous treatment is administered without suspecting Tsutsugamushi disease and complication with DIC occurs, this is potentially a very dangerous situation. It should be emphasized that the prognosis of Tsutsugamushi disease depends on the competence of physicians.

c. *Diagnosis*

1) Definitive serodiagnosis

In diagnosing Tsutsugamushi disease, it is necessary, as previously stated, to have mastered the characteristic clinical symptoms (clinical diagnosis) and to provide a definitive diagnosis. As will be detailed in Chapter 6, the definitive diagnosis of Tsutsugamushi disease consists of isolation of the infecting *R. tsutsugamushi* and detection of *R. tsutsugamushi* DNA and specific antibodies to *R. tsutsugamushi*. However, we shall focus here on the evaluation of serological diagnosis methods.

Serological methods for the diagnosis of Tsutsugamushi disease began with the Weil-Felix (WF) test (Weil and Felix, 1916). Various other methods have been used, including the complement fixation test, indirect immunofluorescence (IF), and the indirect immunoperoxidase (IP) test. There has been a call for evaluation of these diagnostic methods and a decision as to which method should be selected for the routine diagnosis of Tsutsugamushi disease worldwide. It is necessary for the definitive serological diagnostic method to be simple, easy, and rapid, as well as being capable of determining IgM and IgG antibody titers in order to distinguish initial infections from reinfections. To achieve this objective, a meeting of the Task Force of the WHO Regional Office for the Western Pacific was held in Okinawa, Japan, on November 24, 1986 (Regional Office for the Western Pacific of the WHO, 1987). As a result of this meeting, the indirect IF (Iida, *et al.*, 1966a; Kawamura and Aoyama, 1983) and the IP test (Suto, 1982; Yamamoto and Minamishima, 1982) methods were recommended by the Task Force. These recommendations read as follows.

"(1) The Weil-Felix (WF) test should not be used for the diagnosis of Tsutsugamushi disease if more sensitive methods such as the IP test or indirect IF are available.

(2) Use of the WF test should be discouraged, but not abandoned, while, concomitantly, the acquisition and utilization of the IP test or indirect IF should be promulgated in areas within the Region where the more specific methods (the IP test or indirect IF) are currently not available.

(3) For the routine diagnosis of Tsutsugamushi disease, the IP test should be adopted and its use standardized throughout the Region, in preference to the indirect IF, since the IP test is currently available in a test kit form from at least two sources within the Region, it is less expensive and requires less sophisticated equipment, and it provides a permanent record of serum reactivity, while concurrently affording an equivalent specificity and an increased degree of sensitivity.

(4) Commercial production of an inexpensive and readily available the IP test kit should be encouraged.

(5) Enzyme-linked immunosorbent assays (ELISA), immune adherence hemagglutination (IAHA), and other assays using biotin-avidin-immunofluorescence (BA-IF) and similar amplifying complexes should be further explored and modified to enhance their usefulness in rural settings for the rapid, simple, and inexpensive diagnosis of Tsutsugamushi disease.

(6) Efforts should be undertaken to raise the general awareness of Tsutsugamushi disease among providers of health care, to determine its incidence and, where appropriate, to determine the socio-economic impact of the disease in endemic areas within the Region.

(7) An organized effort should be encouraged to further evaluate both currently available and developmental diagnostic tests and to support the development of improved diagnostic methods that can be made readily and economically available throughout the Region.

(8) A mixture of three prototype antigens plus, where appropriate, one or more local non-prototype antigens should be utilized in preference to purified strain-specific polypeptides in the routine diagnosis of Tsutsugamushi disease.

(9) Both, but separately measured, IgM and IgG reactivity with *R. tsutsugamushi* antigens should be used as the basis (as is the case with both the IP test and indirect IF) of routine serological diagnostic methods for Tsutsugamushi disease.

(10) Basic research efforts to identify and characterize both

group- and strain-specific epitopes should be encouraged and supported.

(11) Methods to stabilize the antigenic identity of various polypeptides, so that they may be utilized in field adaptable diagnostic kits, are to be encouraged.

(12) An open interregional exchange of *R. tsutsugamushi* isolates should be encouraged, supported, and promulgated.

(13) Promotion of the ideas of test availability and relative standardization of serological test methods for the diagnosis of Tsutsugamushi disease should be expedited by the exchange and multilaboratory evaluation of new isolates, isolate specific sera and various new diagnostic methodologies."

2) Isolate types and serotypes of patients

As stated in the WHO Task Force recommendations (8), the definitive serodiagnosis of Tsutsugamushi disease in Japan utilizes six strains as antigens, the Shimokoshi, Kawasaki, and Kuroki strains, in addition to the three prototype strains, regardless of whether the IP test on indirect IF is used. As a result, the serotypes of patients in certain areas are frequently expressed with a systematic bias. In particular, in a long-term study, there is a strong tendency for the infecting *R. tsutsugamushi* serotypes to become localized. These phenomena have been reported by many researchers since the time that complement fixation test became available (Kawamori *et al.*, 1992; Shishido, 1962a).

Aside from the case in which only a specific antibody to a certain *R. tsutsugamushi* type remains for a long period, would it be possible to specifically identify the *R. tsutsugamushi* type or epidemic *R. tsutsugamushi* type infecting patients from the serotypes of paired sera obtained from the acute and recovery stages in the patients? An indirect IF study of Tsutsugamushi disease patients in Chiba Prefecture, Japan, by Kaiho *et al.* (1993), using a monoclonal antibody, identified the type of isolates from patients with a high anti-Gilliam antibody to be a Kawasaki type. Consequently, it appears that there are further issues remaining to dertermine the epidemic type of *R. tsutsugamushi* solely from patient serotype.

3) Detection of *R. tsutsugamushi* DNA by polymerase chain reaction (PCR)

As stated previously, further studies are necessary before serotypes can be used for the type-specific diagnosis of infecting *R.*

tsutsugamushi. However, it takes a considerable time to isolate and type *R. tsutsugamushi* for the diagnosis of Tsutsugamushi disease. Today, however, it is possible to type infecting *R. tsutsugamushi*, using nested PCR, by extracting *R. tsutsugamushi* DNA from patients' blood. This method will be most useful in diagnosing, in particular, inapparent infections caused by *R. tsutsugamushi* as well as typical Tsutsugamushi disease. For details, see Chapter 6 (Furuya and Yoshida, 1992; Furuya *et al.*, 1991a; Furuya *et al.*, 1993; Yoshida *et al.*, 1994).

d. Treatment

Before the advent of the antibiotic age, typical Tsutsugamushi disease in Japan had a very high fatality rate and was called a disease of terror. With the advent of the antibiotic age, which began with penicillin, rickettsioses in which the fatality rate was high, such as Tsutsugamushi disease, Rocky Mountain spotted fever, and typhus, have become simple diseases that are easy to treat and in which rapid recovery occurs. Today, people are not even interested in the names of rickettsiae, which symbolize the sacrifices made in the past by the many researchers who elucidated these pathogens.

Drugs with a specific action against *R. tsutsugamushi*, which consequently are especially effective against Tsutsugamushi disease, include antibiotics of the tetracycline family [tetracycline (TC), demethylchlortetracycline, doxycycline (DOXY), minocycline, and others]. Their minimum inhibitory concentration (MIC) against *R. tsutsugamushi* grown in cell culture ranges from 0.39 to 0.05 μg/ml. Quinolones, including the new and old types, have an MIC range of 2.5–3.12 μg/ml against *R. tsutsugamushi*, and exhibit moderate efficacy. However, the beta-lactam antibiotics, the penicillins, and the first through third generation cephems are all completely ineffective, with MIC values of >1000 μg/ml (Brown *et al.*, 1978; Miyamura *et al.*, 1985; Miyamura *et al.*, 1989; Tamiya, 1962; Urakami *et al.*, 1988a). However, there are differences in the action and efficacy of quinolones and beta-lactams in *R. tsutsugamushi* and other rickettsiae. For example, the MIC for other rickettsiae ranges from 3.12 to 0.09 μg/ml, while the MIC for *R. tsutsugamushi* is 25 μg/ml for benzyl penicillin, 100 μg/ml for ampicillin, and (≥1000 μg/ml for other penicillins) (Miyamura *et al.*, 1989). It is thus evident that the susceptibility of *R.*

tsutsugamushi to these antibiotics is fundamentally different from that of other rickettsiae (see Chapter 2).

Regarding the administration of effective antibiotics, Katsura *et al*. reported, as cited in a monograph by Tamiya (1962), that low-dose, long-term use is effective and prevents resurgence of the disease. For example, in classical Tsutsugamushi disease, 50 mg TC is given twice a day, the amount being halved after the fever subsides, with twice-daily administration to a total of 1.5 g. In new type Tsutsugamushi disease, they state that a total of 0.5–1.0 g is sufficient.

In contrast, Brown *et al*. (1978) reported that one dose of 200 mg DOXY cured Tsutsugamushi disease without resurgence, and they stated that this regimen also served as a prophylactic against Tsutsugamushi disease. Irrespective of the method used, Tsutsugamushi disease is now virtually completely curable when treatment is given after clinical diagnosis alone or after a definitive serodiagnosis is obtained.

In cases complicated with DIC, in addition to the use of *R. tsutsugamushi*-specific antibiotics, it is necessary, of course, to administer a drug to cure the hemorrhagic tendency and to energetically perform platelet transfusion and heparin therapy.

4

Behavior of Trombiculid Mites

1. Species of Vector Mites

The determination of vector mites in Japan was reviewed in Chapter 3. The methods used for this determination were epidemiological association, determination of a human preference in mite species, and the isolation of rickettsiae both from mites recovered from sentinel animals and unfed larvae, the unfed larvae being collected directly from the soil by plate setting or by the Tullgren funnel method (Tamiya, 1962).

Apart from the studies noted above, there have been many reports on the isolation of rickettsiae from mites recovered from wild rodents caught in endemic areas; these studies were carried out to determine vector species in these endemic areas. All the investigators assumed that these mites may have harbored rickettsiae while feeding on rickettsemic wild animals, as well as vertically transmitted rickettsiae. Since experiments indicated that the possibility of acquiring rickettsiae under field conditions was low, it was also assumed that larval mites from wild animals were materials to determine the source of infection. The reports summarized below are results of the efforts made by many investigators since 1955 to determine the vector species in Japan by detecting rickettsiae in mites obtained from wild animals and by studying the human preferences of mites. Since the mites obtained from animals could approximately be regarded as a source of infection, the vector species determined by these efforts were similar to those determined in studies detecting rickettsia from unfed larval mites, as indicated in Section 4 below.

Mite species as possible vectors in countries other than Japan are listed in Table 5, although the reliability of the findings is not clear.

a. Vector mites in Japan

1) Conditions under which trombiculid mites are vectors to humans

Infection of Tsutsugamushi disease in humans is initiated by the infestation and biting of trombiculid mites harboring *Rickettsia tsutsugamushi*. Therefore, the species of vector mite and its epidemiological role as a transmitter are determined by studying (1) the infection rate of *R. tsutsugamushi* in a suspected mite species and (2) the behavior of mites that have a predilection for and bite humans.

Of more than 100 species of trombiculid mites listed from mammals, birds, and reptiles, in Japan (Takada, 1990), only several species of larval mite are known to fulfil the above conditions to qualify as a vector of *R. tsutsugamushi*.

The original hosts of trombiculid mites are vertebrates, especially wild rodents living in the endemic areas. For example, the number of mites collected from three *Apodemus speciosus* caught at South Izu, Shizuoka Prefecture, in February 1960 was 1,201, an average of 400.3/rat. These mites belonged to six species (Asanuma *et al.*, 1962a). The number of mites collected from seven *A. speciosus* caught at Chichibu, Saitama Prefecture, in October 1985 was 3,402, an average of 486.0/rat. These mites belonged to five species (Takahashi *et al.*, 1993b). Wild rodents may be repeatedly infested by a tremendous number of trombiculid mites, possibly totaling in excess of 10,000 over the entire lifetime of the animal.

The stage of the life cycle (which develops from egg to larva, nymph, and adult) in which trombiculid mites infest humans and rodents and transmit rickettsiae is the larval stage. The mite's need for feeding on the tissue fluid of vertebrates is limited to the unfed larval stage, immediately after the larvae have hatched from the egg. In general, this occurs only once in the mite's life, for a period of a few days, or a week at most. Mites in stages other than the larval stage, *i.e.*, nymphs and adults, are free-living and are predators in the soil. Therefore, the unfed larvae already harbor *R. tsutsugamushi*, which is transmitted vertically from infected female mites before the larvae hatch from the egg stage.

It is an interesting and important question whether *R. tsutsugamushi* is a symbiont of mites, or whether the mite acquires the rickettsial agent from host aminals from time to time. This question will be discussed in Chapter 5.

For actual infections to occur in humans, including inapparent infections due to the bite of vector mites, various factors are necessary. Factors to be considered in regard to the characteristics of human behavior are whether and how frequently the subject has entered and passed through "mite islands" (Audy, 1961) in endemic areas in the epidemic season, and how long the subject stayed in the area of risk. Among the factors that determine the chance of human infection are the proportion of mites harboring rickettsiae, the density of infective mites, and the frequency with which they bite humans.

As was described in Chapter 3, the number of species that serve as sources of infection is small, and even among individuals in the same species, infective mites are limited in number. Therefore, if a person in an endemic focus is bitten by a trombiculid mite, this does not always lead to infection. However, in the same area, wild rodents may be infested with large numbers of mites, and they are considered to have a far greater chance of being infected than humans. For this reason, survey data on *R. tsutsugamushi* infection in wild rodents are also an important indicator of the occurrence of human infections in survey areas.

A research group for scrub typhus in Japan, chaired by the late Dr. T. Tamiya, carried out intensive surveys on the infection of wild rats throughout Japan in the period from 1954 to 1960. A total of 511 strains of *R. tsutsugamushi* were isolated from 5,807 wild rats, and infested foci of *R. tsutsugamushi* were demonstrated in 46 prefectures (Tamiya, 1962). These results suggested the possibility of human infection in almost all areas of Japan. Nevertheless, it was not easy to determine the vector species of trombiculid mite in each endemic area.

2) Isolation of *R. tsutsugamushi* from larval mites collected from wild animals in Japan

Many studies in Japan have been performed to isolate *R. tsutsugamushi* from the larvae of trombiculid mites collected from wild rodents, the main emphasis being determination of the vector mite in each endemic area.

These studies were based on experiments which had shown that rickettsiae were generally not transmitted to unfed mites feeding on rickettsemic animals, or, if they were transmitted, that this occurred in very low numbers (Fukuzumi, 1953; Ito and Obata, 1961; Miura and Kawai, 1968; Toyokawa, 1972; Traub *et al*., 1975). However, more recent studies have indicated that rickettsiae are transmitted in large numbers to the unfed larvae of some species while they feed on highly rickettsemic mice (Kaneko *et al*., 1987; Takahashi *et al*., 1990a, 1994a).

Such high rates of transmission of rickettsiae to feeding mites may be realized only under specially designed experimental conditions; in the field, transmission of rickettsiae to the mites may not be so frequent from wild rodents, which usually show low levels of rickettsemia. In any case, data based on the isolation of rickettsia from larvae collected from wild animals should be regarded as reflecting the rates in unfed mites originally harboring the rickettsiae, together with (as a minor component) the rate at which rickettsia-negative unfed larvae acquired rickettsia from wild rodents.

For the determination of vector mites in many localities in Japan, Dr. Tamiya's group examined a large number of engorged larvae for *R. tsutsugamushi*. More than 200,000 live mites of approximately 30 species were identified immediately after collection from animals, and isolation of *R. tsutsugamushi* was attempted by the mouse passage method. Sixteen species belonging to six genera were confirmed to harbor rickettsiae, as shown in Table 1.

As can be seen in this table, *R. tsutsugamushi* was detected quite

Table 1. Species of Larval Trombiculid Mites Detected with *Rickettsia tsutsugamushi* at Different Localities in Japan; Mostly Engorged, but Including a Few Unfed Larvae

Species[a]	Area of mite collection	Authors
1. *L. akamushi*		
	Niigata	Asanuma, 1983; Fukuzumi, 1953; Ito and Obata, 1961; Kitaoka *et al*., 1967; Shishido, 1964; Tamiya, 1962; Asanuma, 1986
	Akita	Kitaoka *et al*., 1967; Kitaoka and Asanuma, 1968
	Yamagata	Asanuma, 1983
2. *L. pallidum*		
	Aomori	Takada, 1982
	Akita	Kitaoka *et al*., 1967, 1976; Kitaoka and Asanuma, 1968

	Niigata	Murata *et al.*, 1986; Asanuma *et al.*, 1961; Asanuma *et al.*, 1964a,b; Asanuma, 1983, 1986; Fukuzumi, 1953; Kawamura, 1926; Kenmotsu *et al.*, 1979; Kitaoka *et al.*, 1967; Shishido, 1964
	Toyama	Ishikura *et al.*, 1985
	Tokyo	Shishido, 1964
	Kanagawa	Asanuma *et al.*, 1960, 1962a,b,c; Kitaoka *et al.*, 1967; Shishido, 1964; Tamiya, 1962
	Gumma	Oyama *et al.*, 1983
	Shizuoka	Asanuma *et al.*, 1960, 1962a,b,c; Kawamori *et al.*, 1992; Kitaoka *et al.*, 1967; Tamiya, 1962
	Saitama	Murata *et al.*, 1986; Takahashi *et al.*, 1986a, 1993b
	Nagano	Kumada *et al.*, 1986
	Gifu	Kasuya *et al.*, 1985
	Kyoto	Matsuno *et al.*, 1990
	Fukui	Tanaka *et al.*, 1987
	Oita	Kitaoka *et al.*, 1967; Umeki *et al.*, 1970
3. *L. scutellare*		
	Tokyo	Asanuma *et al.*, 1958; Asanuma, 1983; Kawamura, 1953; Kitaoka *et al.*, 1953b;
	Chiba	Asanuma *et al.*, 1959c, 1962b,c; Tamiya, 1962
	Shizuoka	Asanuma *et al.*, 1974; Kawamori *et al.*, 1993
		Noguchi *et al.*, 1953
4. *L. murotoense*		
	Oita	Asanuma, 1983; Kitaoka *et al.*, 1967; Umeki *et al.*, 1970
5. *L. tosa*		
	Kochi	Asanuma, 1983; Nakaya, 1957
6. *L. kitasatoi*		
	Oita	Asanuma, 1983; Umeki *et al.*, 1970
7. *L. palpale*		
	Oita	Asanuma, 1983; Kitaoka *et al.*, 1967; Umeki *et al.*, 1970
8. *L. kawamurai*		
	Hokkaido	Asanuma, 1983; Kitaoka *et al.*, 1967, 1973; Shishido, 1964

9. *L. intermedium*		
	Niigata	Saito and Otsuru, 1959
10. *N. pomeranzevi*		
	Hokkaido	Asanuma, 1983; Kitaoka *et al.*, 1973
11. *N. japonica*		
	Kanagawa	Asanuma, 1983
12. *N. sadoensis*[b]		
	Niigata	Saito and Otsuru, 1959
13. *C. ikaoensis*		
	Shizuoka	Asanuma *et al.*, 1974; Asanuma, 1983; Kitaoka *et al.*, 1967; Shishido, 1964
14. *H. miyagawai*		
	Niigata	Asanuma, 1983; Saito and Otsuru, 1959
15. *G. saduski*		
	Oita	Asanuma, 1983; Kitaoka *et al.*, 1967; Umeki *et al.*, 1970
16. *W. masoni*		
	Niigata	Saito and Otsuru, 1959

[a] L, *Leptotrombidium*; N, *Neotrombicula*; C, *Cheladonta*; H, *Helenicula*; G, *Gahrliepia*; W, *Walchia*.
[b] *N. sadoensis* is often regarded as a synonym of *Eltonella ichikawai*.

often in *Leptotrombidium akamushi*, *L. scutellare*, and *L. pallidum*. As *L. tosa* was suspected to be a vector mite from the epidemiological point of view, repeated attempts were made to isolate *R. tsutsugamushi* from that species by Kawamura *et al*. (1952), but they were not successful. Later isolation was successful only once, from 31 larval *L. tosa* collected from rodents by Nakaya (1957). Mite species in which *R. tsutsugamushi* is detected do not always play a role in transmitting rickettsiae to humans.

3) Positive rates of rickettsiae in larval mites in Japan

In a study in Gosen, Niigata Prefecture (Asanuma, 1983), the isolation of *R. tsutsugamushi* from individual unfed larvae of *L. akamushi* collected by the plate method was successful in one of 93 mites (1.08%), by the mouse passage method (Table 2).

Isolation of *R. tsutsugamushi* from individual engorged mites by mouse passage was attempted in *L. akamushi*, *L. scutellare*, and *L. pallidum* at various localities in Japan. In *L. akamushi*, positive rates were 2.08% (5/240) and 1.67% (4/240) in Gosen and 0.82% (1/122) in Nagaoka, Niigata Prefecture. The positive rate in *L. pallidum* was

0.32% (1/314) in Gosen City. In *L. scutellare,* none was isolated (0/200) in Shirahama, Chiba Prefecture and 0.28 (1/360) on Izu Ohima Island, Tokyo (Asanuma, 1983, Table 2).

Of 148 pools consisting of 13,039 engorged larvae of *L. scutellare* collected in the 11 years from 1960 to 1970, only two pools were positive for *R. tsutsugamushi.* The minimum positive rate (MPR) was based on the assumption that one positive mite was involved in each positive pool of mites, and the MPR was thus calculated by the equation: number of positive pools of mites/total number of mites examined. In this case, the MPR was 0.02% (2/13,039) (Asanuma *et al.*, 1974).

Monthly surveys were conducted in Gosen, Niigata Prefecture, to isolate rickettsiae from the engorged larvae of trombiculid mites collected from wild voles, *Microtus montebelli.* The number of mites collected from 192 voles was 14,292; the mites were of four species. Rickettsiae were isolated from a total of 13,786 *L. akamushi, L. pallidum, L. palpale,* and *G. saduski* larvae. Of 940 pools of mites, 71 were positive for *R. tsutsugamushi.*

The mites species that were positive for *R. tsutsugamushi* were *L. akamushi* and *L. pallidum*; results were positive in 32 of 291 and in 39 of 639 larvae, respectively. The MPR in *L. akamushi* was markedly higher than that in *L. pallidum*, ranging from 0.63% to 3.32% (average 1.94%) in the period from June to October, while the MPR in *L. pallidum* ranged from 0.06% to 1.09% from April to December (average 0.33%), excluding negative results in July and November

Table 2. Isolation of *Rickettsia tsutsugamushi* from Individual Engorged Larvae of Trombiculid Mites Collected from Wild Rodents

Species	Collection area	No. of mites examined	No. *Rt*-positive	Positive rate (%)
L. akamushi	Niigata (Gosen)	240	5	2.08
	Niigata (Gosen)	240	4	1.67
	Niigata (Nagaoka)	122	1	0.82
	Niigata (Gosen)	93[a]	1	1.08
L. scutellare	Chiba (Shirahama)	200	0	0
	Tokyo (Oshima)	360	1	0.28
L. pallidum	Niigata (Gosen)	314	1	0.32

[a] Unfed larvae.
Source: Asanuma (1983).

Table 3. Isolation of *Rickettsia tsutsugamushi* in Monthly Surveys, from *L. pallidum* and *L. akamushi* Collected from *Microtus montebelli* in an Area Endemic for Classical Tsutsugamushi Disease, Gosen, Niigata Prefecture

	L. akamushi			*L. pallidum*		
Month	No. of mites examined (pools)	No. of positive pools	Minimum positive rate	No. of mites examined (pools)	No. of positive pools	Minimum positive rate
Jan.				16 (1)	0	0
Feb.				10 (1)	0	0
Mar.				298 (127)	0	0
Apr.				1554 (291)	1	0.06
May				7612 (155)	27	0.35
Jun.	211 (8)	7	3.32	183 (4)	2	1.09
Jul.	728 (26)	10	1.37	46 (2)	0	0
Aug.	160 (160)	1	0.63	337 (13)	1	0.30
Sep.	512 (96)	14	2.73	353 (11)	3	0.85
Oct.	36 (1)	0	0	1090 (22)	4	0.37
Nov.				225 (5)	0	0
Dec.				203 (7)	1	0.49
Total	1647 (291)	32	1.94	11927 (639)	39	0.33

Source: Asanuma, 1983.

(Table 3). These results suggested that if the inhabitants of Gosen had an equal chance of being bitten by *L. akamushi* or *L. pallidum*, the possibility of infection would be much higher if they were bitten by *L. akamushi* (Asanuma, 1983).

In *L. scutellare*, although there was one successful isolation from a single mite at Izu Oshima (Table 2), results were negative in about 1,400 larval *L. scutellare*. In the same species at Shirahama, Chiba Prefecture, of 3,548 larvae in 270 pools one pool was positive (MPR 0.03%); and in the Higashi-Fuji Camp area, in more than 13,000 larvae in more than 560 pools three pools were positive (MPR of approximately 0.02%) (Asanuma, 1983). Such a low MPR in *L. scutellare* is assumed to be caused by the use of conventional mice for passage, and suggests that the rickettsiae harbored by *L. scutellare* have low pathogenicity in conventional mice (Kawamori *et al.*, 1992; Kawamura *et al.*, 1980; Kobayashi *et al.*, 1978; Misao *et al.*, 1967).

The *R. tsutsugamushi*-positive rates of trombiculid mites in endemic areas examined by the same mouse passage method was highest in the order of *L. akamushi*, *L. pallidum*, and *L. scutellare*, and generally their respective MPR were approximately 1%, 0.2%, and 0.02% (Asanuma, 1983). However, in one limited area where mite islands were found by chance, the MPR of *L. pallidum* was 1.65% [6 pools/363 mites in 7 pools at Tokamachi, Niigata Prefecture (Asanuma, 1983)], and the positive rate determined by rickettsial isolation from individual mites at Chichibu, Saitama Prefecture, was 60.7% (17/28) (Takahashi *et al.*, 1993b). However, there are many areas in which mites of the same species are entirely negative.

Of the 16 species of candidate vector mites listed in Table 1, apart from the three species *L. akamushi*, *L. pallidum*, and *L. scutellare*, it is necessary to consider other species as vector mites; these species are listed in Table 4, with their positive rates. The positive rates were calculated only for areas in which at least one positive result was achieved. As shown in Table 4, *L. kawamurai* had a high positive rate (2.05%), whereas other species showed positive results in only one pool of mites. More than 10,000 larvae each of *L. palpale* and *G. saduski* were examined in many other areas, but there were no positive results (Asanuma *et al.*, 1983).

L. kawamurai harbored rickettsiae at a high rate in Hokkaido, and although this species has no preference for humans and there was no human Tsutsugamushi disease in that locality, it is possible that this

Table 4. Positive Rates of Trombiculid Mites Harboring *R. tsutsugamushi*, as Observed in Engorged Larvae of Species Other than *L. akamushi*, *L. pallidum*, and *L. scutellare* Collected from Wild Animals (Mostly Rodents) throughout Japan

Species of trombiculid mite	No. of pools positive for rickettsia	No. of pools examined for rickettsia	Total no. of mites in examined pools	Minimum positive percentage[a]
L. kawamurai	7	37	342	2.05
L. murotoense	1	79	4,169	0.02
L. kitasatoi	1	18	1,618	0.06
L. palpale	1	16	1,912	0.05
N. pomeranzevi	1	5	370	0.27
G. saduski	1	41	5,431	0.02
C. ikaoensis	1	30	3,755	0.03

After Asanuma (1983), with corrected species name.

[a] No. of positive pools / total no. of mites in pools examined, based on the assumption that at least one rickettsia-positive mite was involved in a positive pool.

species could be a transmitter in wild rodents. Indeed, in Hokkaido, *R. tsutsugamushi* was isolated from *L. kawamurai* (Kitaoka *et al.*, 1973) and from wild rodents in June, the most prevalent season for *L. kawamurai* (Takahashi *et al.*, 1981).

Laboratory animals used as sentinels so far have been mice, white rats, chickens, and the vole, *M. montebelli*. *L. akamushi* has been confirmed as a vector (Kitaoka and Asanuma, 1968). *L. pallidum* (Kitaoka *et al*, 1976; Takahashi *et al.*, 1990b) and *L. scutellare* (Asanuma, 1959; Asanuma *et al.*, 1959c; Asanuma *et al.*, 1962a) have also been determined as vectors by the use of sentinel animals.

4) Mite species feeding on, and actual vector mites in, humans

Of the 16 species of mites in which *R. tsutsugamushi* was detected, epidemiologically and in practice four species of mites are suspected of transmitting rickettsiae to humans, *i.e.*, *L. akamushi*, *L. pallidum*, *L. scutellare*, and *L. kawamurai*.

However, to date, it has been confirmed that, in Japan, the larvae of seven species bite human skin in the natural environment, *i.e.*, *L. akamushi* (Asanuma, 1959; Ito and Obata, 1961; Kitaoka *et al.*, 1974), *L. pallidum pallidum* (Asanuma, 1959; Asanuma *et al*, 1962b; Kawamura, R., 1926), *L. pallidum burnsi* (Suzuki *et al.*, 1958), *L. scutellare* (Arai, 1955; Asanuma, 1959, 1962b; Hayashi and Tanaka, 1955), *L. palpale* (Asanuma, 1959; Kawamura, R. 1926), *E. wichmanni* (Asanuma, 1959; Kitahara, 1952; Sasa, 1956), and *Shoengastia hanmyaensis* (Suzuki, 1976).

Since there is no record of *L. kawamurai* biting humans, nor of *E. wichmanni* transmitting disease to humans (Asanuma, 1959, 1983; Sasa, 1956), taking into consideration the mite species harboring *R. tsutsugamushi*, the principal vector species that actually transmit rickettsiae to humans in Japan are considered to be the three species *L. akamushi*, *L. pallidum*, and *L. scutellare*. The human preference of these mites is highest in the order of *L. akamushi*, *L. scutellare*, and *L. pallidum*, and the infection rate is highest in the order *L. akamushi*, *L. pallidum*, and *L. scutellare*.

In oriental Siberia, however, *N. japonica*, *N. mitamurai*, and *N. pomeranzevi* were reported to feed on humans (Kulagin *et al.*, 1967, 1968; Shubin *et al.*, 1970).

In regard to the regional and seasonal distribution of the above three vector species in Japan, the main vector in endemic areas in the three northeast prefectures (Akita, Niigata, and Yamagata) in the summer season is *L. akamushi*. In other endemic areas in Japan, including the above-mentioned areas, the vectors in the season from autumn to the next spring are *L. pallidum* and *L. scutellare*, depending on the locality.

b. Vector mites outside Japan
Outside Japan, *R. tsutsugamushi* in local chiggers has been detected by mouse passage or directly by immunofluorescence (IF), and these results, together with epidemiological considerations, have led to the determination of vector species in various localities. The 45 confirmed or suspected vector species, including 8 unidentified species, belonging to 13 genera thus determined are distributed widely in Southeast Asia and in the southwest Pacific islands (Table 5).

Whether those species suspected as the vectors to humans are actually the culprits should be studied further, considering their predi-

Table 5. Chigger Mites Confirmed or Suspected as Vectors of Scrub Typhus in Various Areas of the World Excluding Japan

Species[a]	Area	*R. tsutsugamushi*-positive	Authors
L. deliense	Burma	+	Mackie *et al.*, 1946ab
		+	Audy, 1949
		+	Audy *et al.*, 1947
		+	Traub, 1949
	China	+	Yu and Lin, 1957
		+	Yu and Wu, 1959
			Hsu *et al.*, 1959
			Fan *et al.*, 1987
			Walker and Fishbein, 1991
		+	Wang *et al.*, 1965
		+	Chao *et al.*, 1953
		+	Ch'iu *et al.*, 1962
	India	+	Mackie *et al.*, 1946ab
		+	Krishnan *et al.*, 1949
		+	Kalra, 1959
	Malaysia	+	Philip *et al.*, 1949
		+	Audy and Harrison, 1951
		+	Shirai *et al.*, 1978, 1981b
		+	Dohany *et al.*, 1980
	New Guinea	+	Kohls *et al.*, 1945

		+	Philip and Kohls, 1948
	Indonesia	+	Blake *et al.*, 1945
	Australia	+	Campbell and Domrow, 1974
		+	Shirai *et al.*, 1982a
	Pakistan		Traub *et al.*, 1967
		+	Nur Ahmad and Burney, 1962
	Pescadores	+	Cooper *et al.*, 1964
		+	Lien *et al.*, 1967
		+	Shirai *et al.*, 1982b
		+	Olson *et al.*, 1978
	Philippines		Philip *et al.*, 1946
	Thailand	+	Trishnananda *et al.*, 1966
		+	Shirai *et al.*, 1981d
L. fletcheri	Malaysia	+	Philip *et al.*, 1949
		+	Rapmund *et al.*, 1969
		+	Audy and Harrison, 1951
		+	U.S. Army Med. Res. Unit, 1969
		+	Shirai *et al.*, 1981b
	New Guinea	+	Blake *et al.*, 1945
		+	Kohls *et al.*, 1945
	Philippines		Philip *et al.*, 1946
	Indonesia		Gispen, 1950
		+	Blake *et al.*, 1945
	Melanesia	+	Shirai *et al.*, 1981c
L. arenicola	Malaysia	+	U.S. Army Med. Res. Unit, 1960
		+	Traub, 1960, 1962
		+	Traub and Wisseman, 1968b
		+	Rapmund *et al.*, 1972
		+	Roberts *et al.*, 1972
			Upham *et al.*, 1971
	Indonesia	+	Dennis *et al.*, 1981
		+	Hadi *et al.*, 1979
	Thailand	+	Shirai *et al.*, 1981d
L. pallidum	Primorye	+	Tarasevich, 1964, 1969
		+	Kudryashova and Tarasevich, 1964
		+	Kulagin *et al.*, 1967

		+	Schluger and Kudryashova, 1967
		+	Rehacek and Tarasevich, 1988
		+	Kulagin *et al.*, 1968
	Korea	+	Jackson *et al.*, 1957
		+	Ree *et al.*, 1991a
L. pavlovskyi	Primorye	+	Tarasevich, 1969
		+	Kudryashova and Tarasevich, 1964
		+	Kulagin *et al.*, 1967
		+	Schluger and Kudryashova, 1967
		+	Kudryashova *et al.*, 1968
		+	Kulagin *et al.*, 1968
		+	Rehacek and Tarasevich, 1988
L. palpale	Primorye	+	Kudryashova *et al.*, 1967, 1968
		+	Kulagin *et al.*, 1968
		+	Rehacek and Tarasevich, 1988
L. orientale	Korea	+	Schluger and Kudryashova, 1967
		+	Kulagin *et al.*, 1967, 1968
		+	Rehacek and Tarasevich, 1988
	Primorye	+	Schluger and Kudryashova, 1967
L. scutellare	China		Fan *et al.*, 1987
			Walker and Fishbein, 1991
		+	Xiangrui *et al.*, 1991
			Walker *et al.*, 1990
		+	Wang *et al.*, 1983
	Malaysia	+	Shirai *et al.*, 1981b
	Thailand	+	Shirai *et al.*, 1981d
L. vivericola	Malaysia	+	Dohany *et al.*, 1980
		+	Shirai *et al.*, 1978
L. bodense	Malaysia	+	Shirai *et al.*, 1981b
L. keukenschrijveri	Malaysia	+	Shirai *et al.*, 1981b
L. umbricola	Malaysia	+	Shirai *et al.*, 1981b
L. arvinum	Thailand	+	Shirai *et al.*, 1981d
L. sp. A	Thailand	+	Shirai *et al.*, 1981d
L. sp. B	Thailand	+	Shirai *et al.*, 1981d

L. imphalum	Thailand	+	Tanskul *et al.*,1994
L. sp.	Thailand	+	Tanskul *et al.*, 1994
L. paniculatum	Thailand	+	Shirai *et al.*, 1981d
L. gaohuensis	China		Fan *et al.*, 1987
			Walker and Fishbein, 1991
		+	Wei *et al.*, 1985b
		+	Wei *et al.*, 1985a
		+	Wei *et al.*, 1987
L. insulare	China		Walker and Fishbein, 1991
			Walker *et al.*, 1990
L. jishoum	China		Walker and Fishbein, 1991
			Walker *et al.*, 1990
L. waiganmensis	China		Wei *et al.*, 1983
		+	Fan *et al.*, 1987
L. tachensis	China		Wei *et al.*, 1983
		+	Fan *et al.*, 1987
L. nangii	China		Wei *et al.*, 1983
		+	Fan *et al.*, 1987
L. pulchra	Tajik SSR		Fetisova *et al.*, 1968b
A. indica	Sumatra	+	Tarasevich, 1960
A. audyi	Malaysia	+	Traub *et al.*, 1950
N. japonica	Primorye	+	Kudryashova *et al.*, 1967
		+	Shubin *et al.*, 1970
		+	Kulagin *et al.*, 1967, 1968
		+	Rehacek and Tarasevich, 1988
N. mitamurai	Primorye	+	Kudryashova *et al.*, 1967
		+	Shubin *et al.*, 1970
		+	Kulagin *et al.*, 1967, 1968
		+	Rehacek and Tarasevich, 1988
N. pomeranzevi	Kurile	+	Shubin *et al.*, 1970
N. tamiyai	Primorye	+	Rehacek and Tarasevich, 1988
N. monticola	Tajik SSR		Fetisova *et al.*, 1968[b]
N. minuta	Tajik SSR		Fetisova *et al.*, 1968[b]
Neoshoengastia sp	China		Wei *et al.*, 1983
		+	Fan *et al.*, 1987
E. rotundata	Tajik SSR		Fetisova *et al.*, 1968[b]
E. indicum	China		Wei *et al.*, 1983

		+	Fan *et al.*, 1987
		+	Yu and Lin, 1957
Et. wichmannni	Thailand	+	Shirai *et al.*, 1981d
M. chamlongi	Thailand	+	Shirai *et al.*, 1981d
Odontacarus sp.	Thailand	+	Shirai *et al.*, 1981d
S. oudemansi	Tajik SSR		Fetisova *et al.*, 1968[b]
Leeuwenhoekia sp.	Tajik SSR		Fetisova *et al.*, 1968[b]
Acomatacarus sp.	China	+	Yu and Lin, 1957
			Wei *et al.*, 1983
		+	Fan *et al.*, 1987
Walchia sp.	China	+	Yu and Lin, 1957
W. chinensis	China		Wei *et al.*, 1983
		+	Fan *et al.*, 1987
G. ligula	Pakistan		Traub *et al.*, 1967 Traub and Wisseman, 1968a,b, 1974b
	Malaysia		Traub and Wisseman, 1974b
	India	+	Kalra, 1959 Traub and Wisseman, 1968a,b

[a] *L, Leptotrombidium* ; *A, Ascoschoengastia* ; *N, Neotrombicula* ; *E, Euschoengastia* ; *Et, Eutrombicula* ; *M, Machiena* ; *S, Shunsennia* ; *G, Gahrliepia.*

[b] From a review by Rehacek and Tarasevich (1988).

lection for humans and their transmission capability, in terms of their infection rates. Of these species, six — *L. deliense*, *L fletcheri*, *L. arenicola*, *L. pallidum*, *L. pavlovskyi*, and *L. scutellare* — are regarded as the main vectors of Tsutsugamushi disease in all areas (Traub and Wisseman, 1974b).

L. deliense is the main vector and is distributed widely in Southeast Asia and the southwest Pacific islands; it causes severe infestations in humans (Audy, 1961; Traub and Wisseman, 1974b). In China also, *L. deliense* is the main vector in many regions, including Guangdong, Fujian, Zhejiang, Guangxi, Yunnan, Hunan, Sichuan, Tibet, Shandong, Hainan, and Jiangsu. Transovarian transmission of rickettsiae in this species has been confirmed in laboratory experiments (Davis *et al.*, 1947; Krishnan *et al.*, 1949; Mackie *et al.*, 1946 a,b; Rai and Bandopadhyay, 1978; Yu and Wu, 1959), and *R.*

tsutsugamushi has been detected in the eggs, nymphs, and adults (Audy, 1961; Wang *et al*., 1965).

L. fletcheri is the vector species distributed widely from Malaysia to Melanesia, and transovarian transmission in the species has also been confirmed (Rapmund, 1984; Rapmund *et al*., 1969; Shirai *et al*., 1982c). The species is also confirmed to transmit rickettsiae to mice, monkeys, and humans (Shirai *et al*., 1982c,d; Twartz *et al*., 1982).

L. arenicola, found principally on the sandy beaches of peninsular Malaysia (Traub, 1960; Upham *et al*., 1971) and Indonesia (Hadi *et al*., 1979) had been considered at first only as a potential vector. In this species, transovarian transmission of rickettsiae has also been confirmed by laboratory experiments (Rapmund *et al*., 1972; Roberts and Robinson, 1977; Shirai *et al*., 1982c). When larvae fed on humans, they were fully engorged in several days (Shirai *et al*., 1982d; Traub and Wisseman, 1974b). Successful transmission of Tsutsugamushi disease to human volunteers via the bites of an infected colony of *L. arenicola* has been reported (Shirai *et al*., 1982d). In Thailand, Shirai *et al*. (1981d) detected *R. tsutsugamushi* in the larvae of this species directly by the IF method.

L. pallidum is the main vector in Korea and in the Primorye region, Primorskiy Kray, near Vladivostok, Russia (Table 6). *R. tsutsugamushi* has also been detected in the nymphs of this species (Kulagin *et al*., 1967; Schluger and Kudryashova, 1967; Tarasevich, 1969).

L. pavlovskyi is also considered to be a vector in the Primorye region of Russia, and *R. tsutsugamushi* has been detected in the nymphs (Kudryashova and Tarasevich, 1964). In the same region, *L. palpale*, *L. orientale*, *N. japonica*, and *N. mitamurai* have been suggested as possible vectors (Kudryashova *et al*., 1967; Kulagin *et al*., 1967, 1968; Schluger and Kudryashova, 1967; Tarasevich, 1969). In the former Tajik Soviet Socialist Republic, six species, including *L. pulchra*, are thought to be possible vectors (Fetisova *et al*., 1968; Rehacek and Tarasevich, 1988).

L. scutellare is suspected to be the vector in Shandong, China (Fan *et al*., 1987; Walker and Fishbein, 1991; Xiangrui *et al*., 1991) and in Fujian (Fan *et al*., 1987; Wang *et al*., 1983); in both these regions. *R. tsutsugamushi* has been detected in patients and in wild rodents

(Xiangrui *et al.*, 1991). *R. tsutsugamushi* has also been detected in *L. scutellare* in Malaysia (Shirai *et al.*, 1981b) and Thailand (Shirai *et al.*, 1981d).

The other suspected vectors in China are *L. gaohuensis* in Zhejiang, *L. insulare* in Zhejiang, and *L. jishoum* in Hunan (Fan *et al.*, 1987; Walker and Fishbein, 1991; Walker *et al.*, 1990; Xiangrui *et al.*, 1991). Transovarian transmission (Wei *et al.*, 1985a,b, 1987) and feeding on humans have been confirmed (Wei *et al.*, 1985c) in *L. gaohuensis*.

Besides the above species, it has been reported that rickettsiae were detected at low rates in *L. waiganmensis*, *L. tachensis*, *L. nangii*, *Eushoengastia indicum*, *Acomatacarus* sp., *Neoshoengastia* sp., and *Walchia chinensis* (Fan *et al.*, 1987; Wei *et al.*, 1983).

In Pakistan, the possibility of transmission to humans was reported in six species: *L. subintermedium*, *L. dihumerale*, *L. rupestre*, *L. jayewickremei*, *L. gliricolens*, and *L. irregulare* (Traub and Wisseman, 1968b, 1974b; Traub *et al.*, 1967).

Extensive surveys have been made to detect *R. tsutsugamushi* efficiently by IF in individual unfed larvae collected by the black plate method directly from the soil surface. Thus, *R. tsutsugamushi* was detected in seven species, *L. vivericola*, *L. bodense*, *L. deliense*, *L. fletcheri*, *L. keukenschrijveri*, *L. scutellare*, and *L. umbricola* in Malaysia (Shirai *et al.*, 1978, 1981b), and in eleven species, *L. deliense*, *L. arvinum*, *L. scutellare*, *L.* sp. A, *L.* sp. B, *L.* sp., *L. imphalum*, *L. paniculatum*, *Eutrombicula wichmanni*, *Microtrombicula chamlongi* and *Odontacarus* sp. in Thailand (Shirai *et al.*, 1981d; Tanskul *et al.*, 1994). Two unknown species "A" and "B" were later named *L. harrisoni* and *L. andrei*, respectively (Tanskul and Gingrich, 1986).

The results of surveys for the detection of *R. tsutsugamushi* in individual mites are listed in Table 6. In the same species, there were large differences in positive rates; this was possibly due to differences in areas in which they were collected and to the different stages of the mites, whether they are unfed or engorged larvae, or in any other stages of development.

Table 6. *Rickettsia tsutsugamushi* Positive Rate in Larval Trombiculid Mites by Individual Examination

Species[a]	Positive rate(%)	Method[c]	Area	Authors
L. bodense	2.6 (2/77)[b]	iFA	Malaysia	Shirai *et al.*, 1981b
L. deliense	4.8 (116/2394)	iFA	Malaysia	Shirai *et al.*, 1981b
	1.8 (10/570)	iFA	Malaysia	Shirai *et al.*, 1978
	5.9 (17/290)	iFA	Malaysia	Dohany *et al.*, 1980
L. fletcheri	3.5 (14/404)	iFA	Malaysia	Shirai *et al.*, 1981b
L. keuken -schrijveri	2.3 (15/646)	iFA	Malaysia	Shirai *et al.*, 1981b
L. vivericola	1.3 (1/80)	iFA	Malaysia	Shirai *et al.*, 1978
	4.2 (15/358)	iFA	Malaysia	Dohany *et al.*, 1980;
L. scutellare	2.6 (6/235)	iFA	Malaysia	Shirai *et al.*, 1981b
L. umbricola	1.9 (15/791)	iFA	Malaysia	Shirai *et al.*, 198lb
L. pallidum	0.4 (2/447)	iFA	Korea	Ree *et al.*, 1991a
	30.0 (12/40)	iFA	Primorye	Kulagin *et al.*, 1967
	26.7 (12/45)	iFA	Primorye	Rehacek and Tarasevich, 1988
L. orientale	45.5 (5/11)	iFA	Primorye	Kulagin *et al.*, 1967
	35.3 (6/17)	iFA	Primorye	Rehacek and Tarasevich, 1988
L. pavlovskyi	64.3 (9/14)	MP	Primorye	Kulagin *et al.*, 1968
	36.5 (73/200)	iFA	Primorye	Kulagin *et al.*, 1967
	24.1 (77/320)	iFA	Primorye	Rehacek and Tarasevich, 1988
L. palpale	36.8 (7/19)	MP	Primorye	Kulagin *et al.*, 1968
	7.8 (9/116)	iFA	Primorye	Rehacek and Tarasevich, 1988
N. japonica	21.4 (3/14)	MP	Primorye	Kulagin *et al.*, 1968
	16.3 (14/86)	iFA	Primorye	Kulagin *et al.*, 1967
	13.7 (20/146)	iFA	Primorye	Rehacek and Tarasevich, 1988
N. mitamurai	20.0 (1/5)	MP	Primorye	Kulagin *et al.*, 1968
	33.3 (1/3)	iFA	Primorye	Kulagin *et al.*, 1967
	18.2 (4/22)	iFA	Primorye	Rehacek and Tarasevich, 1988
N. tamiyai	25.0 (1/4)	iFA	Primorye	Rehacek and Tarasevich, 1988

[a] *L, Leptotrombidium*; *N, Neotrombicula.*
[b] No. of positive mites/no. of mites examined.
[c] iFA, indirect immunofluorescence; MP, mouse passage.

2. Human Preferences of Larval Mites and Their Bites

a. Species of larval trombiculid mites that bite humans in Japan

When larval mites bite humans, some cause only pain and itching on the skin; others infect with *Rickettsia tsutsugamushi*. Of the more than 110 species of trombiculid mites (Takada, 1990) in Japan, to date, seven species — *Leptotrombidium akamushi*, *L. scutellare*, *L. pallidum pallidum*, *L. pallidum burnsi*, *L. palpale*, *Eutrombicula wichmanni* and *Schoengastia hanmyaensis* — have been found to bite humans. However, another species, *Gahrliepia saduski*, has now also been recognized as a human biter (Takahashi *et al.*, unpublished data), and it can be assumed that, with further surveys, more species that bite humans will be identified. Mites that bite humans usually have a wide range of host preferences, and the above seven species do not specifically prefer humans.

b. Reactions at bitten sites on skin

Skin reactions at the biting site differ depending on the mite species and depending on whether or not *R. tsutsugamushi* was transmitted. When rickettsiae are transmitted by mite bites, the skin manifestations seen differ according to the mite species, as will be described below, but in all cases a small papule appears and an eschar, a characteristic ulcer with a hard black scab, is formed at the biting site; a high fever and the characteristic widespread skin rash are manifested clinically, as described in detail in Chapter 3.

When bitten by *L. akamushi*, victims feel as if a tiny thorn has penetrated and stayed in the skin, and the area is painful when rubbed with clothing or the hand.

Inhabitants of endemic areas in Japan call this sensation "ira" in the local dialect; most people who are bitten have this "ira" sensation, which has also been confirmed by volunteers who were bitten (Ito and Obata, 1961; Obata and Aoki, 1958; Takahashi *et al.*, 1991b).

In the experimental bites, it was reported that the "ira" sensation appeared 10–20 h after the bite the bitten site exhibited an inflammatory exanthem (Ito and Obata, 1961). Stylostome formation by larval *L. akamushi* is assumed to be the cause of the "ira" sensation (Hase *et al.*, 1978; Ito and Obata, 1961; Obata and Aoki, 1958; Schumacher and Hoeppli, 1963).

Inhabitants of endemic areas in Japan long ago associated this painful skin symptom and the onset of Tsutsugamushi disease with the Akamushi (red mite). This is why *L. akamushi* was the first identified vector of Tsutsugamushi disease. There are many records of bites by *L. akamushi*, mainly in Niigata Prefecture, as shown in Table 7.

The skin manifestations caused by bites of *L. palpale* are reported to be almost as painful as those caused by *L. akamushi* (Kadosaka, unpublished data).

The bite of *L. scutellare*, which occurs on Hachijo Island in autumn and winter, causes mild skin manifestations, usually an itch, and is often not recognized by the victim. In volunteer human subjects, careful observation showed small papules or elevated exanthemas at the bitten sites (Arai, 1955; Sasa, 1956; Toriyama *et al.*, 1988).

Suspicion of *L. scutellare* as a vector mite of Tsutsugamushi disease on Hachijo Island increased when *R. tsutsugamushi* was successfully isolated from *L. scutellare* collected from a house rat in December 1952 (Kitaoka *et al.*, 1953b). Kitaoka *et al.* attempted to confirm *L. scutellare* as a transmitter, placing 15 larvae on the skin of a human volunteer. Three of 15 larvae became attached to the skin, but no Tutsugamushi disease was manifested.

Hayashi and Tanaka (1954) collected unfed larvae of *L. scutellare* by the plate method on Hachijo Island and in Chiba Prefecture, and placed these larvae on human skin. Of 336 larvae in a glass ring cover, 64 (17.5%) bit the skin.

The biting of *L. scutellare* on human skin was more precisely confirmed by exposing 35 volunteers to mites by having them sit on the ground in a mite habitat on Hachijo Island for 1 h. Twenty hours later the skin was examined for the presence of mites, and 100 mites were recovered from 21 persons. The mites were all identified as *L. scutellare* (Arai, 1955).

Under almost the same conditions, 67 and 83 bites each were found on two researchers after they had collected *L. scutellare* in a mite habitat on Hachijo Island for 2 h daily for 2 consecutive days (Sasa, 1959); this finding indicated that many inhabitants in the area of *L. scutellare* may have been bitten by these mites without noticing it.

In the Izu Peninsula, 30 unfed larvae of *L. pallidum*, *L. fuji*, and *L.*

Table 7. Trombiculid Mites That Bite Humans in Japan

Species	Natural conditions	Experimental infestation
Leptotrombidium akamushi		
	Niigata Prefecture	
	Asakawa and Miyajima, 1905	Obata and Aoki, 1958
	Ukai, 1906	Ito and Obata, 1961
	Hayashi, 1906, 1907, 1909	Takahashi *et al.*, 1991b
	Miyajima, 1908	
	Kawamura *et al.*, 1920	
	Kawamura, 1925	
	Katsura, 1953	
	Yamagata Prefecture	
	Nagayo *et al.*, 1920	
	Akita Prefecture	
	Kitaoka *et al.*, 1974	
L. scutellare		
	Hachijo Island (Tokyo)	
	Kitaoka *et al.*, 1953a	Kitaoka *et al.*, 1953a
	Asanuma *et al.*, 1958	Sasa *et al.*, 1953
	Sasa, 1959	Hayashi and Tanaka, 1955
	Kitaoka, 1959	Arai, 1955
	Tamiya, 1962	Toriyama *et al.*, 1988
	Nagasaki Prefecture	
	Toriyama *et al.*, 1988	
L. pallidum pallidum		
	Hachijo Island (Tokyo)	Kitaoka *et al.*, 1953b
	Tamiya, 1962	
	Niigata Prefecture	
	Kawamura, 1926	
L. pallidum burnsi		
	Hachijo Island (Tokyo)	
	Suzuki *et al.*, 1958	
L. palpale		
	Niigata Prefecture	
	Kawamura, 1926	
Eutrombicula wichmanni		
	Hachijo-Koshima (Tokyo)	
	Sasa and Kano, 1950	
	Sasa *et al.*, 1958	
	Kuroshima Island (Kagoshima Prefecture)	
	Kitahara, 1952	
Schoengastia hanmyaensis		
	Amami Island (Kagoshima Prefecture)	
	Suzuki, 1976	

kitasatoi, collected by the black plate method, were placed on the forearm of a volunteer researcher. The mites that bit the skin were *L. pallidum* (8 mites), and the researcher was infected with Tsutsugamushi disease after 15 days; however, *R. tsutsugamushi* was not isolated in the engorged mites (Kitaoka *et al.*, 1953a). In one of the above-mentioned researchers who was severely bitten by *L. scutellare* on Hachijo Island, a larva of *L. pallidum burnsi* was also collected (Suzuki *et al.*, 1958).

However, the clinical signs resulting from the bites of *L. pallidum*, *L. intermedium*, and *S. hanmyaensis* are generally very mild, and people hardly notice their bites. In experimental infestation with *L. pallidum* and *L. intermedium*, mild skin reactions lasted for several days and the mites dropped off. In allergic persons, however, an itchy exanthem persisted for more than a month after the bite of *L. pallidum*. Infestations of *E. wichmanni*, appearing on the islands of Hachijo and Aogashima (Tokyo) and Kuroshima, Kagoshima Prefecture, are widespread in rats, birds, and small lizards, and this mite also causes severe bites in humans in the summer. The inhabitants of these areas suffer from itchy papules caused by the bite of this mite, these being more painful than those caused by *L. scutellare*. The bites of this mite have been known in these areas for many years. As there has been no record of Tsutsugamushi disease in this season, this species is not considered to be associated with the transmission of Tsutsugamushi disease, although the itch caused by its bites is severe (Sasa, 1956). Once, by chance, a researcher was bitten by *S. hanmyaensis* while he was collecting the mites in the nest of a white-faced Shearwater, *Colonectris leucomelas* (Suzuki, 1976). This bite did not appear to be associated with the transmission of *R. tsutsugamushi*.

c. *Species harboring* R. tsutsugamushi *but not biting humans*

There has been no report so far of *L. kawamurai* biting humans. In Hokkaido, the positive rate of *R. tsutsugamushi* in this species was as high as 2.05% (Asanuma, 1983), and *R. tsutsugamushi* was also detected at a high rate in wild rodents in the season during which *L. kawamurai* was prevalent (Takahashi *et al.*, 1981). Since this species is regarded as a potential transmitter to humans, the species should be observed more carefully whether it bites humans.

d. Duration of feeding and feeding ratio of infesting mites

In experimental infestations of *L. akamushi* and *L. scutellare* on human skin, the time taken after mites are placed on the skin until they start feeding is about 1 h. The reported duration of feeding is approximately 30–60 h, *i.e.*, 2–3 days, this duration varying somewhat depending on the species (Arai, 1955; Kitaoka, 1959; Obata and Aoki, 1958; Takahashi *et al.*, 1991b; Toriyama *et al.*, 1988). This feeding period is similar to that reported in experimental animals such as the rat and the mouse (Asanuma, 1959; Takahashi *et al.*, 1991b).

In human subjects exposed to *L. akamushi*, Obata and Aoki (1958) and Takahashi *et al.* (1991b) found that the feeding ratio, *i.e.*, the number of mites feeding/number of mites placed on skin, were 42.9% (15/35) and 15.2% (5/33), respectively. These ratios for *L. scutellare* were 20.0% (3/15), 15.0% (9/60), 17.5% (64/336) and 40.0% (8/20), as determined by Kitaoka *et al.* (1953a), Sasa *et al.* (1953), Hayashi and Tanaka (1955), and Toriyama *et al.* (1988), respectively.

e. Regions on body surface bitten by mites

The regions on the body surface that were bitten by larval trombiculid mites were studied mainly with *L. akamushi* in areas endemic for classical Tsutsugamushi disease and with *L. scutellare* on Hachijo Island, since the biting sites of these mites were well identified by the painful or itchy skin sensation. The regions bitten were similar, regardless of the mite species and the presence or absence of *R. tsutsugamushi* in the mite (Katsura, 1953; Sasa, 1956).

The regions bitten were frequently the folds of soft skin in the axilla, upper leg, and abdominal skin, but bites were not limited to these regions, occurring also in other regions, *e.g.*, the head and the lower and upper extremities (Arai, 1955; Asakawa and Miyajima, 1905; Ito and Obata, 1961; Katsura, 1953; Kawamura, 1926; Kitaoka, 1959; Sasa, 1956; Ukai, 1906). In an experimental infestation in human volunteers, the mites released on the arm became attached to the skin in the axilla and on the abdomen (Takahashi *et al.*, 1991b).

The number of sites bitten by *L. akamushi* was studied by Katsura (1953) in Niigata Prefecture, who found that 87.6% (247/282) of all victims had one site, and the maximal number of bites on a person was seven. Other researchers reported similar observations (Asakawa and Miyajima, 1905; Kitaoka, 1959; Miyajima, 1908; Ukai, 1906). In a mite habitat on Hachijo Island, the number of sites bitten by *L. scutellare* was mostly in the range of 1–3 among children living there and in subjects voluntarily exposed to the mites (Arai, 1955; Tamiya, 1962).

f. Ratio of infecting bites to the total number of bites

Since the sites bitten by *L. akamushi* are readily observed due to the characteristic pain, and inapparent infection due to the bite of *L. akamushi* is rare, the ratio of infecting bites, recognized by eschar formation and the onset of Tsutsugamushi disease, to the total number of painful bites has been well studied. This ratio also corresponds with the ratio of *R. tsutsugamushi*-positive mites to the total number of mites. Therefore, the *R. tsutsugamushi*-positive ratio of *L. akamushi* was well known for many years before the causative agent of Tsutsugamushi disease was identified. The infection rate observed by early research, and by one more recent group, varies from 2.0% to 11.7% (Table 8).

An early report by Asakawa and Miyajima (1905) of observation at the Agano river basin in Niigata Prefecture showed that the bites of the red mite (*L. akamushi*) began in June and peaked in July and

Table 8. Early Reports and a More Recent Report in Japan of the Relationship between *R. tsutsugamushi* Infection and Bites of *L. akamushi* in Humans

Prefecture	No. of subjects bitten	No. of mites recovered	No. of patients	Infection rate (%)	References
Niigata	24	13	1	4.2	Asakawa and Miyajima, 1905
Niigata	14	19	0	0	Ukai, 1906
Niigata	30	50	1	2.0	Hayashi,1906
Niigata	—	30	0	0	Hayashi, 1907
Niigata	212[a]	50	17	8.0	Hayashi, 1909
	365[a]	50	29	7.9	Hayashi 1909
Niigata	36	28	2	5.6	Miyajima, 1908
Niigata	—	33	1	3.0	Kawamura, *et al.*, 1920
Yamagata	—	37	—	0	Nagayo *et al.*, 1920
Akita	386	93	45	11.7	Kitaoka *et al.*, 1974

[a] Number of sites bitten.

August. These investigators collected 13 red mites from 24 human subjects who had been bitten and found that only one of the 24 manifested Tsutsugamushi disease. This finding demonstrated, for the first time, the presence of harmless red mites that were not bearing the causative agent of Tsutsugamushi disease. In contrast, Hayashi (1906) and Miyajima (1908) found that when the bitten site from which a red mite had been removed developed into a small ulcer and formed an eschar, then the victim manifested Tsutsugamushi disease. By this experience, the red mite was determined to be the transmitter of the disease.

In more recent years, Kitaoka *et al.* (1974) clearly demonstrated the relationship between the bite of *L. akamushi* and the development of Tsutsugamushi disease. In Akita Prefecture, during the period from 1956 to 1970, 93 red mites were recovered from 386 human subjects who had been bitten. Of these 93 mites, 87 that were identified were all *L. akamushi*. Of the 386 subjects, 45 (11.7%) developed Tsutsugamushi disease, and each had only one eschar. Of seven subjects who had only one biting site from which *L. akamushi* was removed, one manifested Tsutsugamushi disease 10 days after removal of the mite, confirming that *L. akamushi* was the transmitter of the disease. The infection rate of *L. akamushi* in this study was 2.5% (11/446), close to the 2.3% (10/435) infection rate reported in the mites recovered from wild rodents in neighboring areas (Kitaoka *et al.*, 1974).

g. Mite species biting humans in countries other than Japan

Many species of mites that bite humans have been reported in other parts of the world. Similarly to *E. wichmanni*, a mite that causes severe bites in humans in Japan, chiggers belonging to the genera *Eutrombicula*, *Neotrombicula*, or *Schoengastia* also cause itchy bites, and it seems significant that those species involved in biting humans normally infest birds or reptiles rather than mammals (Audy, 1951, 1968). Mites belonging to the genus *Eutrombicula* that cause severe bites in humans are widespread in both North and South America. In Europe, *Neotrombicula autumnalis*, the harvest mite, is well known to cause severe bites in humans. Biting mites are found worldwide, although those in Africa are not well known; 46 species belonging to 13 genera have been reported (Table 9).

In Southeast Asia, vector mites such as *L. fletcheri* and *L. deliense*

Table 9. Mite Species That Bite Humans: Geographic Distribution Outside Japan

Species	Locality	References
Acomatacarus barrinensis	Australia	Wharton and Fuller, 1952
A. australiensis	Australia	Wharton and Fuller, 1952 Clifford, 1983
Apolonia tigipioense	Brazil	Wharton and Fuller,1952
Blankaartia acuscutellaris	Southeast Pacific region	Wharton and Fuller, 1952 Vercammen-Grandjiean, 1968; Wen, 1984
Euschoengastia guyanensis	South America	Wharton and Fuller, 1952
Eus. nunezi	Mexico	Wharton and Fuller, 1952 Fuller, 1952
Eutrombicula alfreddugesi	South and North America	Wharton and Fuller, 1952 Fuller, 1952 Clifford, 1983
E. batatas	South and North America	Wharton and Fuller, 1952 Fuller, 1952 Clifford, 1983
E. belkini	North America	Wharton and Fuller, 1952
E. goldii	Brazil, Colombia, Panama	Wharton and Fuller, 1952 Fuller, 1952
E. hirsti	Southeast Pacific region	Wharton and Fuller, 1952 Domrow and Lester, 1985
E. lahillei	Argentina	Wharton and Fuller, 1952
E. samboni	Australia	Wharton and Fuller, 1952 Fuller, 1952 Domrow and Lester, 1985 Clifford, 1983
E. sarcina	Australia	Wharton and Fuller, 1952 Clifford, 1983 Domrow and Lester, 1985
E. splendens	North America	Wharton and Fuller, 1952 Clifford, 1983
E. wichmanni	Southeast Pacific region	Wharton and Fuller, 1952 Fuller, 1952; Vercammen-Grandjiean, 1968; Wen, 1984; Clifford, 1983

E. vanommereni	New Guinea	Fuller, 1952
Gahrliepia ligula	Southeast Asia	Traub and Wisseman, 1974b
Helenicula kohlsi	China	Wen, 1984
Leptotrombidium deliense	Southeast Pacific region	Walch and Keukenschrijver, 1924a,b; Philip *et al.*, 1949; Wharton and Fuller, 1952; Fuller, 1952; Audy, 1961; Traub and Wisseman, 1968b, 1974b Shirai *et al.*, 1982b; Wen, 1984; Domrow and Lester, 1985
L. keukenschrijveri	Indonesia	Wharton and Fuller, 1952; Walch and Morawa, 1924
L. pallidum	Korea	Wharton and Fuller, 1952; Traub and Wisseman, 1974b
L. scutellare	China	Wharton and Fuller, 1952; Wen, 1984
L. fletcheri	Southeast Pacific region	Philip *et al.*, 1949; Fuller, 1952; Audy, 1961; Traub and Wisseman, 1968b, 1974b; Shirai *et al.*, 1982d
L. subintermedium	Pakistan	Traub and Wisseman, 1974b
L. arenicola	Malaysia	Traub and Wisseman, 1974b; Shirai *et al.*, 1982d
L. gaohuensis	China	Wei *et al.*, 1985c; Wei *et al.*, 1987
Neotrombicula autumnalis	Europe	Wharton and Fuller, 1952; Fuller,1952 Clifford, 1983
N. mackayensis	Australia	Domrow and Lester, 1985
N. japonica	Primorye	Shubin *et al.*, 1970
N. mitamurai	Primorye	Shubin *et al.*, 1970

N. pomeranzevi	Kuriles	Shubin *et al.*, 1970
N. desaleri	Austria	Fuller, 1952
Odontacarus australiensis	Southeast Pacific region	Wharton and Fuller, 1952; Fuller, 1952
Schoengastia schueffneri	New Guinea	Wharton and Fuller, 1952; Fuller, 1952; Clifford, 1983
S. vandersandei	New Guinea	Wharton and Fuller, 1952; Fuller, 1952 Vercammen-Grandjiean, 1968; Clifford, 1983
S. katonis	Palau	Wharton and Fuller, 1952; Fuller, 1952
S. blestowei	New Guinea	Blake *et al.*, 1945
S. pusilla	New Guinea	Blake *et al.*, 1945
S. psorakari	Southeast Pacific region	Vercammen-Grandjiean, 1968; Clifford, 1983
Trombicula canis	South America	Wharton and Fuller, 1952
T. japa	Peru	Wharton and Fuller, 1952
T. landazuri	South America	Wharton and Fuller, 1952
T. rara	Indonesia	Walch and Morawa, 1924; Wharton and Fuller, 1952
T. buloloensis	New Guinea	Blake *et al.*, 1945
Walchiella oudemansi	India, New Guinea, Sumatra	Fuller, 1952

have been known to cause severe bites in humans since the time that early researchers were attempting to identify vector mites, using human volunteers who were exposed in fields in Malaysia (Audy, 1961; Philip *et al.*, 1949; Shirai *et al.*, 1982d; Smadel *et al.*, 1949, 1950; Traub and Frick, 1950; Traub and Wissemann, 1974b).

In general, however, members of the subgenus *Leptotrombidium*, which ordinarily infest small mammals, do not cause severe itching in humans. This has been noted for *L. deliense*, *L. fletcheri* (Fuller,

1952; Philip *et al.*, 1949; Traub and Wisseman, 1968b; Walch and Keukenschrijver, 1924a,b), *L. arenicola*, and *L. subintermedium* (Traub and Wisseman, 1974b).

The sites bitten in humans by the above-mentioned mites are areas of soft skin; as with mites in Japan, the body regions bitten are described as the webs between the fingers, the popliteal area behind the knee, folds of skin of the genitalia or "abdomen," the skin under the breasts, and skin beneath areas that are constricted by clothing such as garters, belts, or brassieres (Philip *et al.*, 1949).

3. Rearing and Life History

a. Rearing of trombiculid mites

1) History of laboratory rearing

The laboratory rearing of trombiculid mites is important for elucidating the behaviors of vector mites, such as seasonal development, reproduction, longevity, and other features, since these behaviors are closely associated with the seasonal prevalence of human Tsutsugamushi disease. Research of biological and medical importance is required to elucidate morphological differences at each stage in the various species; differences in the responses of mites to such environmental factors as temperature, humidity, and length of daytime; and the vertical and horizontal transmission of *R. tsutsugamushi*. These features have been studied by the successful rearing of succeeding generations.

The life cycle of trombiculid mites was first clarified by the studies of Miyajima and Okumura (1916), Nagayo *et al.* (1916), and R. Kawamura and Yamaguchi (1916). Despite their important discovery of the life cycle of the mites — *i.e.*, their development from egg to larva, nymph, and adult — the fundamental biological characteristics of reproduction and longevity were not understood, because the feeding habits of the free-living stages of nymphs and adults living in the soil were not known at that time.

The key issue in successful laboratory rearing was the discovery of the most appropriate food for the mites. Many types of feed have been used since Ewing's attempts (1944), as shown in Table 10. In the first attempts, the feces of springtails, millipedes, or chickens was mixed with soil as nutrients and a few adult mites were raised by this means; however researchers were not successful in rearing succeeding generations of trombiculid mites at this time (Ewing, 1944;

Melvin, 1946; Michener, 1946a).

Wharton and Carver (1946) were successful in rearing *Eushoengastia indica* to the adult stage by giving the eggs of mosquitoes and *Drosophila* to deutonymphs as soon as they emerged, and Jayewickreme and Niles (1946), Jenkins (1947) and others showed clearly that mites were successfully reared by feeding with mosquito eggs. Besides mosquito eggs, Lipovsky (1951) used collembolan eggs, successfully rearing 25 species, belonging to eight genera, to the adult stage.

Ito and Obata (1961) could not rear *L. pallidum* with mosquito egg feed, but had excellent results on feeding with the eggs of a dragonfly, *Sympetrum frequens*. They collected a large number of these eggs in autumn, stored the frozen eggs and used them after thawing, the whole year round. This method, however, was not practical, since they encountered serious difficulties in collecting and storing the eggs until the following autumn, and if the frozen eggs deteriorated once, the whole mite population was damaged.

Takahashi *et al.* have been utilizing collembolan eggs since 1988 (Table 10), and many species of the genus *Leptotrombidium* were reared successfully due to the simplicity of culturing collembola and the continuous availability of fresh eggs the whole year round. *Gahrliepia saduski*, however, did not eat collembolan eggs but ate the just-hatched larvae. *Helenicula miyagawai*, which infests the wild hare at very high rates, ate neither collembolan eggs nor the hatching larvae. Thus the feeding habits of mites differ depending on the species (Takahashi *et al.*, 1986b).

Many types of containers have been used for rearing trombiculid mites: a wide-mouth bottle approximately half full of soil (Melvin, 1946), a filter paper cell (Jones, 1950), a hollow glass block containing damp cellulose wadding (Jayewickreme and Niles, 1946), and bottles lined on the bottom with a thick layer of plaster of Paris to which charcoal has been added (Wharton and Carver, 1946).

Various jars and vials have been used that contained modified plaster of Paris to which charcoal powder had been added (Hyland, 1951, 1961; Jenkins, 1947; Lipovsky *et al.*, 1957; Michener, 1946a; Sasa and Miura, 1953; Takahashi *et al.*, 1986b, 1988a, 1993a).

At the Institute for Medical Research in Malaysia, mass culture was achieved in small unglazed clay pots placed on a shelf. The bottoms of the pots were kept moist by placing them on a strip of wet

Table 10. Feed Used for Rearing Nymphs and Adults of Chigger Mites in the Laboratory

Authors	Type of feed
Ewing, 1944	Feces of springtails and millipedes
Melvin, 1946; Michener, 1946a	Chicken manure
Wharton and Carver, 1946	Eggs of mosquitoes (*Culex quinquefasciatus, C. jepsoni,* and *Aedes aegypti*), flour beetles (*Tribolium* sp.) and flies (*Drosophila*)
Jayewickreme and Niles, 1946	Eggs of mosquitoes (*Mansonia uniformis*, *Anopheles subpictus*, and *A. vagus*)
Jenkins, 1947	Eggs of mosquitoes (*Anopheles albimanus* and *Aedes aegypti*)
Jones, 1950, 1951	Mixture of moist chicken feces, agar, yeast, and molasses
	Exuded contents of the eggs of *Aedes aegypti*
Lipovsky, 1951; Lipovsky *et al.*, 1957	Collembolan eggs
Sasa and Miura, 1953	Eggs of mosquito (*Culex pipiens*)
Hsu, 1959	Eggs of mosquitoes, fruit flies, fleas, and springtails
Miura, 1960	Eggs of mosquitoes (*Culex* and *Aedes*), dragonflies, and collembola
Neal and Barnett, 1961	Eggs of collembola (*Sinella curviseta*)
Ito and Obata, 1961	Eggs of mosquito (*Culex*) and dragonfly (*Sympetrum frequens*)
Wang *et al.*, 1965	Eggs of flea (*Xenopsylla cheopis*)
Shirasaka and Sasa, 1967	Eggs of colembolla
Nadchatram, 1968	Eggs of mosquitoes (*Culex fatigans*) and collembola (*Sinella curviseta*)
Rapmund *et al.*, 1969	Eggs of mosquito
Roberts *et al.*, 1977	Eggs of mosquito (*Culex fatigans*)
Roberts and Robinson, 1977	Eggs of mosquito (*Culex fatigans*)
Liao *et al.*, 1981	Eggs of flea (*Leptopsylla segnis*)
Takahashi *et al.*, 1986b	Larvae of collembola (*Sinella curviseta*)
Takahashi *et al.*, 1988b,c	Eggs of collembola (*Sinella curviseta*)

filter paper the other end of which was submerged in water in a large Petri dish under the shelf (Dohany *et al.*, 1977; Nadchatram, 1968; Roberts and Robinson, 1977; Roberts *et al.*, 1977;).

2) Rearing methods

Although each group of researchers may have their own methods for rearing trombiculid mites, we have found the methods described below, those improved and employed by Takahashi *et al.* (1988b, Table 10), successful for rearing *L. akamushi*, *L. pallidum*, *L. intermedium*, *L. fletcheri*, *L. arenicola*, *L. deliense*, *L. fuji*, *L. scutellare*, *L. miyazakii*, *L. miyajimai*, *Eltonella ichikawai*, and *Gahrliepia saduski*. Strains of the first six of the above species have been maintained in the laboratory.

(a) Containers

A plastic vial 60 mm in diameter and 37 mm high with a tightly sealed lid was used. A mixture of plaster of Paris and active charcoal (9 : 1) was moistened with water and placed at the bottom of the vial to a depth of 5 mm. After the plaster had hardened, the containers were closed tightly by placing a sheet of pharmaceutical wrapping paper between the vial and lid to prevent the mites from escaping as well as to retard or prevent the loss of moisture. Since larvae often enter holes and become lost, or die in cracks between the edge of the substrate and the vial wall, these cracks are carefully filled with the plaster mixture.

While the mites are being cultured, the plaster mixture begins to dry out; its color changes from near-black to gray. Whenever this occurs, a few drops of distilled water are added to prevent the culture from drying out and to keep the inside of the container humid enough. Tiny water droplets that condense on the vial wall and fungus proliferating on the surface of the substrate are cleaned off with a fine paint brush.

(b) Culture procedure

Eight to ten fully engorged larvae in a group were placed in a culture vial. When larvae climbed up the vial wall and formed a cluster, they were returned to the substrate, using a paint brush.

The engorged larvae in the vial stop moving and develop into the protonymph within several days. Daily observation is necessary for the maintenance of the protonymph; water is added to moisten the substrate and to remove fungus, which is harmful to the mites and tends to proliferate easily around immobile protonymphs and on the substrate.

Deutonymphs shed from the protonymphs should be transferred daily to new culture vials; otherwise, the deutonymphs eat the protonymphs. Deutonymphs are given fresh, shiny, round collembola eggs (five eggs per mite). Old collembola eggs distorted before hatching should not be given to the mites. The remaining collembolan eggs and other debris should be removed every day, and the paper between the vial and lid replaced. Any torn paper is also replaced; otherwise deutonymphs enter the slit, are trapped in the narrow space, and die.

When deutonymphs develop into immobile tritonymphs, the latter are transferred into a new culture vial and are maintained in the same way as the protonymphs.

When an adult casts off the tritonymph, it is transferred into a new vial. In one vial, ten adults are reared, at an approximate ratio of four males to six females. Fresh collembolan eggs are given to the adult mites at a daily rate of ten eggs per adult, or more when necessary, and the vials are kept clean, as they are for the rearing of the deutonymph. Water droplets should be removed to prevent the mites from drowning.

Males lay spermatophores along cleavages of the substrate or on the vial wall. In mating experiments, only males are kept in a culture vial at first; after the spermatophores have been deposited, appropriate females are placed in the same vial. The females lay eggs after about 10 days.

To determine the sex of the adult mite, the mite is placed, lying on its back, in the depression of a depressed glass slide. A cover slip is placed over the mite, which is observed under a microscope with $40\times$ magnification. The presence of male genital setae (Jenkins, 1949; Wharton and Fuller, 1952; Wormersley, 1952) distinguishes males from females. *L. akamushi* have four pairs of male genital setae, and *L. pallidum* have three pairs.

Newly laid eggs of trombiculid mites are round, with a shiny surface. After one week their shape changes; they develop into the deutovum stage, and then become cone-shaped and orange-colored on one side. Eggs of this shape are in the stage immediately before hatching. About 100 eggs of this stage are harvested and transferred to a clean container to prepare for hatching.

(c) Larvae after hatching

After hatching, the larvae form a cluster in a cleavage of the substrate or at the corner of the lower surface of the lid, and they remain still. *L. scutellare* form tighter aggregations in a cluster than *L. akamushi* and *L. pallidum*.

If the lid of the vial is opened carelessly, the larvae start moving actively, stimulated by human breath, and easily escape from the vial beyond the control of the researcher, who is thus exposed to a high risk of bites at this time.

The mites immediately after hatching do not bite an animal host, possibly due to the accumulation of nutrients in the body; they appear to aggressively bite after 2 weeks.

(d) Methods of attaching unfed larvae to host animal

For unfed larvae of the genus *Leptotrombidium*, hairy ddY mice have generally been used as an appropriate experimental host for the attachment of unfed larvae. These mice are not always appropriate hosts, however, being poor hosts for common pest species such as *Eutrombicula alfreddugesi* and *E. splendens*, whereas hamsters make fairly satisfactory hosts (Wharton and Fuller, 1952).

To transfer larvae to the mouse ear, 100 unfed larvae are placed on the water surface in a Petri dish. The floating larvae gradually gather to form a cluster. The extremities of a ddY mouse are pinched loosely with laundry clips and the mouse is fixed by the abdomen to a small board and placed under a stereomicroscope.

The ear lobe is turned inside out, and a loop made of 2 cm of cotton thread is placed in the deeper portion of the inner auricle. A cluster of mites on the water surface is transferred, with a fine paint brush, into the middle of the looped thread.

Water is absorbed by the cotton thread, enabling the mites to bite the skin readily. Larvae two weeks after hatching are an appropriate age to be attached to the mouse skin; and with the above-mentioned procedures, most larvae bite within 30 min. The appropriate number of larvae to release in one ear lobe is about 100.

To prevent the larvae from escaping from the inner auricle, immediately after they are released inside the loop, the ear lobe is rolled along the long axis and sealed with cellophane tape, leaving the top portion open. If the auricle is completely sealed, the inside becomes wet and all the larvae will die.

In another method of transferring larvae, a fine wooden stick is sharpened to make a spatula, and this is used in place of the fine paint brush. Instead of using the mouse ear as the site of attachment, the fur on the back is shaved and larvae are enclosed in a capsule made of various materials. For attachment to the mouse, in some cases a capsule was made from the end of a toothpaste tube; in others it was made of glass, which allowed for continuous observation of the attached chiggers (Baker *et al.*, 1968). Some workers use Nembutal for anesthetizing the mice while attaching unfed larvae. However, it is not easy to control the dosage so as to keep the mouse alive in an appropriate condition.

(e) Recovery of engorged larvae from the mouse

The mice to which the larvae are attached are kept in an incubator at 25°C; the cellophane tape is removed after 6 h, and the fixed extremities are released after 4 more h. If the mouse scratches its ear, since the foot pads are swollen, the larvae are not scratched off. Each mouse is placed in a stainless wire cage (50 × 45 × 8 mm) that is set on a large Petri dish half full of water (Takahashi *et al.*, 1990a), and fed with fresh mouse pellets and water. Fully engorged larvae falling on the surface of the water are collected with a paint brush and placed in a rearing container. Although the period during which the larvae feed on the mouse is only 2–3 days, it takes about 7 days until no more larvae fall down onto the water. Most of the larvae released in the ear lobe are collected by this process.

3) Life cycle

(a) Discovery of life cycle

The life cycle of *L. akamushi* was first observed by releasing engorged larvae on the soil surface in a container, and was confirmed by observations of the development from one stage to the next, made nearly simultaneously by Miyajima and Okumura (1916), Nagayo *et al.* (1916), and Kawamura and Yamaguchi (1916). Later, the development of *L. pallidum* was observed by R. Kawamura (1940), who used a flowerpot with soil for observation, and its life cycle was shown to be the same as that of *L. akamushi*.

Improvements in methods for the laboratory rearing of trombiculid mites (Ewing, 1944; Jenkins, 1947; Melvin, 1946; Michener, 1946a; Wharton and Carver, 1946) led to clarification of the life cycle of the harvest mite, *Eutrombicula autumnalis* (= *Neotrombicula autumnalis*) and that of many other species of mite (Fuller, 1952; Jayewickreme and Niles, 1946; Melvin, 1946; Michener, 1946c; Wharton, 1946; Wharton and Fuller, 1952; Wormersley, 1952). The discovery of the spermatophore and the elucidation of its morphology by Lipovsky *et al.* (1957) was a noteworthy contribution to the study of the trombiculid mites; by elucidating the method of fertilization, which had hitherto been unknown, Lipovsky *et al.* (1957) found that these mites did not mate directly but that a peculiar indirect insemination occurred by which the male laid spermatopheres on the substrate and the female took these in for fertilization. This process was found in *Eutrombicula splendens* in North America, and in four other species, including *L. pallidum*, in South Korea. Later, Wen (1958, 1959) reported the indirect mating process and the process of transferring the spermatophore in *Acomatacarus yosanoi*.

In Japan, *L. akamushi* and a few other species were reared in the laboratory (Ito and Obata, 1961; Sasa and Miura, 1953; Shirasaka and Sasa, 1967; Takahashi *et al.*, 1988b). Three important species which are vectors to humans, *L. akamushi*, *L. pallidum*, and *L. scutellare*, have been successfully reared in culture vials exposed to a natural outdoor climate the whole year round (Takahashi *et al.*, 1993a, 1994b, 1995); and the seasons for oviposition and hatching, the speed of development, and the stage that survives in the winter have been elucidated.

(b) Morphological characteristics of each stage

The life cycle of trombiculid mites observed in culture vials is shown in Fig. 2 of Chapter 3, and the morphological characteristics of each stage are summarized in Table 11. The life cycle is classified into seven stages: egg, unfed larva, engorged larva, protonymph, deutonymph, tritonymph, and adult (Goff *et al.*, 1982).

Egg : Eggs immediately after oviposition are spherical. As the egg develops, the eggshell is separated into halves, and the germinal cells encapsulated by the inner egg membrane are exposed to the exterior. This developed stage of the egg is the deutovum.

Unfed larva: Larvae immediately after hatching have three pairs of legs and move around actively.

Engorged larva: Unfed larvae infest the host animal and feed on it. They have three pairs of legs and move slowly. After becoming engorged on the body fluid of the host, they become detached from it.

Protonymph: Engorged larvae become static; at this stage, four pairs of legs develop inside the integument. Molting starts at the end of this stage.

Deutonymph: In this stage shedding from the protonymph occurs; the deutonymph has four pairs of legs, is motile, and actively eats collembolan eggs.

Tritonymph: This is a static stage after the deutonymph has become motionless. At the end of this stage, an adult with four pairs of legs emerges by molting.

Table 11. Characteristic Features of Developmental Stages in the Life Cycle of Trombiculid Mites

Stage	Characteristic features
Egg	Spherical; laid singly on moist soil; many small pits on the surface
Deutovum	Quiescent in the egg membrane after the egg shell is broken; dorsal spine; no setae; unsegmented legs
Larva	
Unfed larva	Active; six legs; setae on the body and legs
Engorged larva	Active; fully engorged with the hosts body fluid; six legs; setae on the body and legs
Protonymph[a]	Quiescent; found in the dead larval integument; four pairs of leg sheaths; dorsal spine; unsegmented legs; no setae
Deutonymph	Active; eight legs; numerous plumosa setae on the body; two pairs of genital suckers
Tritonymph[a]	Quiescent; found in the dead deutonymphal integument; four pairs of leg sheaths; dorsal spine; unsegmented legs; no setae
Adult	Active; eight legs; many plumosa setae on the body; three pairs of genital suckers; large gnathosoma

[a] Resting stages.

Adult: This is the sexual stage after the second molting. The adult moves actively and eats collembolan eggs. The male deposits spermatophores; the female takes these into her body for indirect fertilization, then lays eggs.

Parthenogenesis has been reported in *L. arenicola* (Kaufman and Traub, 1966). This was the first such report for a trombiculid mite, and the progeny were found to be either male or female. Adult mites which shed from the females with a split at the posterodorsal integument tended to be male adults (Mitchell and Nadchatram, 1969).

An exceptional life cycle has been reported in *Babiangia* (*Vatacarus*) *ipoides*, which infests the air sac of the sea snake. In this mite, the active nymphal stage (deutonymph in other species) is bypassed, and larvae give rise to adults with only a single intermediate molting stage. Lavae of two sizes emerge; small bright orange larvae develope into males, and large light orange ones into females. This suggests that sex differentiation is determined at the larval stage, although this is not apparent in the other trombiculid species (Nadchatram and Audy, 1965).

(c) Behavioral characteristics of some stages

Females of *L. pallidum* lay individual eggs separately in the tiny pores or in the cleavage of the substrate. The same distribution of laying eggs was observed in *L. fuji* and *G. saduski*, in *Trombicula alleei* (Michener, 1946c), in *Ascoshoengastia indica* (Wharton, 1946), in *L. akamushi* (Ito and Obata, 1961; Sasa and Miura, 1953), and in *L. fletcheri*, *L. deliense*, and *L. arenicola* in Malaysia (Neal and Barnett, 1961). On the other hand, clusters of 25 and 50 eggs have been observed in *T. attenuata*, and sometimes in the above listed species (Michener, 1946c).

The shape of eggs immediately after oviposition is usually spherical, irrespective of species. However, in *Guntherana kallipygos* the egg is wider on both sides (Wharton and Fuller, 1952).

The color of the eggs differs according to species, being light yellow in *L. pallidum*, *L. fuji*, *L. intermedium*, *L. deliense*, and *L. arenicola*; white in *G. saduski*; and orange in *L. akamushi* and *L. fletcheri*; the coloration appears to be similar to that of the adult. Such coloration of adult mites is closely associated with the surrounding environment, and the color is, to a great extent, dependent on the biotope of the mites (Nadchatram, 1970).

In many species in Japan, and in *Ascoschoengastia indica* (Wharton, 1946), *E. splendens*, *E. alfreddugesi*, and *E. batatus* (Jenkins, 1947), the egg develops into a cone-shaped deutovum.

Immediately after hatching, the larvae become active as the body surface dries. The longevity of unfed larvae differs depending on the species; at temperatures below 25°C, it is about 1 month in *L. fletcheri*, *L. deliense*, *L. arenicola*, and *L. akamushi*; 4–5 months in *L. pallidum*; approximately 6 months in *L. intermedium*; and several months in *L. scutellare*. Once the larvae bite the host, they continue sucking the body fluid until they are completely engorged. In a rare case, with *L. akamushi*, two feedings on the host were observed (Kawamura, R. and Ikeda, 1936).

The feeding period also differs according to the species. It is short, 2–4 days, in *L. akamushi* and the Malaysian species, such as *L. fletcheri*, *L. deliense*, and *L. arenicola*; generally 3–5 days in *L. pallidum*, *L. intermedium*, and *L. fuji*; and longer, 4–7 days, in *G. saduski*. It has also been reported that *A. indica* fed on a rat for as long as 10–32 days (Wharton, 1946). The structure of the stylostome appears to be a factor in the differences in feeding periods.

Unfed larvae in a culture vial form clusters of 50 to 100 individuals in a pore of the substrate. When the lid is opened, the larvae start moving, especially under light, showing negative phototaxis. Tanaka *et al.* (1955) found that the cluster-forming larvae of *L. scutellare* did not start moving on stimulation by light or sound, or when the substrate was turned upside down if they were not exposed to human breath. These investigators then confirmed that the stimulant was carbon dioxide in the expired human breath.

All stages, from engorged larvae to adults, stay in clusters in the cleavages or pores in the substrate in vials. In the natural environment, they would also stay in clusters in similar conditions, such as under fallen leaves or in rotting wood. Even with a Tullgren funnel, collecting mites in the soil is not easy, especially in the immobile stages, the protonymphs and tritonymphs (Takahashi, 1988a). A new method is necessary for collecting the free-living phase in the soil.

(d) Temperature and speed of development

An outbreak of Tsutsugamushi disease is closely associated with the size of the population of newly hatching larvae. Therefore, the speed at which the mites develop, the number of times that larvae hatch in a year, and the number of generations arising in a year are important behavioral factors in the endemicity of Tsutsugamushi disease.

It has long been known that various environmental factors limit the reproductive period of the mites. The limiting factors are probably temperature in temperate climates and humidity in tropical climates (Wharton and Fuller, 1952). In laboratory rearing, temperature is the most important factor.

The entire life cycle from larvae to adults in most species can be repeated in the laboratory at temperatures of 23–28°C. At this temperature range, the higher the temperature, the shorter the duration of each developmental stage. At temperatures lower than 20°C, a long time is required for the mites to develop into the next stage even though they may be alive. The speed of development differs greatly for individual mites, some of which are unable to complete normal development (Table 12).

The time required for engorged larvae to develop into adults at

Table 12. Days Required for Metamorphosis of Trombiculid Mites Reared in the Laboratory at Various Temperatures

Species	Temperature (°C)	EL	PN	DN	TN	References
L. akamushi	23	18.4	14.0	27.2	15.0	Sasa and Miura, 1953
	28	7.3	8.3	25.3	8.3	Sasa and Miura, 1953
L. pallidum	15		32.0			Jameson, 1968
	20		13.4		14.0	Jameson, 1968
	23	15.8	15.8	11.2	27.0	Sasa and Miura, 1953
	25		9.3		11.8	Jameson, 1968
	25	17.6	12.8	25.2	12.7	Takahashi, 1987
	28			25.0	19.6	Liao *et al.*, 1981
	28	3–5	6–9	48.0		Sasa and Miura, 1953
	30		7.0		6.8	Jameson, 1968
L. scutellare	28	8.9	23.5	21.0	10.0	Sasa and Miura, 1953
	28			24.6	19.7	Liao *et al.*, 1981
L. fletcheri	27	4	9	14	10.0	Neal and Barnett, 1961
	NT			25.5	10.9	Dohany *et al.*, 1977
L. deliense	20		21.8			Jameson, 1968
	30		7.9			Jameson, 1968
L. fuji	10		190.0			Jameson, 1968
	15		38.1		34.8	Jameson, 1968
	20		14.0		17.3	Jameson, 1968
	23	29	18	29	16	Sasa and Miura, 1953
	25		10.2			Jameson, 1968
	30		7.9			Jameson, 1968
L. kitasatoi	28	9.5	6.5	21.6	13.2	Sasa and Miura, 1953
L. palpale	15		32.0		31.0	Jameson, 1968
	20		12.7		15.8	Jameson, 1968
	23	10.5	15.5			Sasa and Miura 1953
	25		8.9			Jameson, 1968
	28	7.8	10.0			Sasa and Miura, 1953
	30		7.6			Jameson, 1968
L. intermedium	25	5.6	8.9	12.9	11.8	Takahashi *et al.*, 1988c
	28	9.5	9.5	5.7	12.5	Sasa and Miura, 1953
L. miyazakii	10		101.5			Jameson, 1968
	15		25.9		29.0	Jameson, 1968
	20		15.2		16.1	Jameson, 1968
	25		10.6		18.2	Jameson, 1968
	25	3.6	11.8	27.9	19.3	Takahashi *et al.*, 1988c
	28	13	6		13	Sasa and Miura, 1953

	30		8.8			Jameson, 1968
L. miyajimai	20		25.7			Jameson, 1968
	25		19.8			Jameson, 1968
	28	9	13			Sasa and Miura, 1953
	30		10.3			Jameson, 1968
L. tenjin	23	27	19	39	19	Sasa and Miura, 1953
L. teramurai	23	13.5	12.0	26	16	Sasa and Miura, 1953
	28	7.0	10.0	35		Sasa and Miura, 1953
L. tosa	23–28	19.2	21.2	18.0	11.5	Sasa and Miura, 1953
G. saduski	20		18.0			Jameson, 1968
	23	16.0	23.5			Sasa and Miura, 1953
	25		14.0			Jameson, i968
	28	9	4			Sasa and Miura, 1953
	30		7.2			Jameson, 1968
E. masoni	25–30	2	6	9	6	Jenkins, 1947
E. alfreddugesi	25–30	2	6	11	7	Jenkins, 1947
E. batatas	25–30	2	6	15	6	Jenkins, 1947
E. wichmanni	23	21.1	9.9	20.4	8.8	Sasa and Miura, 1953
D. okabei	28	15	17			Sasa and Miura, 1953

NT, natural environmental temperatures; *L, Leptotrombidium*; *E, Eutrombicula*; *D, Doloisia*; *G, Gahrliepia*; EL, engorged larva; PN, protonymph; DN, deutonymph; TN, tritonymph.

23°C is 75 day for *L. akamushi*, 70 days for *L. pallidum*, and 92 days for *L. fuji* (Sasa and Miura, 1953). At 25°C, this duration is 68 days for *L. pallidum* and 39 days for *L. intermedium* (Takahashi, 1987; Takahashi *et al.*, 1988c). This duration in *L. fletcheri* colonies at 27°C is 37 days (Neal and Barnett, 1961), whereas the duration in infected colonies at 25.6°C averages 54 days (Dohany *et al.*, 1977).

The high speed of development at the higher temperature indicates that in humid tropical and subtropical areas, mites develop in an unsynchronized manner, producing several generations in a year. The occurrence of human patients the whole year round also suggests manner of larval shedding noted above.

In temperate areas, as in Japan, where there are four distinct seasons, eggs are laid mostly in the summer, as noted in Section 3 in this chapter. There are differences in longevity of unfed larvae according to species, therefore there is a clear seasonal occurrence of larvae, as observed by the collection of larvae from wild rodents.

b. Life cycle of chigger mites

Since humans are infected with Tsutsugamushi disease by the bite of vector species of larval mites that harbor *R. tsutsugamushi*, the prevalent season of human Tsutsugamushi disease is closely associated with the occurrence of specific larval mites. Studies of the seasonal prevalence of Tsutsugamushi disease at different localities in Japan have shown that Tsutsugamushi disease caused by the same vector species exhibited change in its prevalent season in various localitities due to different seasonal occurrences of the same mite (Sasa, 1956; Tamiya, 1962).

The larval stage of mites is easily observed by collecting them from small mammals, especially small rodents, but the other stages in the life cycle — *i.e.*, the egg, nymph, and adult — are difficult to observe, since they are free-living in the soil. Some stages are predatory and are difficult to observe due to the lack of collection or observation methods.

Since these difficulties have not yet been overcome, the seasonal development of chigger mites, which governs the seasonal occurrence of the mite species, has not yet been completely elucidated, even though the number of species acting as vectors to humans is limited. Takahashi *et al.* (1988b) were successful in rearing chigger mites in the laboratory by feeding them with collembolan eggs. Using the same feeding method, Takahashi *et al.* (1993a, 1994b, 1995) successfully reared engorged specimens of the three main vector mites in Japan, *i.e.*, *L. akamushi*, *L. scutellare*, and *L. pallidum*, in outdoor conditions exposed to the natural seasonal changes in climate. The seasonal development of these three species, in conjunction with their seasonal occurrence, was thus made clear.

1) Seasonal occurrence of larval mites of the three main vectors for *R. tsutsugamushi* in Japan

The seasonal occurrence of chigger mites has been observed in many localities in Japan by collecting engorged mites from small rodents captured in each area. The typical seasonal occurrence of the three main vector mites is shown in Fig. 1.

L. akamushi shows one peak in the summer, on the banks of large rivers in Akita (Teramura, 1954), Yamagata (Nagayo *et al.*, 1921), and Niigata Prefectures (Asanuma, 1986; Ito and Obata, 1961;

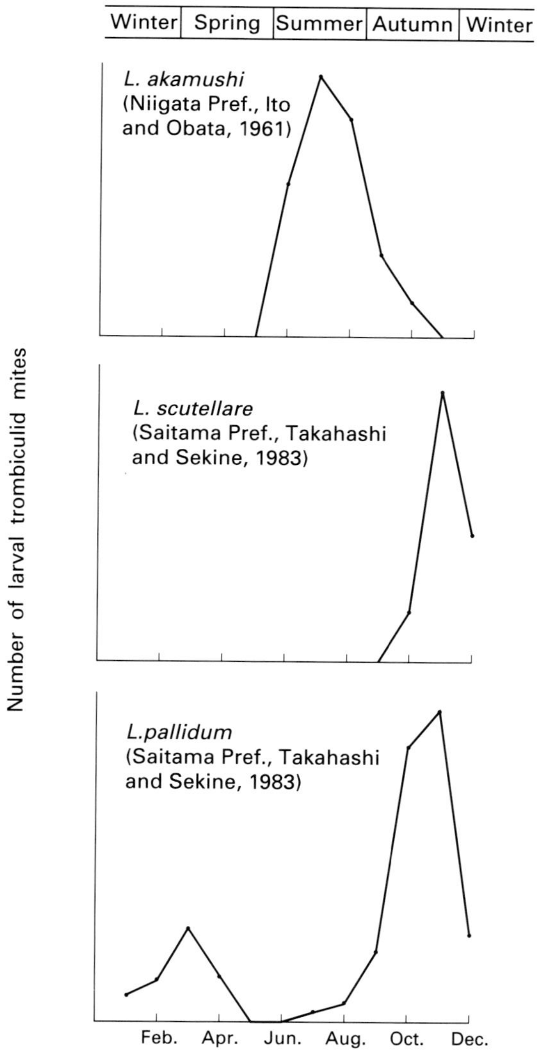

Fig. 1. Seasonal fluctuations in the number of larval trombiculid mites, *L. akamushi*, *L. scutellare*, and *L. pallidum*, the main vector of Tsutsugamushi disease, found on rodents in Japan.

Kawamura, 1926; Kenmotsu *et al.*, 1979) in the northeastern part of Honshu.

The seasonal occurrence of *L. scutellare* has been studied in many parts of Japan; in the prefectures of Yamagata (Nagayo *et al.*, 1921), Niigata (Asanuma, 1983; Kawamura, 1926; Kenmotsu *et al.*, 1979; Tamiya, 1962), Gumma (Oyama *et al.*, 1982), Saitama (Takahashi and Sekine, 1983), Kanagawa (Tamiya, 1962), Shizuoka (Asanuma *et al.*, 1974; Kawamori *et al.*, 1992), and Chiba (Asanuma *et al.*, 1959c; Sasa, 1956; Tamiya, 1962); on Oshima Island, Tokyo (Tamiya, 1962), on Hachijo Island, Tokyo (Ueno, 1956), and in Gifu (Iwasa *et al.*, 1990), Fukui (Ohse *et al.*, 1958), Miyazaki (Sasa, 1956), and Kagoshima Prefectures (Yamamoto, 1961). These observations have shown that this species is distributed widely, but in a spotty fashion, from the northeastern region of Honshu to Kyushu in the season from autumn to winter, occurring in one peak, at different months according to the locality. The more southern the locality, the later the peak is observed in the autumn.

The occurrence of *L. pallidum*, larvae, observed by collection from rodents, shows two peaks, one each in the autumn and spring at some localities, and one peak in the autumn or winter in other areas. Two peaks were observed in cold areas such as Aomori (Takada, 1976), Akita (Teramura, 1954), Yamagata (Nagayo *et al.*, 1921), Niigata (Asanuma *et al.*, 1961; Kawamura, 1925, 1926; Kenmotsu *et al.*, 1979; Tamiya, 1962), Toyama (Kamimura *et al.*, 1972), Gumma (Oyama *et al.*, 1982), Saitama (Takahashi and Sekine, 1983; Takahashi *et al.* 1993b), Nagano (Uchikawa and Kumada, 1986), and Gifu (Iwasa *et al.*, 1990).

One peak was seen in areas with a moderate winter, such as Kanagawa (Asanuma *et al.*, 1962a,b; Obata *et al.*, 1952; Tamiya 1962), Chiba (Sasa, 1956), and Kagoshima Prefectures (Yamamoto, 1961).

2) Seasonal development in cultures maintained in the natural environment

The method of rearing mites in plastic containers has been described in detail above. Engorged larvae collected from wild rodents were reared in conditions corresponding to the seasonal occurrence of the same species in the natural environment. Dishes were kept in boxes placed on the ground at selected locations near our laboratory where environmental conditions were similar to those in the original habitat of the larval species. Mobile and predatory stages of the mite were fed with collembolan eggs.

(a) *L. akamushi*

In early behavioral studies of *L. akamushi*, mites were reared successfully from one stage to the next, but the results were fragmentary; however, entire life cycle was inferred from these results (Kawamura and Yamaguchi, 1916; Miyajima and Okumura, 1916; Nagayo *et al.*, 1916). R. Kawamura and Ikeda (1936) found that adult *L. akamushi* lived in the soil the whole year round, especially in the autumn; in the summer, they observed oviposition by females that they had placed in glass vials, and they found that mites survived the cold winter in the protonymph and adult stages. Rearing *L. akamushi* in the soil in a flowerpot for a longer period, R. Kawamura (1940) found unfed larvae to be prevalent in the summer, while adults survived for two winters and laid eggs in two consecutive summers. These early observations of mite development were confirmed by later experiments in which individual mites were reared in vials or dishes, by feeding them with the eggs of mosquitoes, dragonflies, or collembola (Asahina, 1952; Ito and Obata, 1961; Sasa *et al.*, 1951).

In our studies on the rearing of *L. akamushi* in the natural environment (Takahashi *et al.*, 1995), the culture was begun in July and October, corresponding to the peak and the late seasons, respectively, with larvae collected from rodents *Microtus montebelli* in the field, in Jumonji, Akita Prefecture. The larvae were reared in vials in a natural environment at Kawagoe, near Tokyo, and the following results were obtained.

In the culture begun in July 1991, engorged larvae developed rapidly into protonymphs after several days, and developed into adults in late August. The females laid eggs in September, when the atmospheric temperature was 23.1°C. The population peak of unfed larvae occurred in October. Adults that survived the cold winter laid eggs again in the period from early May to late June (Figs. 2, 3).

In parallel with the above experiments, ten male-female pairs were reared in individual vials for follow-up studies. Of the ten females, six laid eggs in two consecutive summers. The average number of eggs laid was 106.3 and 26.8 per female, respectively, in the first and second year, with a hatching rate that did not differ greatly in the two years, being 72.1% and 64.6%, respectively.

In this study, larvae hatching from eggs showed a population peak in early October of the first year and in early July of the second year,

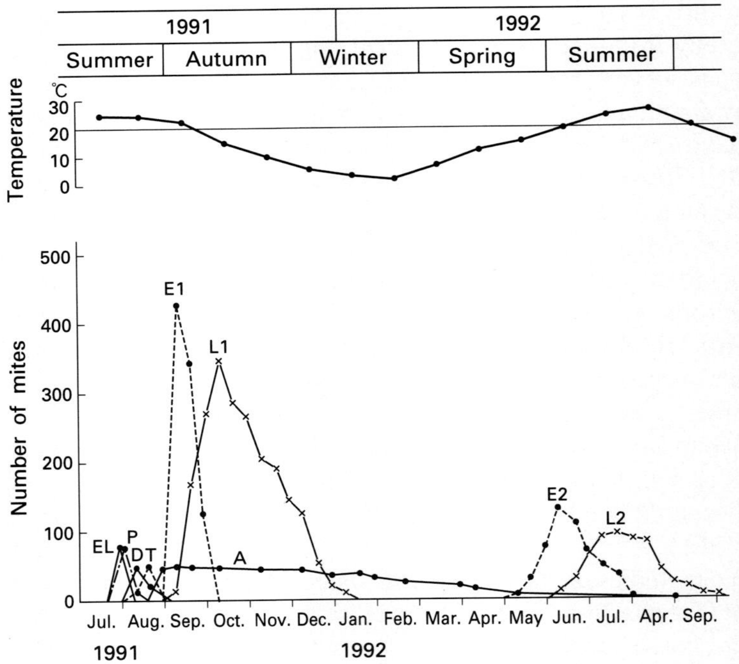

Fig. 2. Development of engorged *L. akamushi* larvae reared under field conditions
EL : engorged larva; P : protonymph; D : deutonymph;
T : tritonymph; A : adult; E1, E2 : eggs of succeeding generations; L1, L2 : unfed larvae of succeeding generation.

died off gradually, and had almost disappeared by the end of December. Hatching started in early July within a short period (3 weeks) after oviposition, and the average longevity of the unfed larvae was about 2 months.

In the culture begun in October 1990, engorged larvae developed into deutonymphs by December, survived the cold winter in a dormant state, developed into tritonymphs in May of the following spring, and then developed into adults.

The deposition of spermatophores was seen from late May to the middle of October, and females laid eggs, at an average rate of 351.8 per female, from the middle of June to late August, when the average temperature was 24.9°C. Larvae hatched from early July, with the

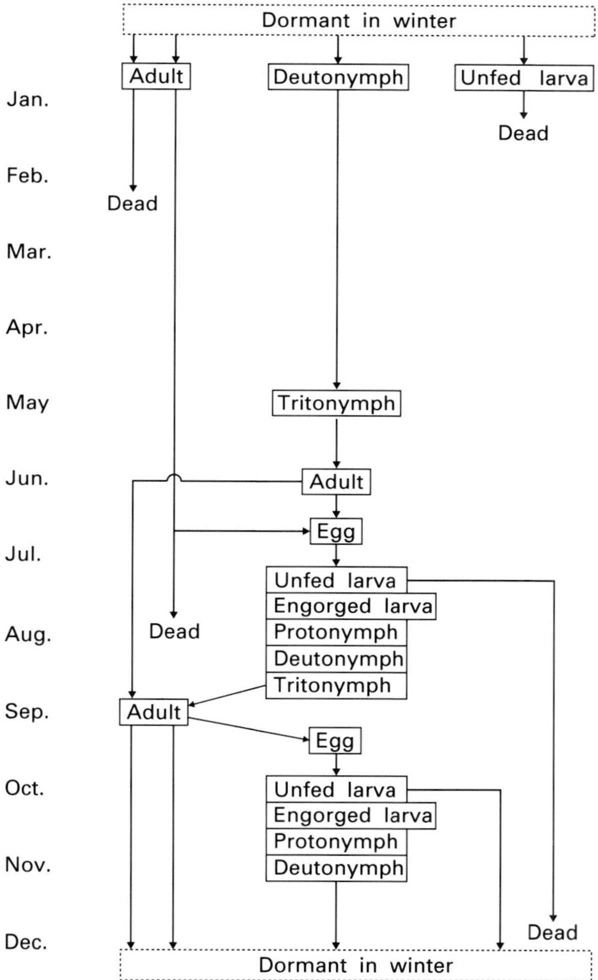

Fig. 3. Life history of *L. akamushi* in natural conditions in Saitama Prefecture

hatching rate being 71.3% in the 2,814 eggs laid in the summer, The population peak of 2,006 occurred in late August, after which time the mites died off; they were all dead by the end of December. After oviposition, females survived the winter and were alive until the following February, with the maximum period of longevity being 9 months (Fig. 3).

(b) *L. scutellare*

The rearing of this species has been difficult in the past, only one adult having been developed by feeding with mosquito eggs (Sasa *et al.*, 1953b). Once feeding with collembolan eggs was successful, the entire life history was elucidated (Takahashi *et al.*, 1994b).

Larval *L. scutellare* were collected from *Apodemus speciosus* in Okegawa, Saitama Prefecture, in November 1988 and reared in a natural environment at Kawagoe for about 3 years until June 1991. Culture was begun in November, corresponding to the peak season of larval *L. scutellare* in the natural environment. Apart from these larvae, engorged larvae collected in November were kept at 4°C in a refrigerator, and experimental cultures were begun in May and August of the following year in seasons when no larvae of this species were found in the field.

In the culture begun in November 1988, engorged larvae developed into protonymphs by the end of the year, and were dormant during the winter. In the second year, in the spring, the larvae developed into deutonymphs. They reached the tritonymph stage from the middle of May to the middle of July, and the adult stage from early June, the peak adult population occurring in the period from late July to early September. The number of engorged larvae that completed development to the adult stage was 89 (57.8%).

The deposition of spermatophores was observed from early July to the middle of October. Oviposition continued from late July to late September, when the average temperature was 24.9°C. During this season, females laid 359 eggs at an average daily rate of 1.1 eggs, the maximum being 5. Adults survived after oviposition and were dormant in the winter.

In the third year, the males deposited spermatophores from May to October, and the females laid 838 eggs from the middle of May to late September. In general, females seemed to lay eggs in the consecutive summers of years 2 and 3, and the greatest longevity of the adult was 24 months in the natural environment.

From the 359 eggs laid in the second year, 214 larvae (59.6%) hatched; the larval population reached a maximum in late November, after which larvae gradually died off: the last larva survived until March of the third year. From the 838 eggs laid in the third year, 285 larvae (34.0%) were hatched; the maximal population occurred in November of the third year, and the last larva survived until

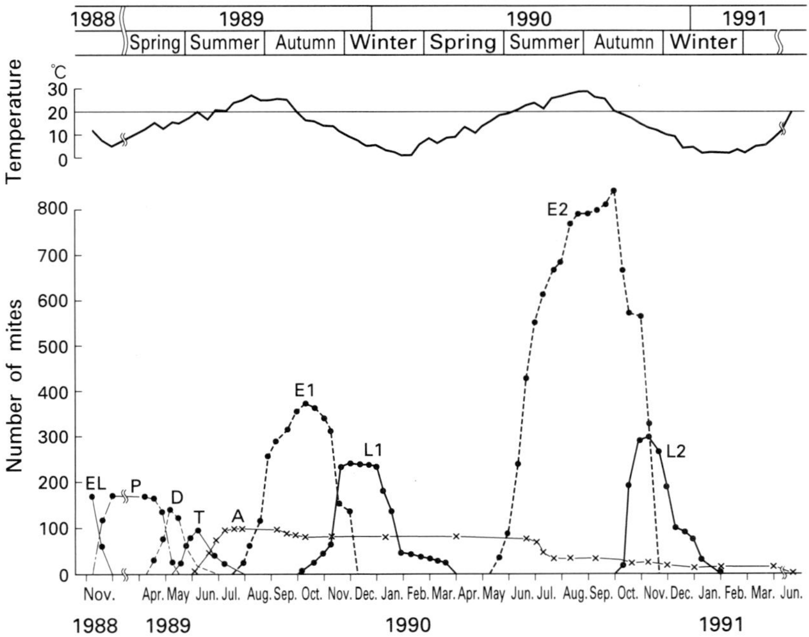

Fig. 4. Development of engorged *L. scutellare* larvae reared under field conditions

March of the fourth year. Figure 4 shows the *L. scutellare* culture graphically.

The engorged larvae in the culture that was begun in May 1989 developed into protonymphs after several days; later development was synchronized with the mite stages cultured from November in the previous year.

In the culture begun in August 1989, larvae developed into deutonymphs, tritonymphs, or adults before winter, and these stages were able to survive the cold winter in a dormant state. After developing into adults in the following spring, the females laid eggs for the 1st time in the summer of the second year.

The ten females individually reared in the culture begun in November 1988 laid eggs in two consecutive summers, in the second and third years. The larvae hatched in early October, 3 months after oviposition. The fecundity and hatching rate were higher for the first than for the second oviposition. In the cultures begun in three different months *i.e.*, May, August, and November, the speed of develop-

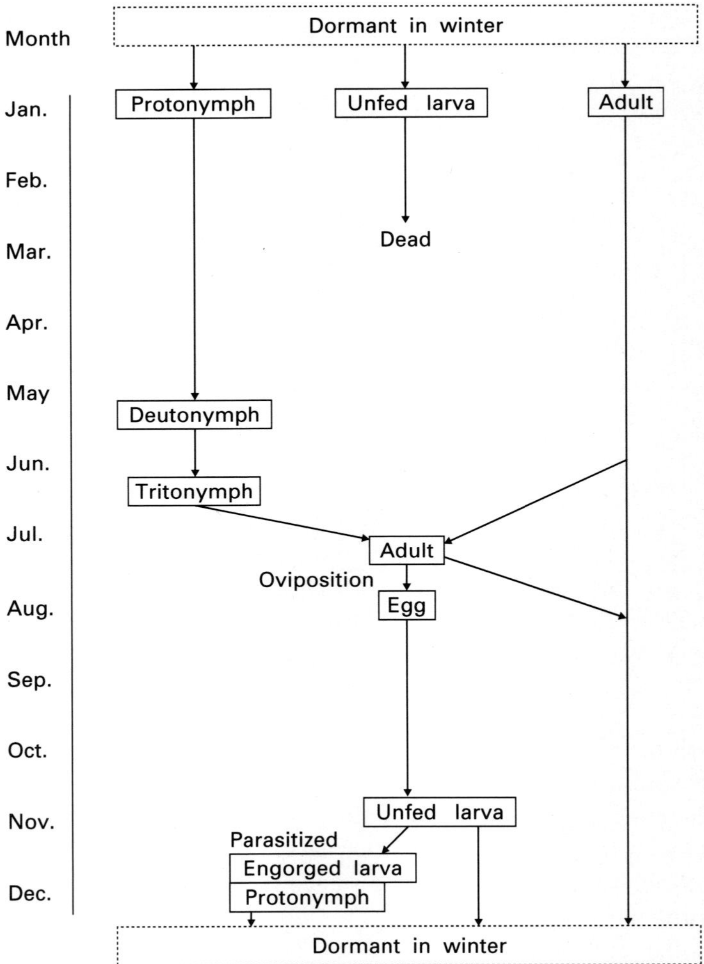

Fig. 5. Life history of *L. scutellare* in natural conditions in Saitama Prefecture

ment to the adult stage differed greatly, and females laid eggs in July and August (summer), with later development being synchronized with the development that began in November, irrespective of the time the culture was begun. Observation of 19 females indicated that the appropriate temperature for oviposition was 20.0–24.4°C.

For a reference study of the life cycle and seasonal prevalence of *L. scutellare* in soil, mites were directly collected from soil, using a Tullgren funnel, on the banks of the Arakawa river at Okegawa,

Saitama Prefecture. The unfed larvae were collected from October to the following March, primarily in November. Deutonymphs were observed only in May and June, and adults were found throughout the year, but particularly in August. These findings agreed well with the results of the culture begun in November. The seasonal development of this species observed in culture, which may reflect that in the natural environment, is shown in Fig. 5. The life cycle shown in this figure is generally observed in Saitama Prefecture, near Tokyo, and may differ to some extent in different localities in Japan.

(c) *L. pallidum*

The laboratory rearing of this species has not been successful, as it was difficult to maintain colonies in succeeding generations by feeding them mosquito eggs (Sasa and Miura, 1953). Successful rearing was first achieved by feeding with collembola or dragonfly eggs (Ito and Obata, 1961; Miura, 1960).

The prevalent season for larval *L. pallidum* is late autumn; in some areas the larvae are again prevalent in spring. In accordance with the seasonal occurrence of chigger mites, cultures were begun in October and November 1985 and in April 1986, with engorged larvae collected from *A. speciosus* at Hitsujiyama Park, Chichibu, at each of these times (Takahashi *et al.*, 1993a). The mites collected in October were kept in a refrigerator at 4°C and reared from June and August in the following year; during these months no larval *L. pallidum* are found on wild rodents.

October group: In the culture begun in October, engorged larvae soon stopped developing and became dormant during the cold winter. The development began again in April, the larvae developing into protonymphs in May, deutonymphs in June, tritonymphs in July, and adults in August. The deposition of spermatophores was observed from early August to early October. Females laid eggs from the middle of August to the middle of September, when the average temperature was 23.3°C. Larvae began hatching in September and showed a population peak in November, after which time their number decreased as they died off; some remained alive until April of the following year (Figs. 6, 7).

November group: The development of larvae in the culture that was begun in November was similar to that in the October group. Although the development into protonymphs was somewhat delayed compared to that in the October group, the time course of their devel-

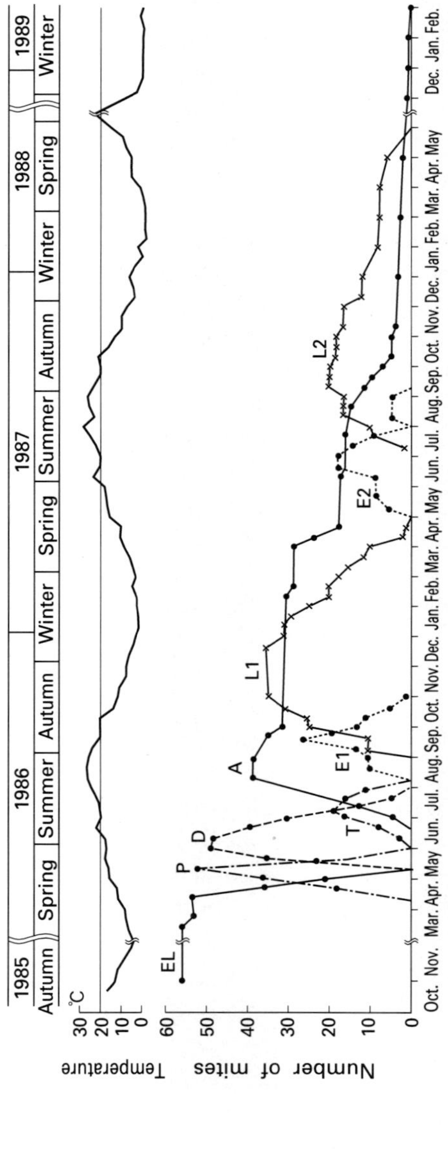

Fig. 6. Development of engorged L. pallidum larvae reared under field comditions

opment was similar, except that oviposition by the females began one month earlier in the October group.

April group: Larvae in the culture begun in April developed quickly into protonymphs, and later development was synchronized with the November group. The larvae developed into adults in August, as did the larvae in the two autumn groups, and larval hatching began in September, one month later than in the November group.

June group: Rearing of the engorged larvae kept in the refrigerator began in June. Larvae developed into protonymphs, deutonymphs, and tritonymphs comparatively rapidly, developing into adults in September. Adults passed through winter in a state of dormancy without the occurrence of oviposition, laying eggs for the first time in the summer of the following year.

August group: The engorged larvae removed from the refrigerator in August developed into protonymphs in September and then slowly developed, most into deutonymphs and some into tritonymphs or adults, before the winter. They became dormant at different stages in the winter, and all had developed into adults by the following May. Oviposition was markedly delayed; it began in July or August.

The maximum longevity of *L. pallidum* observed in these rearing experiments was 970 days. The average temperatures at which oviposition took place were 21.6 to 26.1°C. Unfed larvae hatching from eggs showed a population peak in the autumn, with the population subsequently being reduced by death in the cold winter, although some remained alive until the end of the following spring, in May.

As a reference study for the seasonal development observed in cultures, different stages of *L. pallidum* in the soil were collected at Hitsujiyama Park with a Tullgren funnel (Takahashi *et al.*, 1988a). Unfed larvae were collected in winter, spring, autumn, and summer, from June to August, being most abundant in September. Deutonymphs were collected only in May and June, and adults were collected the whole year round, with especially large numbers being collected in August. This fragmented collection corresponded with the seasonal development of larvae in the cultures begun in October and November. Thus, the November group appears to represent the main life history of this species in the natural environment, as shown in Fig.7.

3) Different seasonal occurrence of mites associated with characteristic development in cultures

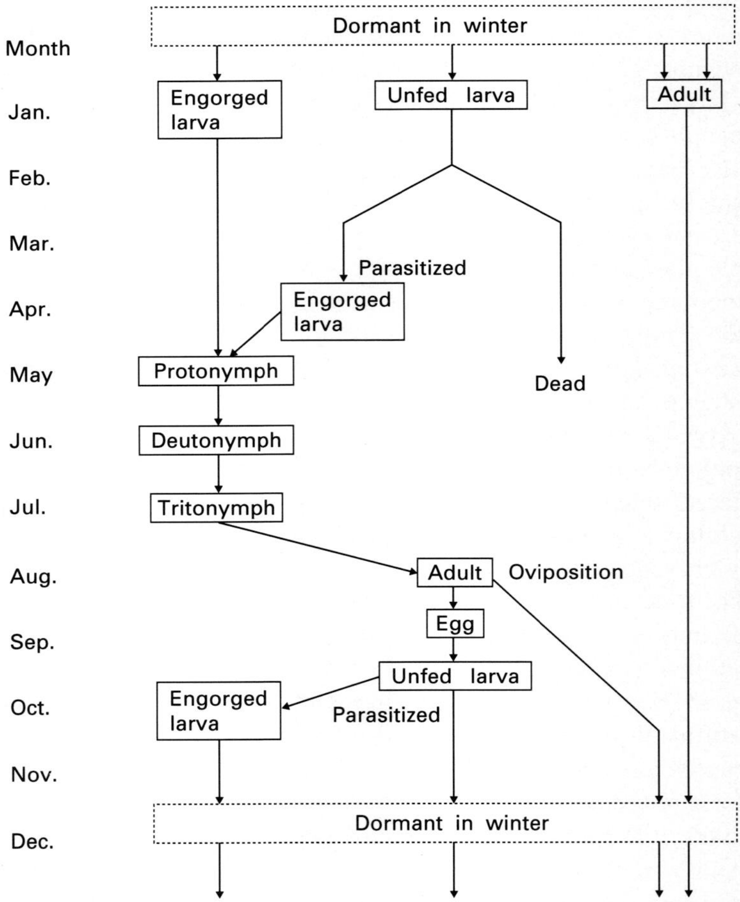

Fig. 7. Life history of *L.pallidum* in natural conditions in Saitama Prefecture

The rearing of mites in the natural environment showed that the seasonal prevalence of larval mites differed greatly depending on the species. This difference appears to be associated with certain characteristics of their life cycle observed in culture, such as the period of incubation of the eggs, the speed of development of the larval and nymphal stages, and the longevity of unfed larvae and their resistance to cold in the winter. These parameters are listed in Table 13.

Table 13. Parameters of Life History of *L. akamushi*, *L. scutellare*, and *L. pallidum* Reared Experimentally

Species	*L. akamushi*	*L. scutellare*	*L. pallidum*
Incubation period of eggs (days)[a]	20. 3 ± 1.56[b] (n = 140)	51.9 ± 3.42 (n = 165)	26.0 ± 3.41 (n = 150)
Survival period of unfed larvae (days)[a]	30.7 ± 7.05 (n = 50)	56.6 ± 4.88 (n = 48)	143.7 ± 24.36 (n = 52)
Susceptibility to cold	Sensitive	Moderate	Insensitive
Speed of development	Rapid	Slow	Moderate

[a] Incubation and survival periods were examined in mites reared in incubator at 25°C.
[b] Standard deviation.

L. akamushi: In the rearing experiments with *L. akamushi*, adults and deutonymphs that survived the cold winter lay eggs in early summer, the incubation period being 3 weeks, much shorter than the periods of 6 and 10 weeks for *L. pallidum* and *L. scutellare*, respectively. The unfed larvae showed a population peak in July, earlier than that in the other two species.

It was unique in *L. akamushi* that larvae hatching in the early summer became attached to wild rodents and developed quickly into adults in August. They soon laid eggs, and the hatching larvae showed another population peak in October. Therefore, the seasonal occurrence of larvae, which appears to consist of one population peak in the summer, is actually a compound of two peaks occurring in July and October, as noted above.

Due to their short survival period of 2 months, much shorter than the 4 and 6 months in *L. scutellare* and *L. pallidum*, respectively, and their sensitivity to the cold, the peak population of *L. akamushi* was reduced gradually, and most unfed larvae died before winter. The culture studies showed that the unfed larvae constituted one population peak (actually a compound of two peaks) in mid-summer in the natural environment. Thus, human infections correspond to this larval peak (Ito and Obata, 1961; Kitaoka *et al.*, 1974; Tamiya, 1962).

After a period of engorgement from July to October, the larvae developed into adults within 2 months, the developmental period being short at each stage. Adults developed from the engorged larvae in early summer, and larvae of the next generation developed into deutonymphs in late summer, with both adult parents and deutonymphs surviving the cold winter. This represents the life history of *L. akamushi* in the soil, as determined from the culture studies.

L. scutellare: In culture, females laid eggs in July and August, and the unfed larvae hatched from eggs showed a population peak in November. Unfed larvae alive before winter became inactive and gradually died off in the cold winter, not remaining alive until spring. This life history observed in the cultures agreed well with the seasonal occurrence of larvae found in wild rodents.

In the natural environment, the population of *L. scutellare* on rodents shows one peak in autumn, is gradually reduced in number in late autumn, and is very low in the winter. This species does not usually return in the spring.

L. pallidum: In experimental cultures, a long survival period of about 6 months, the longest among the three species, was a unique characteristic of the unfed larva of *L. pallidum*. These mites live from early autumn to the following May after surviving the cold winter.

This life history in the culture well reflected the seasonal occurrence of this species, as shown by collection from wild rodents. Essentially, the population peak of larval *L. pallidum* is prolonged over the winter in the natural environment. In autumn, the number of infesting larvae increases, reaching a peak, the population is then gradually reduced during the winter, possibly due to the inactivity of the larvae in the cold conditions. In the spring, when the weather is warm, the surviving larvae become engorged on the wild rodent, producing another small population peak in the rodents, as shown in Fig. 1.

4. Distribution of Trombiculid Mites and Mite Islands

The patchy distribution of Tsutsugamushi disease in areas along large rivers in northeastern Japan has been noted from the earliset times, and although the causative agent was not known, for several centuries local inhabitants had been well aware of the presence of a deadly disease with characteristic clinical manifestations. People called the banks of these rivers *yudokuchi*, literally translated as "presence of poison land." This phrase was later quoted by Asanuma *et al.* (1959b) as "noxious area" in English.

The ancient Japanese living in endemic areas knew that people contracted a deadly disease (Tsutsugamushi), and it appears that their traditional experience led them to suspect that this disease was associated with the bites of the red mites (later identified as *Leptotrombidium akamushi*) that were specific to the noxious areas.

Since the time that US Armed Forces medical personnel detected a new type of Tsutsugamushi disease in Southeast Asia and in regions in the southwest Pacific, it has been noted that the prevalence of the disease was uneven and that there were small pockets of areas where the infection rates in wild rodents were remarkably high (Philip, 1948a; Muur *et al.*, 1975; Traub and Wisseman, 1974b; Traub *et al.*, 1967; Trishnananda *et al.*, 1964).

The uneven distribution of infected and uninfected mites has been confirmed by many methods: by examining wild animals, especially rodents; by the use of sentinel animals; and by collecting the mites on black plates. The findings of studies employing these methods validated the knowledge that had been passed down from ancient times to the inhabitants of the endemic areas.

The discovery of small areas of infected mites — mite islands (Audy, 1949) — led to great progress in the study of the epidemiology of Tsutsugamushi disease and its transmission dynamics. In the mite islands, researchers were successful in determining vector species, both by using sentinel animals and by employing human volunteers (Smadel *et al.*, 1949, 1950), after the curative effects of the tetracycline antibiotics had been demonstrated. The prophylactic use of antibiotics against *Rickettsia tsutsugamushi* was also studied in human volunteers in the infective spots (Philip *et al.*, 1949).

The sentinel animal first used for studies of *L. akamushi* in Japan was the monkey (Kawamura, 1926). Later, other, more economical animals were used: chickens and ducks (Hayashi *et al.*, 1924, 1925), rabbits and rats (Philip *et al.*, 1949; Smadel *et al.*, 1949, 1950; Traub and Frick, 1950), mice, and laboratory-bred voles (Takahashi *et al.*, 1990b).

Sentinel animals and human volunteers (Audy, 1961; Philip *et al.*, 1949; Traub and Frick, 1950) were used for finding infective spots, and also for clarifying the patchy distribution of vector mites in the mite islands. Infected colonies of vector mites could not have been successfully established in the laboratory without knowledge of mite islands.

a. Determination of vector mites in mite islands using sentinel animals

L. akamushi was the first species to be identified as a vector of Tsutsugamushi disease in Japan, based on the relationship between its bite and human clinical manifestations as well as by using monkeys (Kawamura, 1926), chickens, and ducks (Hayashi *et al.*, 1924, 1925) exposed in the noxious areas as sentinel animals. In the latest experiment with *L. akamushi*, Kitaoka and Asanuma (1968) placed laboratory-bred *Microtus montebelli* in noxious areas in which *L. akamushi* were present at Oomagari, Akita Prefecture; *R. tsutsugamushi* was isolated from 11 of 36 pools, a total of 97 larval *L. akamushi* being recovered.

The determination of vectors for the non-*akamushi* type Tsutsugamushi disease that was widely distributed in Japan has not been easy, although local vectors were suspected by epidemiological association. The suspected vector mites are usually distributed widely and in low-density populations, and the rate of infection is low, even in endemic areas. Further, many attempts to isolate in rickettsiae in endemic areas had failed (Jackson *et al.*, 1957; Philip *et al.*, 1949; Rapmund *et al.*, 1969; Traub and Wisseman, 1968b, 1974b). Therefore, it was believed that the mite islands, where mite species may have possibly shown high positivity, would be the appropriate sites to determine which mites were vectors.

Asanuma (1959) and Asanuma *et al.* (1959a, b, c) settled 1055 sentinel animals, including rats, mice, birds, and *M. montebelli*, in many areas in Japan. In their experiment at Shirahama, Chiba Prefecture, in which they placed sentinel animals in a suspected endemic area, four mice, from which four larval *L. scutellare* were recovered, were found to be infected with *R. tsutsugamushi*. This was the first case in which it was determined that *L. scutellare* was a vector of *R. tsutsugamushi*.

Kitaoka *et al.* (1976) settled chickens in a suspected endemic area in Akita Prefecture in autumn, a season when *akamushi*-derived Tsutsugamushi disease was not manifested. *R. tsutsugamushi* was isolated from the livers of the chickens and from larval *L. pallidum* collected from them; *L. pallidum* was thus determined as a vector mite. Takahashi *et al.* (1990b) used laboratory-bred *M. montebelli* as a sentinel animal, and exposed them at a mite island in Chichibu, Saitama Prefecture. Of all mites collected from *M. montebelli* (or sentinel animal), *R. tsutsugamushi* was isolated only from *L. pallidum*. *R. tsutsugamushi* was also isolated from 12 (85.7%) of 14 *Microtus* infested with rickettsia-positive *L. pallidum*. This experiment also confirmed *L. pallidum* as a vector of Tsutsugamushi disease in this area.

b. Efficiency of mite collection in different animals

The species and density of trombiculid mites in a certain area were also studied using sentinel animals, mainly tame laboratory animals such as mice and rats (Asanuma, 1959; Asanuma *et al.*, 1959a,b,c, 1962a,b; Mackie *et al.*, 1946a,b; Philip *et al.*, 1949; Traub and Frick, 1950), or rabbits (Hubert and Baker, 1963a,b). Mites were collected from these animals in anticipation that results would reflect distribution in the fauna and the density in that area.

Asanuma *et al.* (1962a) used a total of 1,204 mice and rats as sentinel animals in the Miura Peninsula and the southern area of the Izu Peninsula, and collected an average of 3.4 mites per animal; the mite species collected from sentinel animals were the same as those collected from wild rodents.

Takahashi *et al.* (1990b) placed 12 laboratory-bred *M. montebelli* and 4 mice in a mite island in Chichibu near Tokyo, exposing the animals for 26 h in November, the time of year when the mites increase their density. From the 12 *Microtus*, they collected 255 *L. pallidum*, 104 *L. fuji*, and 4 *Gahrliepia sadusuki*, an average of 40.3 mites per *Microtus*. No mites were collected from the 4 mice. Wild *Apodemus speciosus* caught in the same area yielded more mite species, *L. miyajimai*, *Neotrombicula japonica*, and *Eltonella ichikawai*, in addition to the above species collected from the sentinel animals.

Thus, it can be concluded that the efficiency of mite collection varies according to the species of sentinel animal. Usually, lower numbers of mites and fewer species are collected from the settled animals than from the wild rodents in the same area, since the sentinel animals are exposed to the natural environment for a limited period, in a small space, and in a limited number of sites in the field.

c. Distribution of larval trombiculid mites on soil surface

The distribution of trombiculid mites has been systematically determined by the black plate method (Hayashi and Suzuki, 1954; Hayashi *et al.*, 1955; Suzuki *et al.*, 1953, 1955). This method, however, is not always applicable to all trombiculid mites, but is particularly suitable for determinig the distribution of specific larval species that lack host specificity and that crawl onto the feet of possible hosts and onto the sampling plate, such as *L. scutellare*, *L. akamushi*, and *E. wichmanni* in Japan and *L. fletcheri* and *L. deliense* in Malaysia.

Although surveys based on mite collection from wild rodents are inefficient, non-systematic, and not subject to control, such surveys were widely used in early studies and were fundamental to later work. Hubert and Baker (1963a) reported that surveys of trombiculid mites in Southeast Asia had been based on the method of wild rodent collection (Audy *et al.*, 1947; Philip *et al.*, 1949; Traub and Frick, 1950). To carry out a systematic survey of the distribution of *L. fletcheri* in Malaysia, Hubert and Baker (1963a) used a simple method, counting mites at points along a transect in a field of Lalang grass (*Imperata cylindrica*), using rabbits as mite collectors. Relatively high chigger populations extended for 3–7 m, with gradually diminishing numbers being found in lower sections. There was a marked seasonal difference in total mite counts, but the relative densities of mites at different sites remained constant.

Further systematic studies of the distribution of mites, conducted in Malaysia (Hubert and Baker, 1963b) using rabbits as the sentinel animal and plate methods for mite collection, confirmed that the habitat of *L. fletcheri* was grassland and that *L. deliense* was found in relatively large numbers in forests. This finding considerably broadened the scope of epidemiological studies of Tsutsugamushi disease in Malaysia. In a two-year distribution study, Dohany *et al.* (1979) used the black plate method in a mature oil palm estate consisting of 200 trees arranged in rows of 20 × 10 trees; *L. deliense*, found in litter piles, was the predominant vector of Tsutsugamushi disease.

In November 1985, Takahashi *et al.* (1990b) settled 12 laboratory-bred *M. montebelli* and 4 mice as sentinel animals in an infected mite island in Chichibu, near Tokyo (Figs. 1, 2). Three hundred and sixty-three larvae were recovered from 9 voles that survived 26-h exposure; 285 of these larvae were examined for the presence of rickettsia

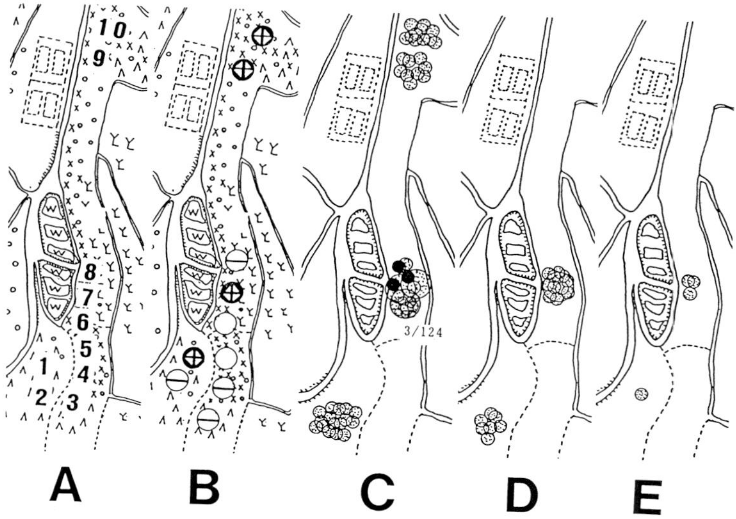

○ One mite
◯ 50 mites
● *R. tsutsugamushi*-positive mite
◍ *Rt*-negative mite
⊕ *Rt*-positive sentinel animal
⊖ *Rt*-negative sentinel animal
○ Not done

Fig. 8. Distribution and density of *R. tsutsugamushi*-positive larval trombiculid mites recovered from sentinel animals placed in an endemic area in Hitsujiyama Park on 4–5th November, 1985. A : location of sentinel animal traps. Nos. 1, 5–7, 9 and 10; *Microtus montebelli*. Nos. 2–4 and 8; ddY mice. B : Sites of sentinel animals whose sera either become *Rt*-positive or remained negative after exposure to trombiculid mites. C–E : spots of *Rt*-positive/negative samples of trombiculid mites. C : *Leptotrombidium pallidum*; D : *L. fuji*; E : *Gahrliepia saduski*.

by a mouse passage method, using one mouse for one mite or pooled mites. Rickettsiae were also detected in dissected larval mites by direct immunofluorescence. The average numbers of mites recovered from a vole and the range (in parentheses) were 1.9 (0–6) for rickettsia-positive *L. pallidum*, 26.4 (2–157) for uninfected *L. pallidum*, 11.6 (0–70) for uninfected *L. fuji*, and 0.4 (0–3) for uninfected *G. saduski*. The number of mites collected from vole no. 7, 157 *L. pallidum* and 70 *L. fuji*, was remarkably high, indicating clusters of two species at this site.

From the 16 points shown in Figs. 8 and 9, 4 points in which there were many infected *L. pallidum* were selected, and a 6 × 6 m quadrat

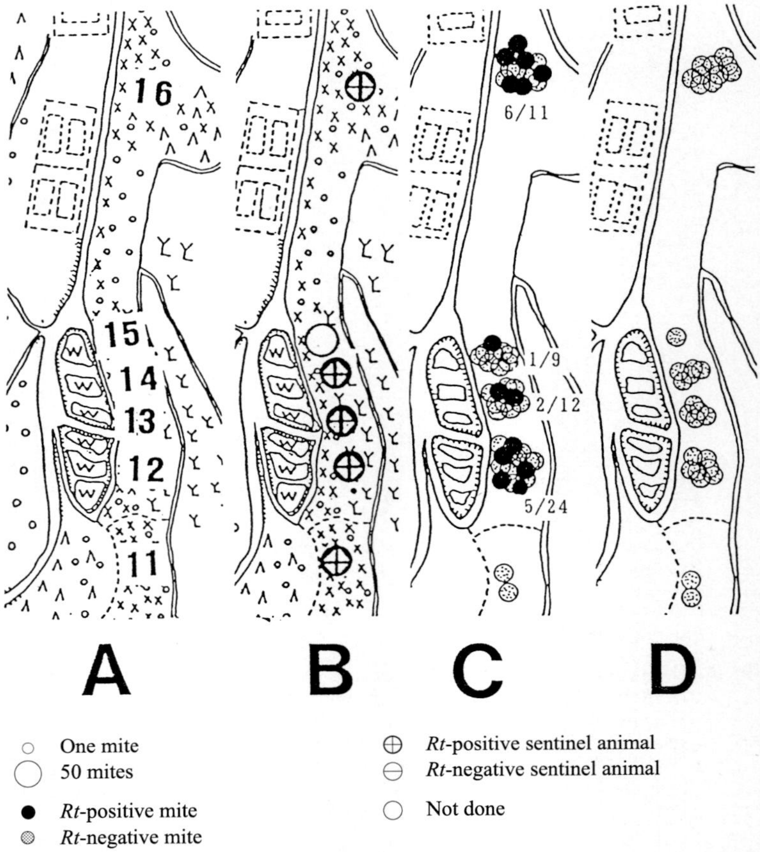

Fig. 9. Distribution and density of *Rickettsia tsutsugamushi*-positive larval trombiclid mites recovered from sentinel animals, *Microtus montebelli*, placed in the same area as shown in Fig. 8 on 13–14th November, 1985.
A: Location of animal traps; B : Spots at which *M. montebelli* (sentinel animals) whose sera either became *Rt*-positive or remained negative after exposure to trombiculid mites. C, D : Spots of *Rt*-positive/negative samples of trombiculid mites recovered from *M. montebelli*; C : *Leptotrombidium pallidum*; D : *L. fuji*.

was marked at each point. Nine sentinel voles were placed in each quadrat and exposed for 26 h. The numbers of mites recovered from these animals are shown in Table 14. The distribution of mites in the 36 voles did not fit a binomial distribution — the uneven distribution of mites was clearly demonstrated by this systematic survey. A vole

Table 14. Number of Larval Trombiculid Mites Recovered from Sentinel Voles *Microtus montebelli* Placed in the Study Area (Squares No. 1–4)

Species	No. of mites recovered					Mean	Range	Range of theoretical distribution[b]
Study area	#1 (9)[a]	#2 (9)	#3 (9)	#4 (9)	Total (36)			
L. pallidum								
infected	3	2	5	4	14	0.4 ± 0.76	0–3	0–2
uninfected	13	4	25	14	56	1.6 ± 2.13	0–9	0–5
L. fuji								
uninfected	65	2	0	3	70	1.9 ± 7.34	0–44	0–5
G. saduski								
uninfected	12	0	0	0	12	0.3 ± 0.75	0–3	0–1
Total	93	8	30	21	152	4.3 ± 8.71	0–51	

[a] No. of quadrats in which sentinel voles were placed (one per quadrat).
[b] $p < 0.01$. Mean (range) 0.4 ± 0.76 (0–3).
Source: Takahashi *et al.* (1990b).

in quadrat no. 1 harbored 44 uninfected *L. fuji*, and it was suspected that this animal had been placed in a site where there was a cluster of mites similar to the cluster of *L. pallidum* and *L. fuji* at the point at which vole no. 7 had been placed (as noted above).

In experiments carried out to determine the distribution of *L. scutellare* on Hachijo Island, Suzuki *et al.* (1953) quantitatively demonstrated uneven distribution. Using rats as sentinel animals, Traub and Frick (1950) also found uneven distribution of mites (*L. fletcheri* and *L. deliense*), one sentinel rat being infested with up to 350 mites. Hayashi *et al.* (1954) used 5 × 5 cm black plates and systematically examined the distribution of larval mites in more detail in 1 × 1 m and 3 × 3 m squares. They found that the distribution pattern differed greatly by species: *L. scutellare* and *L. akamushi* were distributed in aggregations, whereas *E. wichmanni* followed Poisson's distribution. These investigators also reported that the environmental factors that may have controlled the uneven distribution of mites were the ambient temperature and humidity of the atmosphere immediately above the soil surface.

In laboratory cultures of mites, larval *L. pallidum* in vials were active at 100% humidity but died within 5 days at 95% humidity or lower (Takahashi *et al.*, 1988c). The larvae of *L. pallidum*, *L. fuji*, and *G. saduski* formed immobile clusters consisting of 50–100 individuals in cracks in substrate or on the edge of the substrate and on the vial wall at 100% humidity, but they began moving actively when they were exposed to carbon dioxide in expired human breath.

The above results of distribution studies are readily understandable in terms of observations of mite behavior in cultures. The formation of clusters by mites may be associated with pheromones, as has been reported in grain mites (Kuwabara, 1990).

d. Distribution of infected trombiculid mites on soil surface

Once the distribution of most trombiculid mite larvae on the soil surface was demonstrated, the next question to be resolved was the distribution of infected larvae on the soil surface. Traub (1949) examined the rate of *R. tsutsugamushi*-positivity in mites recovered from wild rats at four points along a 21-mile stretch of road in the Ledo region of Assam; the findings showed a wide range of positivity, from 0% to 50%. He also pointed out that the isolations of rickettsial strains were frequent enough to establish that in certain areas the percentage of successful attempts was much greater than in others.

Audy and Harrison (1951) reviewed the epidemiological investigations carried out by an British Army Research Unit on the India-Burma border in 1945–1946. The vector mites there, *L. deliense* and *L. fletcheri*, were found to be distributed only in limited colonies, or in mite islands, forming an irregular pattern on the ground. Only a small proportion of these mite islands appeared to be infected.

Rapmund *et al.* (1969) suggested that an important epidemiological characteristic of the vector mites was their uneven distribution, with relatively large numbers of larvae being present on certain patches of ground and absent or almost absent from others. They questioned the number of infectious mites that were to be found in a mite island, and concluded that, surprisingly, this important epidemiological determinant had not been measured.

The number of infectious mites in a mite island was eventually determined in a study of *L. pallidum*. Takahashi *et al.* (1986a, 1993b) surveyed the infectivity of *A. speciosus*, a wild rodent, and larval mites collected from these rodents in a park in Chichibu, near Tokyo, where humans had been infected with *R. tsutsugamushi*. They found an area that was highly endemic for *R. tsutsugamushi*, *i.e.*, an infected mite island, an area of some 350 × 35 m in a corner

Suzuki, 1953, 1954; Suzuki *et al.*, 1953) as unfed larvae from the ground in Lalang grass (*Imperata cylindrica*) near Kampong Jendram, Selangor, West Malaysia. The colony was maintained in humidified clay pots stored at the natural environmental temperature. The larvae fed on mice, and non-parasitic stages developed after the larvae were fed on mosquito eggs. The transovarian infection rate was 98%, and the filial infection rate was usually 100%.

Rapmund *et al.* (1972) also colonized an infected *L. arenicola* strain. They collected unfed larvae from the ground on black plates on a few meters of sandy beach at Kampong Sri Pantai, near Mersing, Johore State, West Malaysia. Since it was already known that only this species was collected by the plate method there, the collected mites were brought back to the laboratory and fed on laboratory mice either in pools or singly, according to the technique of Baker *et al.* (1968). They were reared in clay pots as described for *L. fletcheri* above. Transovarian transmission through two generations was confirmed. The filial infection rates were 1/39 and 3/42 in the F1 and F2 generation, respectively, and were markedly lower than those in *L. fletcheri*. In F2, one infected male was obtained.

Roberts and Robinson (1977) also colonized an infected strain of the same mite species. They collected 800 engorged or semi-engorged mites of *L. arenicola* from 16 *Rattus jalorensis* in the same areas as that used by Rapmund *et al.* (1972). An infected colony was established from a single infected larva. The transovarian transmission rate was 100% through four generations, and the filial infection rates varied from 20% to 100%, with an overall rate of 97% (see Chapter 5).

For *L. deliense*, Rai and Bandopadhyay (1978) reported that larvae selected from an infected mite group were attached individually to separate mice, one larva to one mouse. After the larvae were collected, they were transferred individually to jars and fed with mosquito eggs through the subsequent stages of development into adults. The mice on which the larvae had fed were monitored to note illness or death, or a state of immunity, confirmed by protection test. The larvae causing the disease in mice were colonized. The progeny in the infected *L. deliense* colony were almost all infected females, although there were some uninfected females and rarely infected males. The male, however, is known to play no role in the vertical transmission of rickettsia, and no parthenogenesis was found.

The successful colonization of infected mites in the three major vectors in the western Pacific region has led to marked progress of studies in various fields, such as the bionomics of mites in culture, the transmission dynamics of *R. tsutsugamushi* within mites and in relation to field rodents, the route of infection, and the distribution of rickettsiae in the mite (Dohany *et al.*, 1970, 1977, 1978; Rapmund *et al.*, 1969, 1972; Roberts and Ram, 1973; Roberts and Robinson, 1977; Roberts *et al.*, 1975a, 1977, 1982; Robinson *et al.*, 1977; Shirai *et al.*, 1982c,d, 1984b; Takahashi *et al.*, 1993c; Traub *et al.*, 1975; Twartz *et al.*, 1975; Walker *et al.*, 1975; Wright *et al.*, 1984).

c. Search for infective spots of L. pallidum

The infectivity of vector mites collected in the field in Japan is very low, and it is almost impossible to establish an infected colony by collecting mites at random, in view of the infection rates of vector mites estimated by Asanuma (1983).

For collecting mites with a high infection rate, the most reliable approach is to find an infective spot, as discussed above. Takahashi *et al.* (1988b) were successful in establishing an infected colony of *L. pallidum*, one of the main vector mites in Japan, by collecting *L. pallidum* mites with very high *R. tsutsugamushi*-positive rates from infective sites located by the methods described below.

The site at which *R. tsutsugamushi* infection was thought to have been acquired in a patient in Chichibu was determined to be a natural park in the city. Wild rodents were captured in the park, and the species and density of mites on the rodents were surveyed. The putative site of infection was identified in a small corner of the park, and the vector was thought to be *L. pallidum*.

Since the method of settling sentinel animals on the ground had been shown to be efficient (Asamuma, 1959) for the detailed survey of the distribution and density of *L. pallidum*, sentinel animals were utilized for further studies. Laboratory-bred *Microtus montebelli* were selected as the uninfected sentinel animals. Six voles (nos. 1 to 6) were enclosed individually in wire mesh cages (9 × 9 × 20 cm) and placed on the ground, 20–30 m apart, in the putative area in the park.

The detection of rickettsia in the engorged mites was performed by mouse passage of homogenized mites or by direct IF in individual mites; the results are shown in Table 15. For mites collected from

Table 15. Isolation of *Rickettsia tsutsugamushi* from *Leptotrombidium pallidum* Larvae Recovered from *Microtus montebelli* Placed as Sentinel Animal on the Ground in the Field

M. montebelli No.	*R. tsutsugamushi*-positive rate[a]				Type of *R. tsutsugamushi*
	IF	Passage	Total	%	
1	1/5	5/6	6/11	54.5	Karp
2[b]	—	—	—	—	—
3	1/5	0/4	1/9	11.1	Karp
4	0/5	2/7	2/12	16.7	Karp
5	2/12	3/12	5/24	20.8	Karp
6	NE	0/2	0/2	0	—

[a] IF, positive detection of *R. tsutsugamushi* from dissected larval mites by direct immunofluorescence;
Passage, successful isolation of *R. tsutsugamushi* from individual mites by mouse passage;
NE, not examined.
[b] This vole died during the time it was on the ground.

vole no. 1, six *L. pallidum* larvae were intraperitoneally inoculated individually to a mouse; five of the six were positive for rickettsia by mouse passage. Of the other five larvae collected from the same vole, one was positive for rickettsia by individual examination with direct IF. Thus, the positive rate for rickettsia in the larvae in vole no.1 was 6/11 (54.5%). The positive rates for rickettsia in voles 3, 4, and 5 were 11.1% (1/9), 16.7% (2/12), and 20.8% (5/24), respectively. This narrow zone was confirmed to be the infective spot for *L. pallidum*.

d. Colonization of infected L. pallidum *strain*

To collect infected larvae efficiently, Takahashi *et al.* (1988b) captured a wild rodent, *Apodemus speciosus*, at the site where vole no.1 had been placed, and subsequently detached all engorged *L. pallidum* larvae from the *Apodemus* and reared these larvae to the adult stage. Male and female pairs were placed in vials, and of 47 pairs, 38 females laid eggs. After the larvae hatched, four or five unfed larvae were removed from each vial, and the presence of rickettsia in the larvae was investigated by mouse passage, injecting ground homogenized mites from each vial to a mouse. Of the progeny of the 38 pairs, the unfed larvae of four pairs were positive for

Table 16. Isolation of *Rickettsia tsutsugamushi* (*Rt*) from Parent Generations of *Leptotrombidium pallidum* That Produced *R. tsutsugamushi*-positive Progeny

Family line	P[a]	Anti-*Rt* antibody titer in passage mice			*Rt* isolation[c] in passage mice								
		Second			First			Second			Third		
		N	K	G	N	K	G	N	K	G	N	K	G
I	M	10>	10>	10>	–	–	–	–	–	–	–	–	–
	F	80	160	80	–	+	–	–	+	–	–	+	–
II	M	10>	10>	10>	–	–	–	–	–	–	–	–	–
	F	40	320≦	160	–	+	–	–	+	–	–	+	–
III	M	10>	10>	10>	–	–	–	–	–	–	–	–	–
	F	160	320≦	160	–	+	–	–	+	–	–	+	–
IV	M	10>	10>	10>	–	–	–	–	–	–	–	–	–
	F	40	160	20(1)	–	+	–	NE			NE		

[a] Parent generation.

[b] Antibodies in mouse sera were titrated and classified by indirect immunofluorescence (IF) against three prototypes of *R. tsutsugamushi*.

[c] The type of *R. tsutsugamushi* was determined by direct IF on peritoneal smears with prototype-specific monoclonal antibodies.

N, Kato type; K, Karp type; G, Gilliam type; (1), antibody titer in the first passage mouse; NE, not examined.

rickettsia. When the adults of these four pairs were examined for rickettsia, all four females were positive, while all males were negative (Table 16).

The remaining unfed larvae from each of these four pairs (infected colonies I to IV in Table 16) were infested individually on the inner auriculae of the four mice for further rearing. To confirm that the unfed larvae attached to the mice were infected, the four mice used for the feeding of the unfed larvae were examined for rickettsial infection by demonstrating rickettsiae in their tissues by showing an elevated level of antibody against rickettsia. Infection was confirmed in all four mice; thus four infected colonies of *L. pallidum* were successfully established.

After the F1 generation, the colonies were maintained to the F3 generation with pairs consisting of an infected female and an infected male or in groups of infected females and males. In the infected colonies of *L. fletcheri*, *L. arenicola*, and *L. deliense* (Rai and Bandopadhyay, 1978; Roberts and Robinson, 1977) almost all the infected adults were female; however, in contrast, adults in the infected *L. pallidum* colony consisted of almost equal numbers of infected females and males (Takahashi, 1990). The transovarian infection rate and filial infection rates in the infected *L. pallidum* colony were both almost 100% (see Chapter 5), and rickettsiae in the males were not transmitted to the next generation, as described in Sections 1 and 2 above. This infected colony reached F15 in June 1994.

6. *Rickettsia tsutsugamushi* Infection and Sex Ratio in Vector Mites

a. Sex ratios in vector mites

As described in detail above, it has been confirmed that *R. tsutsugamushi* in the vector mites *Leptotrombidium fletcheri*, *L. deliense*, *L. arenicola*, and *L. pallidum* is transmitted to the next generation transovarially through infected females. The majority of adults in the infected colonies of these species were females, except in the *L. pallidum* colonies (Table 17) (Rai and Bandopadhyay, 1978; Rapmund *et al.*, 1969, 1972; Roberts *et al.*, 1977; Takahashi *et al.*, 1988b), although both males and females develop in uninfected colonies of these species. Therefore, to maintain those infected colonies, males grown in uninfected colonies should be transferred to infected colonies, or, alternatively, females in the infected colony should be placed in culture containers with spermatophores that have been deposited by male mites (Roberts *et al.*, 1977). This marked difference of sex ratios between infected and uninfected colonies of trombiculid mites has not yet been satisfactorily explained.

b. Sex ratio alteration of L. fletcheri

To examine whether the sex ratios of mites would be altered by killing the rickettsiae in the mites, minocycline hydrochloride (MC) was successfully introduced to the unfed larvae of an infected colony of *L. fletcheri* a vector mite in Southeast Asia, by placing the larvae on mice that had been injected with a high dose of MC.

The fate of the rickettsiae in the infected colony and the sex ratios of the mite progeny were followed up. Table 18 summarizes the major findings of this study (Takahashi *et al.*, unpublished data).

Mice injected with high and low doses of MC were examined to determine whether the drug was transferred to the infesting larval *L. fletcheri*. In the females of the F1 generation of mite exposed to a low dose of MC, live rickettsiae were found, indicating that the low dose had not eliminated the rickettsia in the infected colony. In duplicate experiments with a high dose of MC (mouse no. 2 in Table 18), rickettsia was eliminated from the progency of drug-exposed mites of the infected colony; rickettsia was not detected from F1 to

Table 17. Sex Ratios in the Vector Mites, *Leptotrombidium fletcheri*, *L. deliense*, *L. arenicola*, and *L. pallidum*

Species	No. of generations sampled	Female	Male	References
L. fletcheri				
infected				
	5	98	—	Rapmund *et al.*, 1969
	13	2911[a]	27[b]	Roberts *et al.*, 1977
	1	211	—	Takahashi *et al.*, 1993c
	9	1756	—	Takahashi *et al.*, Unpub.
uninfected	5	1435	624	Roberts *et al.*, 1977
	1	130	272	Takahashi *et al.*, 1993c
	8	1652	960	Takahashi *et al.*, Unpub.
L. deliense				
infected[c]	6			Rai and Bandopadhyay, 1978
uninfected	10	1720	1130	Takahashi *et al.*, Unpub.
L. arenicola				
infected	4	905	1	Roberts *et al.*, 1977
	13	1820	93[b]	Takahashi *et al.*, Unpub.
uninfected	4	203	101	Roberts *et al.*, 1977
	10	1856	1322	Takahashi *et al.*, Unpub.
L. pallidum				
infected	3	72	73[d]	Takahashi, 1990
uninfected	8	686	738	Takahashi *et al.*, Unpub.

[a] More than 10,000 other specimens not sexed individually were apparently all females, since spermatophores from an uninfected colony were invariably required for oviposition to occur.

[b] *R. tsutsugamushi*-negative.

[c] The majority of the offspring were infected females; however, infected male offspring were occasionally produced.

[d] Including six *R. tsutsugamushi*-negative males.

Unpub., Unpublished data.

F5, at the end of the observation period.

A second high-dose experiment was performed (see mouse no. 3 in Table 18), and although a large number of mites that had ingested the drug from this mouse died off gradually before developing into adults, the adult females in the two high-dose experiments (see mice nos. 2 and 3 in Table 18) laid 34.0 and 122.3 eggs per female respectively, in F1. The fecundity of the females in the second high-dose experiment (see mouse no. 3 in Table 18) (122.3 eggs per female) was similar to that of females in uninfected colonies of *L. fletcheri*, which laid 127.9, 134.4, and 133.5 eggs per female, as reported by Dohany *et al.* (1977), Roberts *et al.* (1977), and Takahashi *et al.* (1993c), respectively.

In the two experiments with a high dose of MC, only females ap-

Table 18. Breeding of Succeeding Generations from the Infected Larvae of *L. fletcheri* After They Had Fed on Mice Injected with Minocycline; Detection of *R. tsutsugamushi* in the Mite

Dose of minocycline	Gene-ration	No. of eggs laid	Average no. of eggs per female	No. of larvae hatched (%)	No. of adults raised		*R. tsutsugamushi* in mites[c]	
					Male	Female	Male	Female
Low dose								
Mouse no. 1	P	—	—	—	0	12[b]	—	12[a]/12
	F1	267	44.5	89.5	0	59	—	9/9
High dose	P	—	—	—	0	6[b]	—	0/6
Mouse no. 2	Fl	34	34.0	58.8	0	6	—	0/6
	F2	261	65.3	78.9	35	3	0/35	0/3
	F3	456	152.0	78.9	108	13	0/108	0/13
	F4	1920	147.7	76.5	263	61	0/263	0/61
	F5	1000	111.1	73.0	71	9	0/67	0/9
High dose	P	—	—	—	0	23[b]	—	0/23
Mouse no. 3	F1	978	122.3	59.7	0	90	—	0/90
	F2	2588	35.2	62.1	297	4	0/297	0/4

[a] Not successful in killing rickettsia in mites.
[b] Only the P generation of *R. tsutsugamushi*-infected unfed larvae were fed on a minocycline-treated mouse; larvae of succeeding generations were fed on untreated mice.
[c] Examined by polymerase chain reaction or electron microscopy.
Low dose : 600 μg for first dose, then 360 μg every 12 h for 4 days.
High dose : 6,400 μg for first dose, then 3,400 μg every 12 h for 4 days.

peared in the P and F1 generations, and extremely high male ratios were observed in F2 and later generations, the male and female ratios in F2–F5 being, respectively, 332:7 (47.5:1), 108: 13 (8.3:1), 263:61 (4.3:1), and 71:9 (7.9:1). In another experiment, minocycline was introduced to the unfed larvae of an uninfected colony in the way described above for infected colonies. The drug, however, had no influence on the sex ratio in this colony, the ratio being the same as that in a control non-medicated uninfected colony.

The above findings, that males appeared in the infected colony of *L. fletcheri* after the introduction of MC to infected mites, clearly indicated that *R. tsutsugamushi* in the infected colony influenced the sex ratio of the mites. The occurrence of an extremely high male ratio in F2 and later generations after MC treatment appears to be a unique phenomenon, which has never been observed in insects and Crustacea. In the high-dose experiment (see mouse nos. 2 and 3), although rickettsia was eliminated in F1 generation, only females appeared in this generation, suggesting that the sex of the next generation had already been determined at the larval stage of the parent generation before MC was introduced.

c. Action of bacterial endosymbionts to the host arthropods

In general, rickettsia infecting both cultured cells and mice proliferate in the cells and destroy them, causing not only cell death but also the death of the host animal. However, in trombiculid mites, although *R. tsutsugamushi* proliferates in the cytoplasm of the host cells, the cells are never destroyed, possibly due to some control of *R. tsutsugamushi* proliferation. In this static relationship between the microorganism and the host cells, *R. tsutsugamushi* can be regarded as a symbiont in the mite.

This type of symbiont is well known in some arthropods, particularly in insects. Various types of bacteria and protists co-exist in the cells of such host animals as endocellular symbionts, at times influencing reproduction and sex determination (Table 19) by various modes of action. We carried out an extensive survey of the literature to determine whether a mode similar to that previously shown operated in regard to *R. tsutsugamushi* in trombiculid mites. We noted four modes of action by bacterial symbionts: cytoplasmic incompatibility, male-lethal infection, conversion infection, and parthenogenesis.

1) *Cytoplasmic incompatibility*: In *Drosophila* and mosquitoes this is a well-known example of the above-mentioned symbiosis. A typical consequence is that symbiont-containing males crossed with symbiont-free females produce no viable progeny. However, the reciprocal cross produces a normal number of progeny (Kane and Pierce, 1994). The bacteria responsible for cytoplasmic incompatibility are often in the genus *Wolbachia*, order Rickettsiales (Binnington and Hoffmann, 1989; Hsiao and Hsiao, 1985; Louis and Nigro, 1989; O'Neill, 1989; Rousset *et al.*, 1992; Yen and Barr, 1973), and are sensitive to high temperature and to tetracycline antibiotics (Breeuwer and Werren, 1990; Hoffmann *et al.*, 1986; Trips *et al.*, 1981; Yen and Barr, 1973). The cytoplasmic incompatibility results from bacteria interfering with sperm-derived chromosomes in fertilized eggs by preventing proper condensation (Breeuwer and Werren, 1990; Kane and Pierce, 1994; O'Neill and Karr, 1990).

2) *Male-lethal infection*: Extrachromosomal elements transmitted by females are clearly implicated in distortions of sex ratios in bark beetles, moths, *Drosophila*, lady beetles, and parasitoid wasps, caused by male-lethal infections. The result is a remarkable reduction in the hatching of males due to the death of male embryos (Ebbert, 1993).

In species of the *Drosophila willistoni* group, a spiroplasma and an associated virus kill males early in embryogenesis, and no effect is observed in the females which transmit these agents transovarially, as reported by Williamson and Poulson (1979) and Hackett *et al.* (1986), who cultured the *Drosophila* sex-ratio spiroplasma. In the parasitoid wasp, *Nosonia vitripennis*, a symbiont causes the production of extremely female-biased sex ratios through causing mortality in males (son-killer trait) with some 80% of all male eggs failing to hatch (Huger *et al.*, 1985); the causative agent has been identified by Gherna *et al.* (1991) as *Arsenophonus nasoniae*.

3) *Conversion infections*: In this mode, the infective agent alters the sex of its host. For example, in the amphipod *Gammarus duebeni*, two microsporidians (*Octosporea effeminans* and *Thelohania herediteria*) convert males into functional females, through which the microsporidians are transmitted transovarially (Bulnheim, 1978). The protozoan, *Paramarteilia orchestiae*, has a similar effect in the amphipod, *Orchestia gammarellus* (Ginsburger-

Voger and Desportes, 1979), and a bacteria-like microorganism changes males into females in a strain of the isopod *Armadillidium vulgare* (Martin *et al.*, 1973). In these examples, the sex of genotypic females is unaffected (Huger *et al.*, 1985).
4) *Parthenogenesis* : Parthenogenesis occurs when bacteria prevent the segregation of chromosomes in unfertilized eggs (Stouthamer *et al.*, 1993). In parasitoid wasps — for example, in *Trichogramma deion* and *Muscidifurax uniraptor* — this results in thelytoky, or the production of female progeny only (Kane and Pierce, 1994). This thelytokous parthenogenesis has been tentatively attributed to the presence of a microorganism, since treatment with tetracycline and some other antibiotics, as well as high temperature, induces the recovery of the normal sex ratio (Rousset *et al.*, 1992; Stouthamer, 1991; Stouthamer *et al.*, 1990a,b).

d. Interference of R. tsutsugamushi *with the sex ratio of vector mites*

We examined the sex ratio distortion caused by the symbionts in the infected *L. fletcheri* colony in relation to the above-mentioned four modes of bacterial action, in an attempt to find some similarities. Since no *R. tsutsugamushi*-positive males were available in this infected colony, it was not possible to cross *R. tsutsugamushi*-positive males and *R. tsutsugamushi*-negative females, and it was thus not clear how the distortion in this species was caused by cytoplasmic incompatibility. In experiments with *L. pallidum*, which produced infected males and females at the same ratio, crosses both ways did not suggest cytoplasmic incompatibility (mode no. 1). Individual rearing of *L. fletcheri*, *L. pallidum*, and other *Leptotrombidium* mites has not resulted in parthenogenesis (mode no. 4), except in *L. arenicola*, in which it was rare, as reported by Kaufmann and Traub (1966). If *R. tsutsugamushi* were to have acted as a male-lethal infection (mode no. 2) at the egg stage, the male germ cells therein would have been dead, and only females would have hatched. The hatching rate would thus have been reduced. However, we found no reduction in the hatching rate of eggs in the infected colony of *L. fletcheri* (Table 18) in our culture studies as the causes of sex ratio distortion, referring to the above four modes, following two possibilities are considered.

If the male germ cells had been killed in the ovaries of female

Table 19. Bacterial Endosymbionts Responsible for Various Alterations in Reproduction and Sex Determination

Arthropod (Group)	Host	Effect of bacteria on host[a] (Pathogen)[b]	References
Insecta			
Coleoptera			
(Beetles)	*Hypera postica*	CI (W)	O'Neill *et al.*, 1992 Hsiao and Hsiao, 1985
	Tribolium confusum	CI (W)	O'Neill *et al.*, 1992 O'Neill, 1989; Wade and Stevens, 1985 Rousset *et al.*, 1992
(Bark beetles)	*Orthotomicus latidens*	ML (ECE)	Lanier and Oliver, 1966
(Ladybird beetles)	*Hippodamia quinquesignata*	ML (ECE)	Shull, 1948
	Harmonia axyridis	ML (m?)	Gotoh and Niijima, 1986
	Menochilus sexmaculatus	ML (m?)	Gotoh and Niijima, 1986
Diptera			
(Mosquitoes)	*Aedes albopictus*	CI (W)	O'Neill *et al.*, 1992
	Culex pipens	CI (W)	O'Neill *et al.*, 1992 Rousset *et al.*, 1992 Portaro and Barr, 1975; Fine *et al.*, 1977 Suenaga, 1982, 1992
(Fruit flies)	*Drosophila simulans*	CI (W)	O'Neill *et al.*, 1992 Binnington and Hoffman, 1989 Louis and Nigro, 1989 Nigro and Louis, 1989 Rousset *et al.*, 1992
	D. bifasciata	ML (ECE)	Ikeda, 1970
	D. borealis	ML (ECE)	Carson, 1956
	D. prosaltans	ML (ECE)	Cavalcanti *et al.*, 1957
	D. robusta	ML (S)	Poulson, 1968 Williamson and Poulson, 1979
	D. willistoni	ML (S)	Williamson and Poulson, 1979

			Ebbert, 1991; Hackett *et al.*, 1986
Homoptera			
(Plant-hopper)	*Laodelphax striatellus*	CI(W)	Rousset *et al.*, 1992
Hymenoptera			
(Wasps)	*Muscidifurax uniraptor*	P(W)	Stouthamer *et al.*, 1993
	Trichogramma deion	P(W)	Stouthamer *et al.*, 1990a, 1993
	T. pretiosum	P(W)	Stouthamer *et al.*, 1993
	T. cordubensis	P(W)	Stouthamer *et al.*, 1993; Rousset *et al.*, 1992
	T. oleae	P(W)	Rousset *et al.*, 1992
	Nasonia vitripennis	CI(W)	Breeuwer *et al.*, 1992
		ML (ECE)	Skinner, 1982, 1985 Werren *et al.*, 1986 Huger *et al.*, 1985
	N. giraulti	CI(W)	Breeuwer *et al.*, 1992
	N. longicornis	CI(W)	Breeuwer *et al.*, 1992
Hemiptera			
(Milkweed bugs)	*Oncopeltus fasciatus*	ML(ECE)	Leslie, 1984
Lepidoptera			
(Moths)	*Ephestia cautella*	CI(W)	O'Neill *et al.*, 1992 Kellen *et al.*, 1981
	Epiphyas postvittana	ML(ECE)	Geier and Briese, 1978
(Cotton leafworm)	*Spodoptera littoralis*	ML(ECE)	Brimacombe, 1980
(Caterpillars)	*Estigmene acrea acrea*	ML(ECE)	Earle and MacFarlane, 1968
(Butterflies)	*Hypolimnas bolina*	ML(ECE)	Clarke *et al.*, 1975, 1983
Crustacea			
Amphipoda	*Gammarus duebeni*	CV(ms)	Bulnheim, 1978
	Orchestia gammarellus	CV(pt)	Ginsburger-Voger and Desportes, 1979
Isopoda	*Armadillidium vulgare*	CV(m)	Martin *et al.*, 1973

[a] CI, cytoplasmic incompatibility;
CV, conversion infection;
ML, male-lethal infection (all-female broods);
P, parthenogenesis (all-female broods).

mites (modified mode no. 2), the mites hatching from the eggs would have been all female, and no reduced hatching rate would have been observed. Alternatively, if *R. tsutsugamushi* were to have changed male germ cells into female cells, as occurs in infections of amphipods and isopods (mode no. 3), all larvae would have been female. It is anticipated that further studies will elucidate the actual mechanism whereby entirely female progeny are in produced infected colonies of *L. fletcheri*.

The sex ratio distortion caused by parasitic microorganisms in insects and mites appears to be controlled by the parasitic organisms in the females of the host in order to allow the parasites to persist in succeeding generations of the host animals. Since *R. tsutsugamushi* is not transmitted to the next generation through males (Takahashi, 1990), the production of more females is beneficial to the parasitizing rickettsiae. If we were to look at the distortion in sex ratios in chiggers from this viewpoint, it is possible that some differences would be noticed among mite species.

In our laboratory-reared infected colony of *L. fletcheri*, all the adults in succeeding generations from F54 to F65 were females. In a similar colony, the occurrence of males was reported to be rare, and all the males were free of rickettsiae (Roberts *et al*., 1977).

In an infected colony of *L. pallidum*, in contrast, *R. tsutsugamushi*-positive males were produced at almost the same ratio as females, whereas rickettsia-free males were produced only rarely in infected colonies of *L. fletcheri* and *L. arenicola* (Roberts *et al*., 1977).

7. Detection of *Rickettsia tsutsugamushi* in Mites

Tsutsugamushi disease is transmitted by a trombiculid mite that harbors *R. tsutsugamushi*. The rickettsiae in a mite will then transmit the disease transovarially to succeeding generations. Among the large number of chigger species throughout the world, those species that harbor and transmit *R. tsutsugamushi* are limited in number, and in a

---

[b] ECE, extra-chromosomal elements;
m, microorganism;
m?, possibly microorganism;
ms, microsporidian;
pt, protozoan;
S, spiroplasma;
W, *Wolbachia* sp.

vector species, the proportion of mites that actually harbors *R. tsutsugamushi* is at most, several percent (see Sections 1 and 2 above).

Therefore, for studies on the likelihood of a species of mite transmitting *R. tsutsugamushi* to humans and to wild rodents, and for analyzing the vertical transmission of *R. tsutsugamushi* in a mite species, we must first detect *R. tsutsugamushi* in individual trombiculid mites. Thus far, the five methods outlined below have been used for the detection of *R. tsutsugamushi* in mites.

a. Mouse passage

The mouse passage method has long been used for the detection of *R. tsutsugamushi* in individual mites or pools of mites. In this method, a mite is ground in a small amount of SPG solution, and an emulsion thus made is injected into the peritoneal cavity of a mouse susceptible to *R. tsutsugamushi*. Detection of rickettsiae is then attempted in the tissues of the abdominal cavity, and elevations of antibody levels in the mouse are followed up (Kawamura *et al.*, 1980). Since rickettsiae are not always detected in the first passage mouse, further passages are necessary. Mouse passage is time-consuming, taking 1–3 months for a satisfactory follow-up, and this hampers the development of research. In isolating rickettsiae using mice, when low-pathogenic *R. tsutsugamushi* is targeted, pretreatment with immunosuppressant in conventional mice or the use of nude mice is necessary (Kawamura *et al.*, 1980; Kobayashi *et al.*, 1987). To detect *R. tsutsugamushi* in cells in the omentum and in peritoneal smears, immunofluorescence (IF) or immunoperoxidase (IP) test, using immune sera or monoclonal antibodies, have been used. When indirect serological methods are used for detection, increased antibodies in a passage mouse often suppress the reactions. To avoid this suppression, smear preparations should be rinsed with glycine buffer at pH 3 to remove antigen-antibody complexes. In recent studies (Tamura *et al.*, 1984; Yamamoto *et al.*, 1989), rickettsiae isolated by mouse passage have been placed in cell cultures for proliferation and have been widely used for the antigenic analysis of *R. tsutsugamushi*.

Recent studies of the experimental feeding on rickettsemic mice of trombiculid mites originating from uninfected laboratory colonies have shown fairly high rates of rickettsial transmission to uninfected mites, although the infection was transient (Takahashi *et al.*, 1994a). The same mode of rickettsial infection in mites is also thought to occur in the natural environment. Therefore, if rickettsiae are detected in mites collected from wild rodents, we cannot always determine whether the rickettsiae detected are those originally harbored by the mites. To avoid misleading results in the detection of *R. tsutsugamushi* in mites, unfed mites should be targeted, and earlier studies dealing with rickettsial isolation from mites should be re-evaluated (Takahashi *et al.*, 1994a).

b. Electron microscopy

The distribution of *R. tsutsugamushi* in the tissues of *Leptotrombidium pallidum* in an infected laboratory colony was extensively studied by electron microscopy (Urakami *et al.*, 1994b). The methods used for that study are briefly outlined below.

The infected laboratory colony of *L. pallidum* used in the study originated from engorged mites collected from wild *Apodemus speciosus* in Saitama Prefecture, Japan. This infected colony was established in the laboratory by sibling mating (Takahashi *et al.*, 1988b), and mites of the F8 and F9 generations of this colony were used. To make the mite surface hydrophilic, mites were rinsed successively through serial ethanol solutions of decreasing concentration from 90% to 30%. Then mites were placed in 2% glutaraldehyde (buffered to pH 7.4 with 0.1 M cacodylate solution). Eggs and spermatophores were placed directly in this glutaraldehyde solution without ethanol pretreatment. To gain better penetration of solutions into mite tissues and to improve embedding procedures, the eggs, larvae, and adults were pricked with a fine sharp needle while in the solution. After these materials were fixed in glutaraldehyde for 2 h, they were washed with 0.1 M cacodylate buffer for 1 h. While being treated in glutaraldehyde and in osmic acid, the materials were irradiated in a 500 W microwave oven for 20 sec (Login and Dvorak, 1985). The materials were then stained with 2% uranyl acetate for 20 min and dehydrated by being passed through serial ethanol solutions of increasing concentration, by the routine method, at room temperature. The samples were embedded in an Araldite-Epon mixture and cut into ultrathin sections with a diamond knife. The sections were mounted on grids coated with formvar and carbon. After the sections were subjected to lead staining (Hanaichi *et al.*, 1986), the structures in mites were observed with an electron microscope (JEOL100CX; JEOL, Tokyo, Japan).

c. *Immunofluorescence.*

In immunofluorescence (IF), there are direct and indirect techniques. For our purposes, the direct method, employing fluorescein isothiocyanate (FITC)-labeled antibodies against individual types of *R. tsutsugamushi*, has been utilized, rather than the indirect method, which may involve more unknown factors and a greater number of steps in the procedure. For direct IF, the production of a highly specific antibody at high titers is required.

For the production of antiserum, guinea pigs or rabbits are immunized with a large amount of *R. tsutsugamushi* that have proliferated in cell cultures, in embryonated eggs, or in the spleens of heavily infected mice. The sera with high titers thus produced — or, alternatively, monoclonal antibodies — are used for IF. The production of monoclonal antibodies is described in Chapter 2.

Standardized procedures for labeling antibodies, described in depth by Kawamura and Aoyama (1983), are, briefly:

1. IgG antibodies are separated and purified from the produced antiserum by the ammonium sulfate sedimentation method.

2. FITC, representing the amount of 1/100 total protein of purified IgG, is dissolved in 0.5% carbonate (bicarbonate) buffer representing 1/10 the amount of total protein. This FITC solution is added to IgG solution adjusted to a 2% protein concentration.

3. The mixture is stirred at 7–9°C for 4 h.

4. Unbound FITC is excluded by Sephadex G–25 gelfiltration. FITC-labeled protein, at a binding ratio of fluorochrome to protein (F/P mol ratio) of 1 to 2, is selected by diethyl aminoethyl (DEAE) cellulose chromatography.

5. If any cross-reaction to another rickettsial type is found, the product should be diluted to a level that avoids cross-reaction, or the antibody to the cross-reacting antigen should be added to the labeled antibody to eliminate cross-reactions.

For detecting *R. tsutsugamushi* in a mite, the mite is placed in a drop of 0.5% normal yolk sac solution or phosphate-buffered saline (PBS) on a microscope glass slide. The mite is dissected with two minutin pins under a stereomicroscope. The head of the mite is fixed with a pin, the posterior is pricked with another pin, and the contents of the mite are squeezed out with the pin from the head to the pinhole. The squeezed contents are mixed with the surrounding solution, using the tip of a small round pin, and the mite suspension is transferred to another slide to make smear spots. After being dried in air and fixed with acetone at room temperature for 10 min, the spots on the slide are used as the antigen for IF.

With the antigens and labeled antibodies thus prepared, unfed larvae from infected colonies of *L. fletcheri* and *L. arenicola* were examined individually for rickettsial types with labeled rabbit antibodies against ten rickettsial types (Dohany *et al.*, 1978). In this IF study, the number of larvae reacting with one antibody type was small; most of the larvae reacted with several antibody types. In Malaysia, 4,550 unfed larvae belonging to seven species were collected directly from the soil surface and examined individually for rickettsial type by IF (Shirai *et al.*, 1981). Of the 4,550 larvae, 168 (3.7%) were positive for *R. tsutsugamushi*, and 115 reacted with one antibody; the rest reacted with multiple antibody types.

d. Biotin-avidin immunofluorescence (BA-IF)

In the biotin-avidin complex method, biotin, which has a strong affinity to avidin, a protein, at a binding constant of 10–5 M, is bound to the antibody (biotinylation) and is reacted with FITC-labeled avidin. This reaction is regarded as more sensitive than the routine IF method. *R. tsutsugamushi* in unfed larvae were detected and identified by this technique (Yamamoto *et al.*, 1987). The method used and the results are described below.

Type-specific monoclonal antibodies (Murata *et al.*, 1986) were purified into IgG by filtration on protein A affinity chromatography and biotinylated with biotin succinimide ester (Biosearch, San Rafael, California, U.S.A.) according to the method of Berman and Basch (1980). The concentration of monoclonal IgG was first adjusted to 1 mg/ml, and this was dialyzed in 0.1 M $NaHCO_3$ at pH 8.5 overnight. Immediately before biotinylation, biotin was dissolved in dimethyl sulfoxide (DMSO) at 1.0 mg antibody, and the mixture was then dialyzed in PBS with 0.1% sodium azide overnight.

For labeling avidin with FITC, equal amounts of avidin solution (10 mg/ml) and FITC, dissolved in 0.5 M carbonate-bicarbonate buffer at pH 9.5 at 200 g/ml, were mixed and stirred at room temperature for 60 min. After the labeling procedures, unbound FITC was eliminated by Sephadex G-25 column filtration.

For detecting antigen in mites, a mite was dissected and antigen spots were prepared on a microscope glass slide by the same procedure as that used for IF, noted above.

Technical procedures employed for antigen detection were similar to those for indirect IF. Biotinylated antibody was bound to the antigen spot, after which FITC-labeled avidin was placed on the antibody/antigen spot and incubated for 10–15 min at 37°C or for 15–20 min at 4°C.

If the reaction exceeded 15 min on incubation at 37°C, the fluorescence result was difficult to read. If the reaction was performed with a mixture of biotinylated antibody and FITC-labeled avidin, there was no reactivity until 10 min after mixing. The specificity of biotinylated monoclonal antibodies against rickettsial types was examined with rickettsia-infected L-929 cells and peritoneal smears from infected mice as antigen. The reactions were positive only for homologous types of rickettsiae and were negative for heterologous antigens. The sensitivity and intensity of fluorescence were higher than in routine IF. Results of detecting rickettsiae by this method are shown in Fig. 10.

In the detection of rickettsiae by IF or by BA-IF in the materials squeezed from the mites, attention should be paid to the nonspecific reactions with the tiny granules often found in the mite contents. Another problem with these methods is that antigen materials on the glass slide are easily rinsed off while washing. The addition of bovine serum albumin to antigens as an adhesive paste may solve the problem, ensuring that antigens adhere firmly to the surface of the glass slide.

e. Polymerase chain reaction (*PCR*) *and nested PCR*

The PCR is an *in vitro* method for the enzymatic synthesis of specific DNA sequences, using two oligonucleotide primers. Twenty cycles of PCR yield about a million-fold (2^{20}) amplification.

DNA fragments of *R. tsutsugamushi* in an infected laboratory colony of *L. pallidum* (Takahashi *et al.*, 1988b) were examined by the following methods.

Since the amount of *R. tsutsugamushi* DNA in a mite is rather small, DNA was extracted by alkaline treatment (Kaneko *et al.*, 1989) to prevent loss of DNA during processing. Mites were killed

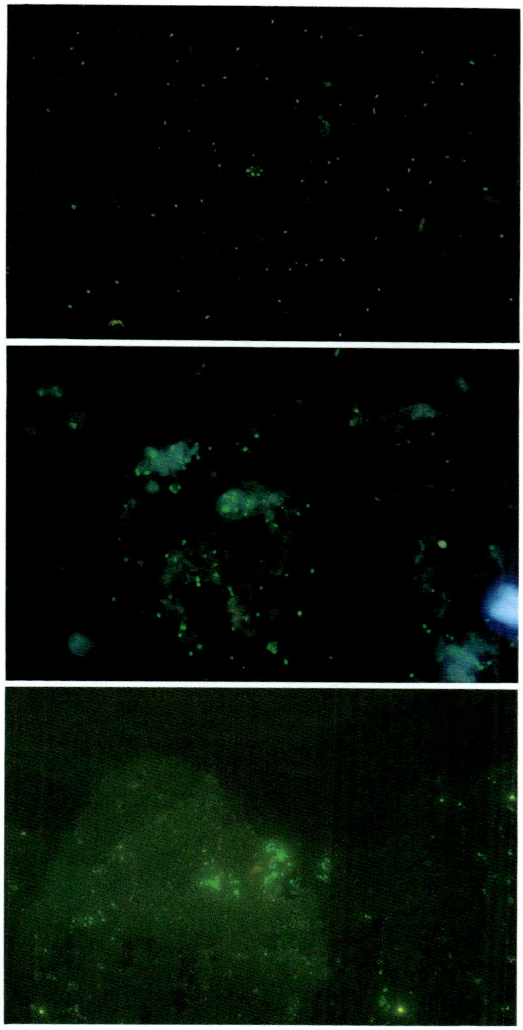

Fig. 10. Detection of *R. tsutsugamushi* by biotin-avidin IF with biotinylated monoclonal antibody against Karp type rickettsia in the materials squeezed from an infected *L. fletcheri* larva (upper), *L. fletcheri* egg (middle), and *L. pallidum* larva (bottom). (Photos by Nogami and Murata.)

in 70% ethanol, and transferred individually to a depression on a glass slide. After the mite was dried in air, the body was disrupted with a tungsten needle and then suspended in 10 μl deionized water (Furuya and Yoshida, 1992). To this suspension, sodium hydroxide was added, at a final concentration of 0.1 M, and the mixture was incubated at 37°C for 1 h. The solution was then neutralized with hydrochloric acid of the same molarity and this was used as the template for PCR.

Nested PCR was performed by carrying out 30 thermal cycles at each step. DNA amplification took place in the samples from mites from the infected colony, PCR was thus determined to be a suitable method for the detection of *R. tsutsugamushi* in the mite. Pairs of primers specific to five types, *i.e.*, Gilliam, Karp, Kato, Kawasaki, and Kuroki, were designed by selecting less homologous areas of the DNA sequence among the five types. The use of these primer pairs as internal primers for nested PCR enabled the identification of the type of *R. tsutsugamushi* in the mite by this method (Furuya *et al.*, 1993).

Of the methods described above, it appears that direct IF and nested PCR will be the principal methods of choice from now on for detecting *R. tsutsugamushi* in the mite.

5

Transmission Dynamics of *Rickettsia tsutsugamushi*

1. Transovarian Transmission

a. Transovarian transmission of Rickettsia tsutsugamushi *in vector mites*

Of the active life stages of the trombiculid mite, the only stage that transmits *R. tsutsugamushi* to wild rodents and humans is the unfed larva. Therefore, *R. tsutsugamushi* harbored by unfed larvae was regarded as originating from eggs laid by the female via transovarian transmission; this was first confirmed by Miyajima and Okumura (1917) and R. Kawamura (1926) in *Leptotrombidium akamushi*. They collected adult *L. akamushi* in the soil and reared them in the labaratory, and the bites of the unfed larvae caused Tsutsugamushi disease in monkeys.

Later Japanese investigators assumed or demonstrated that the same mode of transmission occurred in *L. akamushi* (Asanuma, 1983; Ito *et al.*, 1957; Kawamura, R. *et al.*, 1932; Miura and Kawai, 1968; Tamiya, 1962); in *L. scutellare* (Asanuma, 1983; Asanuma *et al.*, 1962a,b; Tamiya, 1962); and in *L. pallidum* (Asanuma, 1983; Asanuma *et al.*, 1962a; Kumada and Oya, 1968; Miura and Kawai, 1968; Saito *et al.*, 1977; Tamiya, 1962).

Outside Japan, the same mode of transmission was demonstrated in *L. pallidum* in Korea (Jackson *et al.*, 1957); in *L. gaohuensis* in Gaohu village, Zhejiang Province, China (Wei *et al.*, 1985b,c); and in *L. fletcheri*, *L. arenicola*, *L. deliense*, and *L. scutellare* in the western Pacific region (Audy and Harrison, 1951; Davis *et al.*, 1947; Krishnan *et al.*, 1949; Mackie *et al.*, 1946a,b; Traub and Wisseman, 1968b, 1974b).

Infected mites of the species discussed above were colonized, and transovarian transmission was confirmed in succeeding generations by laboratory experiments in *L. deliense* (Rai and Bandopadhyay, 1978; Wang and Wen, 1965); *L. fletcheri* (Rapmund, 1984; Rapmund *et al.*, 1969; Roberts *et al.*, 1977); *L. arenicola* (Rapmund *et al.*, 1972; Roberts and Robinson, 1977; Roberts *et al.*, 1977; Shirai *et al.*, 1982c); *L. gaohuensis* (Wei *et al.*, 1987); and *L. pallidum* (Takahashi *et al.*, 1988b). Recently, infected colonies of *L. imphalum* and another *Leptotrombidium* species were established in northern Thailand, and transtadial and transovarian transmission of the rickettsia by both chigger species were demonstrated in the laboratory (Tanskul *et al.*, 1994).

1) Transovarian and filial infection rates

In their review of the transtadial and transovarian development of disease agents in arthropods, Burgdorfer and Varma (1967) noted two infection rates as indicators of transovarian development; these rates, however, may not bear any relation to each other. One is the transovarian infection rate, which is the percentage of infected females that pass rickettsiae to their progeny, and the other is the filial infection rate, which is the percentage of infected progeny derived from an infected female. These indicators are often used to characterize the infected laboratory colonies of trombiculid mites.

(a) *L. deliense*

Transovarian transmission of *R. tsutsugamushi* was followed up to F2 and F4 in *L. deliense* colonies by demonstrating rickettsia in mice that were bitten by the unfed larvae of two infected colonies (Wang *et al.*, 1965).

Rai and Bandopadhyay (1978) reared larval *L. deliense* from an infected colony in succeeding generations mating five pairs of infected females and uninfected males in each generation, and examining the infectivity of each generation. The transovarian infection rate was 100% (30/30) and the filial infection rates were 95–100% (Table 1). Thus the progeny of an infected female were mostly infected females, as in *L. fletcheri*, but there were a few infected males.

(b) *L. fletcheri*

Rapmund *et al.* (1969) observed transovarian and filial infection rates in *L. fletcheri* by rearing the mites to the F5 generation. Through all generations, infected females produced only female offspring. Therefore, maintenance of the colony required the introduction of males or spermatophores from an uninfected colony. For the

Table 1. Filial Infection Rates in Some Colonies of Vector Mites Established from a Single Mite Naturally Infected with *Rickettsia tsutsugamushi*

Species	Filial infection rate (%)			(Positive no./No. examined)				References
	F1	F2	F3	F4	F5	F6	Total	
L. deliense	100 (75/75)	97 (77/79)	99 (83/84)	99 (87/88)	99 (86/87)	95 (83/87)	98 (491/500)	Rai and Bandopadhyay, 1978[a]
	100 (92/92)	99 (80/81)	100 (85/85)	100 (80/80)	98 (105/107)	100 (84/84)	99 (526/529)	Rai and Bandopadhyay, 1978[b]
L. fletcheri	100 (6/6)	96 (53/55)	90 (455/507)	97 (241/249)	99 (318/322)		94 (1073/1139)	Rapmund *et al.*, 1969
L. arenicola	3 (1/39)	7 (3/42)					5 (4/81)	Rapmund *et al.*, 1972
	100 (4/4)	90 (35/39)	99 (396/400)	95 (441/463)[c]			97 (876/906)	Roberts and Robinson, 1977
L. pallidum	100 (35/35)	97 (115/119)	90 (19/21)				97 (169/175)	Takahashi, 1990
	71 (5/7)	100 (6/6)	100 (3/3)				88 (14/16)	Takahashi, 1990
	100 (5/5)						100 (5/5)	Takahashi, 1990
	67 (4/6)	100 (12/12)	100 (5/5)				91 (21/23)	Takahashi, 1990

[a] Five pairs of infected females and uninfected males were reared in separate jars. After hatching, the larvae were individually fed on mice (one larva for one mouse).

[b] Five infected females from each generation were reared with five uninfected males, and their progeny were observed for infection up to the sixth generation.

[c] Of 22 rickettsia-negative larvae in F4, 16 were the progeny of a single female.

determination of *R. tsutsugamushi* in individual mites performed by feeding the mite on a mouse, only one mouse was used for each unfed larva.

The transovarian infection rate over three generations was 98%; 83 known infected females — 2 in F1, 33 in F2, and 48 in F3 — were reared; only one female, in F3, failed to transmit *R. tsutsugamushi* to her offspring.

Filial infection rates were generally as high as 90% or more in each generation (Table 2). The rates for individual females, however, varied greatly: in 65 females, 51 showed a rate of 100%, 10 a rate of 86–96%, and 4 a rate of 8–29%. Thus, the filial infection rates of mites were classified into three groups: in the first (and commonest), all larval progeny of an infected female are infected; in the second (this group occurring occasionally), infected females produce infected larvae, except for one or two individuals that are uninfected; and in the third (this group also occurring occasionally), infected females produce predominantly uninfected larvae (Table 2).

Roberts *et al*. (1977) reared an infected colony to the F13 generation and acquired 2,938 adults (2,911 females and 27 males). Most of the females were infected with *R. tsutsugamushi*, and all males were uninfected.

When *R. tsutsugamushi* in the females of an infected colony was killed by introducing minocycline (injected to a mouse on which unfed larvae were fed), a number of uninfected males were found (Takahashi *et al*., 1993c). This finding indicates that the sex ratio of mites could be controlled by the rickettsia.

The 27 uninfected males in the study of Roberts *et al*. (1977) were

Table 2. Vertical Transmission of *R. tsutsugamushi* in Five Generations of *Leptotrombidium fletcheri* in an Infected Colony

Generation	Filial infection rate (%)				
F1	100 (1)				
F2	100 (1),	95 (1)			
F3	100 (26),	>95 (3),	29 (1),	22 (1),	8 (1)
F4	100 (10),	93 (1),	86 (2),	17 (1)	
F5	100 (13),	96 (1),	95 (1),	89 (1)	

Note: Numbers in parentheses indicate adult females, each of whose larval offspring was investigated for the presence of *R. tsutsugamushi*.
Source: Rapmund (1984).

produced from two infected females; six males were produced from a female in F4, and 21 males from a female in F13. Initially, the female mite in F13 produced only infected females, but it then underwent a splitting of the posterodorsal integument, or schizeckenosy (Mitchell and Nadchatram, 1969), and produced only rickettsia-negative males. These males were no different from those in an uninfected colony and deposited spermatophores, which were taken in by both infected and uninfected females, producing viable eggs. It was not clear why the infected female suddenly produced uninfected males, but this finding indicated the occurrence of uninfected individuals in an infected colony.

In infected laboratory colonies of *L. fletcheri*, the reported infection rate by Roberts *et al.* (1975a) was 85% (69/81); that reported by Shirai *et al.* (1982c) was also 85% (80/94). Also, as reported by Rapmund *et al.* (1969) and Roberts *et al.* (1977), the progeny of infected females were mostly infected females, and both transovarian and filial infection rates were usually close to 100%, although low rates were rarely observed.

By this mechanism, point foci consisting of virtually 100% infected larval mites could be produced. Further, infected females in the same place could considerably increase the size of the infective spot and could increase the number of infected larval mites in the infective spot, thus accumulating more rickettsiae. The risk of infection for humans exposed to larval mites at such point foci would be extremely high (Rapmund *et al.*, 1969).

(c) *L. arenicola*

In their study of an infected colony of *L. arenicola* reared to the second generation, Rapmund *et al.* (1972) demonstrated a 100% (2/2) transovarian transmission rate and very low filial infection rates: 2.6% (1/39) in F1 and 7.1% (3/42) in F2 (Table 1). However, they were not successful in demonstrating transovarian transmission rates beyond the second generation, since only a single male F2 mite reached the adult stage.

In a successful rearing of an infected colony of the same species to the fourth generation, Roberts and Robinson (1977) found the transovarian infection rate to be 100% (51/51) and the filial infection rates from individual infected females to vary from 20% to 100%; the infection of individual larvae was examined by feeding each larva on a mouse and examining each mouse for infection. The filial infection rate was 100% in the majority of female mites (39/51), but it was 60% (3/5) and 20% (4/20), respectively, from two females at F3. In all, of 906 adult mites reared from 51 infected female mites, 876 (97%) were infected. These high infection rates indicate the maximum vector potential of the species and may not reflect actual rates under field conditions.

In this experiment, 30 chiggers from the colony did not transmit *R. tsutsugamushi* to the mice on which they fed. Of these 30, only 7 (all females) survived to the adult stage, and none laid eggs. This finding, that an infected female sometimes produced uninfected females in the next generation, and that offspring from the latter females were all free of rickettsia, explains the mechanism whereby infective spots naturally disappear in the field.

Roberts *et al*. (1977) found only one uninfected male out of 906 adults in an infected colony of *L. arenicola* reared to the fourth generation. The infection rate in an infected colony of this species examined by Shirai *et al*. (1982c) in 23 familial lines at F11 and F12 was 99% (96/97).

In all the studies of this species, it has been reported that infected females produced mostly infected females in the next generation, even though the filial infection rate was very low in some individual females, as occurred (Rapmund, 1984) in the infected colony of *L. fletcheri*. When infected colonies are reared in succeeding generations in the laboratory, attention should be paid to the time at which males are found in the colony since this is an indication that uninfected individuals are appearing. It is thus possible for the ratio of uninfected mites in such a colony to increase; if this occurs, colonization of an infected family line will be required again.

(d) *L. pallidum*

Infected colonies of *L. pallidum* (Takahashi *et al*., 1988b) were established by mating female-male pairs collected at an infective spot in Chichibu, Japan. Infected pairs were then selected as the parent generation, and succeeding generations were reared by sibling mating, since the male ratio was high in the infected colony of this species.

In four family lines in F1 to F3, the transovarian infection rate in all three generations was 100% (10/10) and the filial infection rate was 97% (209/219), determined by detection of rickettsia by mouse passage. The male : female ratio in the same generations was

51 : 53, almost the same as that in uninfected colonies. All 53 females were positive for rickettsia, whereas 45 of 51 males were positive and 6 were negative.

The infection rate in larvae in F8 and F9 of the above family lines was investigated with electron microscopy by Urakami *et al.* (1994a). The infection rate in F8 and F9 generations was 52% (17/33); this was similar to the rate determined by the mouse passage method, which was 45% (5/11). Compared with the filial rate of 97% at F1 to F3, the rate rapidly dropped in succeeding generations. Electron microscopic observations (Urakami *et al.*, 1994b) revealed that rickettsiae in an infected female did not always invade the oocytes in the ovaries, and this finding clearly indicated why uninfected offspring were produced by infected females.

The occurrence of males and the infectivity of both sexes in infected laboratory colonies of the four species above are shown in Table 3. In the *L. pallidum* colony, there was a high ratio of infected males, in contrast to the other three tropical species, *L. fletcheri*, *L. arenicola*, and *L. deliense*, whose populations were infected females.

2) Transtadial transmission

The isolation of rickettsiae in engorged larvae that are actually

Table 3. Infectivity and Sex Composition of Infected Colonies of Four Species of *Leptotrombidium*

Infected colony	Infected		Uninfected		Reference
	Male	Female	Male	Female	
L. deliense	Rare	Almost all			Rai and Bandopadhyay, 1978
L. fletcheri		Almost all	Rare		Roberts *et al.*, 1977
		All			Rapmund *et al.*, 1969
		All			Takahashi *et al.*, 1993c
L. arenicola	Rare	Almost all			Rapmund *et al.*, 1972
		Almost all	Rare		Roberts *et al.*, 1977
		All?			Roberts and Robinson, 1977
		Almost all	Rare	Rare	Takahashi *et al.*, unpublished data
L. pallidum	Even	Even	Rare		Takahashi *et al.*, 1988b
	Even	Even	Rare	Rare	Takahashi *et al.*, unpublished data

infected is easy; however, isolation becomes very difficult in the free-living stages — *i.e.*, deutonymphs and adults — that have developed from the same group of engorged larvae or that are collected directly in the field. Many investigators have noted this problem (Blake *et al.*, 1945; Fukuzumi, 1953; Ito and Obata, 1961; Kawamura, R. 1926; Mackie *et al.,* 1946a,b; Nagayo *et al.*, 1921; Takahashi *et al.*, 1994a; Traub and Wisseman, 1974b).

In an infected *L. fletcheri* colony established by Rapmund *et al.* (1969) in which both transovarian and filial infection rates were 90% or higher and the same infection rates were anticipated in the postlarval stages, the isolation of rickettsiae by the mouse passage method in the egg, unfed larva, deutonymph, and adult was also reported to be more difficult than in engorged larvae (Roberts *et al.*, 1975a) (Table 4).

In newly molting adult *L. fletcheri*, the isolation rate of rickettsia was as low as 20%, but at the end of their egg-laying period the rate increased to 75% (US Army Medical Research Unit, 1969). This change was considered by the researchers concerned to indicate that rickettsiae were reactivated during the larval feeding stage after being masked or in an occult phase during the other developmental stages (Traub and Frick, 1950). The number of infective rickettsiae increased during the adult stage, at least in females with a 100% filial

Table 4. Transtadial Transmission Determined by Mouse Passage (MP) and Immunofluorescence (IF) in Infected Colonies of *Leptorombidium fletcheri*

Method	Eggs	Deutova	Larvae		Protonymphs	Deutonymphs	Tritonymphs	Adults	References
			Unfed	Engorged					
MP	132	13	59	20	18	19	20	21	ref. 1
	(0)	(8)	(86)	(95)	(94)	(47)	(60)	(19)	
IF	12	—	12	—	13	15	14	15	ref. 2
	(92)	—	(92)	—	(54)	(87)	(86)	(100)	
MP	—	—	—	—	18	19	20	21	ref. 3
	—	—	—	—	(100)	(47)	(60)	(20)	

The numbers examined are shown, and the percentages positive for rickettsia are shown in parentheses.
ref. 1: Roberts *et al.*, 1975a.
ref. 2: Roberts *et al.*, 1975a,b.
ref. 3: U.S. Army Med. Res. Unit, 1969.

infection rate (Traub and Wisseman, 1974b; US Army Medical Research Unit, 1969).

Roberts *et al.* (1975a,b) compared the detection rates of *L. fletcheri* for the mouse passage and IF methods, finding a marked difference in the rates in the egg and adult stages by the two methods, these being 0% and 19% in the egg and female, respectively, by mouse passage, and 92% and 100%, respectively, by IF (Table 4). Based on this result, they considered that rickettsiae in the mites were not masked or in an occult phase, but that the failure to isolate the organisms may have been due to technical factors or may have been related to the number of rickettsiae.

In their observations of transtadial changes of rickettsiae in *L. pallidum* by electron microscopy, Urakami *et al.* (1994a) found that the proliferation of rickettsiae was greatest in the egg-laying female and was also considerable in the unfed larvae. This observation supports the findings and assumptions of Roberts *et al.* (1975a,b) above, since the changes in the proliferation of rickettsiae according to stage would be the same in *L. fletcheri* and *L. pallidum*. The distribution of rickettsiae in the tissues of mites (Urakami *et al.*, 1994a,b; Wright *et al.*, 1984) is discussed in Section 2 below.

3) Role of infected males in the colony

As described in the preceding chapter, fertilization in trombiculid mites does not occur by direct sexual contact, but by the male depositing spermatophores on a surface and the female taking them in through the genital aperture for insemination. It was long assumed that rickettsiae were transmitted from infected males to their progeny.

Rai and Bandopadhyay (1978) found a small number of infected males in their infected colony of *L. deliense*. They mated uninfected females with the infected males individually in separate vials, and five such pairs were followed up to F5. At the same time, five uninfected females were reared in a group together with five infected males; their progeny were examined for *R. tsutsugamushi* up to F6, but no rickettsia was detected in any of the progeny.

Takahashi (1990) reared *L. pallidum* carrying out the following experiments: (a) A pool of spermatophores deposited by an infected male was injected into a mouse for the detection of *R. tsutsugamushi*; a total of 78 spermatophores from 11 infected males were examined, but none of the mice was infected with rickettsia. (b)

Seven pairs of infected males and uninfected females were reared separately, and 227 larvae in the next generation were confirmed to be uninfected. (c) A spermatophore from an infected male was sectioned serially and examined for rickettsia by electron microscopy, but no rickettsia was detected (Urakami *et al.*, 1994b). The findings of these three experiments indicated that there was little possibility that rickettsia was transmitted to the progeny through an infected *L. pallidum* male; these findings were similar to those of Rai and Bandopadhyay (1978), who suggested that infected *L. deliense* males played no role in the transmission of rickettsia other than to provide spermatophores to infected females.

The above findings were supported and more clearly demonstrated by electron microscopy (Urakami *et al.*, 1994b), which showed that, during the process of spermatogenesis in the male mite, rickettsiae were eliminated from the spermatogonia, none finally remaining in the mature sperms.

4) Absence of parthenogenesis in the infected colony

Rai and Bandopadhyay (1978) reared five infected *L. deliense* females separately and another five infected females in a group for two years, and no oviposition by parthenogenesis was observed.

Roberts *et al.* (1977) individually reared 20 unfertilized females from infected colonies of *L. fletcheri* and *L. arenicola* without access to spermatophores. All females failed to lay eggs during an observation period of 60 days. After 60 days, each female was allowed to take up spermatophores and all but 2 then produced viable eggs. Thus, parthenogenesis, as described by Kaufman and Traub (1966) to occur in uninfected colonies, did not occur in this infected colony. In infected colonies of *L. pallidum* (Takahashi *et al.*, 1988b), tritonymphs were kept individually in a vial. After the molting females had been collected and reared separately or in a group without contact with spermatophores. During a three-month observation period, no eggs were laid. After that time, the individually reared females were collected in a group, and infected males were placed in this group and in another group of infected females reared in a pool from the beginning; it was found that oviposition began in both groups. Thus, no parthenogenesis occurred, and the taking of spermathophores by females was confirmed to be essential for oviposition in the infected colony of *L. pallidum*. No parthenogenesis was found in any infected colonies of the four species of

Leptotrombidium discussed in this section.

5) Transmission dynamics of rickettsia in mites and mammals

As stated above, transovarian transmission of *R. tsutsugamushi* from the infected female was demonstrated by rearing infected mites in succeeding generations. Recent electron microscopic studies (Urakami *et al.*, 1988b, 1994a,b) also support this transmission pathway, having detected rickettsiae in germinal cells in the egg immediately before hatching, in unfed larvae immediately after hatching, and in females developing from rickettsia-positive larvae. The same picture has been observed in corresponding stages of infected colonies of *L. fletcheri* and *L. arenicola* (Urakami *et al.*, unpublished data).

As also noted above, it has been confirmed that infected males in laboratory colonies of *L. deliense* and *L. pallidum* played no role in transmitting *R. tsutsugamushi* to the progeny. It can be assumed that infected *L. fletcheri* or *L. arenicola* males in the natural environment similarly play no role in transmission. Thus, we can conclude that the transmission of *R. tsutsugamushi* to the progeny is achieved only through the ovaries of the infected female.

Rickettsiae acquired at a low rate by vector mites while feeding on infected rodents are not considered to be transmitted to the next generation (Fukuzumi, 1953; Ito and Obata, 1961; Takahashi *et al.*, 1994a), and infected males play no role in transmission of rickettsia to the next generation. Thus, rickettsiae in unfed larvae are believed to have no source other than the infected female.

Rickettsiae in unfed larvae are maintained from stage to stage transtadially in the mite, then invade the oocytes in ovaries, and are transmitted in the eggs and larvae successively from generation to generation transovarially. Only the mites act as reservoirs of rickettsia, and the infected unfed larvae, which serve as vectors, cause rickettsial infections in wild animals and humans while feeding on them. Wild rodents are not thus a reservoir, but are only a victim of the infection, similarly to humans.

The transovarian and filial infection rates may offer some explanation, in ecological terms, of the return of rickettsial epidemics every 20–30 years (Kawamura and Tanaka, 1988), although there is, as yet, no biological explanation for this phenomenon. Epidemics would increase when the transovarian infection rate is elevated and when infected larvae are distributed gradually by birds or wild animals to distant localities, and reduced when the filial infection rate is reduced.

b. Electron microscopy of R. tsutsugamushi-*infected* Leptotrombidium

1) Morphology of *R. tsutsugamushi* in mites

A few investigators (Urakami *et al.*, 1994 a,b; Wright *et al.*, 1984) have observed *R. tsutsugamushi*-infected and -uninfected trombiculid mites by electron microscopy. Rickettsiae in mites can be indentified based on morphology identical with rickettsiae in cultured cells, especially in terms of the characteristic structure of the cell walls, which consist of the electron-dense outer leaflet and a less dense inner leaflet. In studies of mites from infected laboratory colonies, many rickettsiae have been observed in various organs and tissues of both larval and adult mites.

The cytoplasm of rickettsia involves ribosomes and DNA fibers, and no other special structures are recognized. However, Wright *et al.* (1984) found bundles of microtubule-like structures in the cytoplasm of some, but not all, rickettsiae in the ovaries of *L. arenicola*. The same structure was observed in rickettsiae in the ovaries of *L. fletcheri*, but not in the microorganisms in *L. pallidum* (Urakami *et al.*, 1994 a, b) (Fig. 1). The tubules were 250–300 nm in length and 18 nm in width, and were located at both sides of the long axis of the rickettsia. Their morphology was similar to the microtubules in eukaryotic cells, but no center hole was recognized. Urakami *et al.* (1994 a,b) attempted to cultivate these tubule-containing rickettsiae in L cell cultures, but none of the rickettsiae seen in the cultured cells contained the tubular structures.

Wright *et al.* (1984) also observed, in a membrane-bound sac in the midgut cells of *L. arenicola*, an aggregate of rickettsia-like structures that had electron-dense cytoplasm a little smaller in size than the normal rickettsia. The structure was surrounded by an envelope morphologically similar to that of *R. tsutsugamushi*, but the relation of these atypical rickettsia-like structures to *R. tsutsugamushi* cannot be clarified unless they are examined by immunoelectron microscopy.

The rickettsia or rickettsia-like structures were mostly cocci-form, and the picture of their binary fission was seldom observed (Urakami *et al.*, 1994b). The bacilli-form of rickettsiae were found in cells in

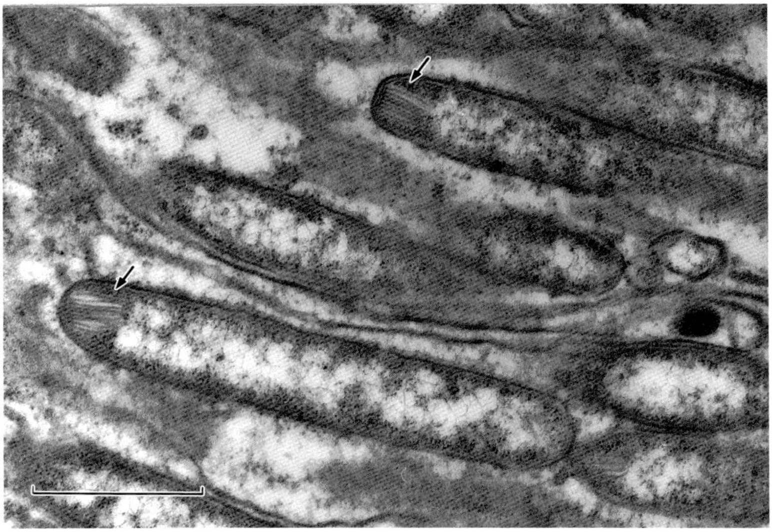

Fig. 1. *R. tsutsugamushi* in ovary of adult *L. fletcheri*. Intracytoplasmic fibrous structures (arrows) are found at the longitudinal ends of rickettsiae. Bar = 1 μm.

the reproductive organs of female *L. pallidum*. These results indicate that the rickettsia multiplies actively in the reproductive organs, but very slowly in other organs and tissues.

2) Distribution of rickettsiae in mites

Roberts *et al.* (1975b) observed rickettsial distribution in *L. fletcheri* in an infected colony by fluorescent microscopy, and reported dense distribution in the salivary gland and midgut of the larvae, and in the ovary of the female, but low density distribution in the excretory bladder and epidermal layer of adults. Wright *et al.* (1984), in their electron microscopic study of *L. arenicola*, reported that rickettsiae were distributed in various organs and tissues, with many in the salivary glands of larvae and the ovaries of females, but none in muscles.

In their electron microscopic study of *L. pallidum* from an infected laboratory colony, Urakami *et al.* (1994a) analyzed the density of rickettsiae in various organs and tissues by counting the number of rickettsiae per 100 μm^2. The results are summarized in Table 5. In the larvae, rickettsiae were distributed most densely in the salivary gland. In the adults, rickettsial density was high in the salivary gland,

Table 5. Density of *R. tsutsugamushi* in Organs and Tissues of Larval and Adult *L. pallidum*

	Organ and tissue										
	SG	TG	MG	EB	BR	MS	EP	RD	OV	TS	ud
Larva	+++	++	+	±	+	±	+	+			+
Adult	+++	+	+	+++	++	+	+++		+++	+++	++

SG, salivary gland; TG, tubular gland; MG, midgut; EB, excretory bladder; BR, brain; MS, muscle; Ep, epidermal layer; RD, rudiment of reproductive organ; OV, ovary; TS, testis; ud, undefined organs.

+++ : 3.0–9.0 rickettsiae/100μm^2 section

++ : 1.0–2.0

+ : 0.3–0.8

± : <0.2

excretory bladder, epidermal layer, and ovary and testis. The ovary and testis in adults contained a number of rickettsiae comparable to that in the salivary gland. Both the midgut, the largest organ in both larvae and adults, and the brain contained a moderate number of rickettsiae. In the muscle, only a few rickettsiae were found in many larvae and adults, while some mites contained moderate numbers of rickettsiae.

Comparison of the distribution in larvae and adults in Table 5 reveals that, in adult mites, the density of rickettsiae was higher in the excretory bladder, epidermal layer, and reproductive organs than in these tissues in larvae. Since all the organs and tissues are much larger in adults than in larvae, the total number of rickettsiae increases with the development of mites from the larval to the adult form. Eggs after oviposition and spermatophores after deposit were observed by the same method, and while a moderate number of rickettsiae were seen in eggs, no one was seen in spermatophores. This observation well supports the evidence that the rickettsiae in infected females are vertically transmitted to the progeny through eggs, whereas those in infected males are not transmitted to the spermatophore (Takahashi *et al.*, 1988b).

The results outlined above indicate the overall tendency of rickettsial distribution; however, the density observed in each organ and tissue differs greatly in individual mites. For example, as shown in Figs. 2a and b, the salivary glands from two different adults exhibit clearly different rickettsial density. In general, in adult mites that have a number of rickettsiae, the density of rickettsiae in the salivary glands is relatively high compared to that in any other organ. This indicates that the total number of rickettsiae in the whole body differs greatly in each mite.

At the cellular level, unequal distribution of rickettsiae is also noticed. As shown in the salivary gland zone of a mite in Fig. 3, many rickettsiae are contained in the cytoplasm of some cells (those marked with stars), but there is none in other cells (those marked with asterisks). Similar results were recognized in the cells of the brain and other organs.

In infected laboratory colonies of *Leptotrombidium*, the efficiency of vertical transmission of rickettsiae from parents to the progeny is generally high, but the production of a few rickettsia-negative progeny has been reported in infected colonies of *L. fletcheri* (Rapmund *et al.*, 1969; Roberts and Robinson, 1977), *L. arenicola* (Roberts and Robinson, 1977), and *L. pallidum* (Takahashi, *et al.*, 1988b).

Recently, Urakami *et al.* (1994a) demonstrated similar evidence by electron microscopy. As mentioned above, the density of rickettsiae differs in individual mites and in individual cells. It is probable that the different concentrations of rickettsiae in the female may cause the reproduction of different ratios of rickettsia-positive and

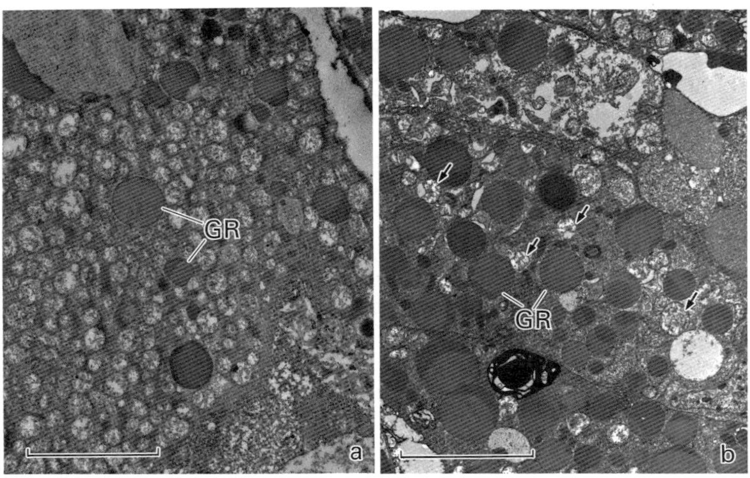

Figs. 2a and **b**. Salivary glands of adult *L. pallidum*. Cytoplasm is filled with rickettsiae in Fig. 2a, but rickettsiae (arrows) are sparsely involved in Fig. 2b. GR: Salivary granules. Bar = 5 μm.

-negative progeny; further, due to the uneven distribution of rickettsiae in oocyte cells, when a female contains only a small number of rickettsiae, the ratio of rickettsia-negative eggs produced would be high, resulting in the production of many rickettsia-negative progeny.

3) Elctron microscopic observation of vertical transmission of rickettsiae

Urakami *et al.* (1994b) carried out an electron microscopic study of rickettsia-infected female *L. pallidum* and demonstrated the vertical transmission of rickettsiae to the eggs. Their findings showed a pair of ovaries, located at the ventral anterior side of the opisthosoma in female mites, containing oogonia of various sizes and oocytes at various stages of oogenesis. The oogonia (Fig. 4) had a small amount of cytoplasm and contained a few rickettsiae, whereas the oocytes at the early stage of oogenesis (Fig. 5) contained a large

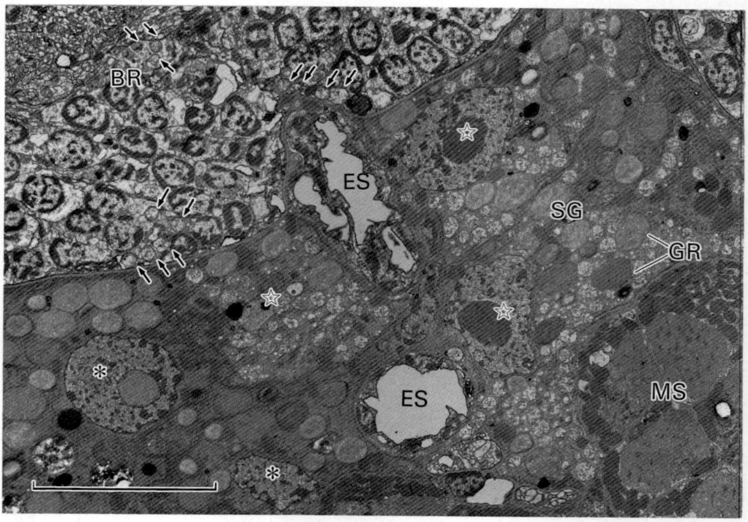

Fig. 3. Anterior part of a larva of *L. pallidum*. Rickettsiae (arrows) are in salivary gland (SG), brain (BR), and muscles (MS). The salivary gland cells indicated by stars, contain a number of rickettsiae, but no microorganisms are in the other cells of the same organ indicated by asterisks. In the brain only some of the cells contain several rickettsiae, while no rickettsiae were found in the majority of the cells. All the rickettsiae in the brain are indicated by arrows. ES: Esophagus, GR: Salivary granules. Bar = 10 μm.

amount of cytoplasm and a number of rickettsiae, suggesting that the rickettsiae were multiplying in the growing oocytes. An incomplete egg shell was then formed around the oocyte at the periphery of the ovary, and the oocytes were shown to contain yolk, vesicles of various sizes, and a number of rickettsiae. These oocytes with an egg shell migrated from the ovary to the posterior part of the opisthosoma, and the shell thickened.

The presence of rickettsiae was also observed in an egg after oviposition (Fig. 6) and in the embryo developing in the egg. In the early stage of development of the embryo, rickettsiae were recognized in the cell layer just under the egg shell, and in the central zone of the egg where many yolk droplets were seen. In embryos at a later stage of development, rickettsiae were seen in various organs and tissues, such as in the immature salivary gland, midgut, and brain (Urakami *et al.*, 1988b).

4) Rickettsiae in the testis of infected male mite

Infected laboratory family lines of *L. fletcheri*, *L. arenicola*, and *L. deliense* produced many female progeny and few, if any, males (Rai and Bandopadhyay, 1978; Roberts *et al.*, 1977). However, it was demonstrated that the infected colonies of *L. pallidum* produced both male and female progeny at a 1 : 1 ratio, and rickettsiae were isolated from both sexes (Takahashi *et al.*, 1988b). Further studies of the vertical transmission of rickettsiae demonstrated that, in females, the transmission of rickettsiae to the progeny occurred commonly, whereas rickettsiae in an infected male were not transmitted to the spermatophore and to the progeny (Takahashi, 1990). In their electron microscopic studies of spermatogenesis in the infected male, Urakami *et al.* (1994b) demonstrated clearly why rickettsiae in the male are not vertically transmitted.

They showed the testis to consist of several morphologically distinguishable parts. In one area of the testis (Fig. 7), the cells, probably spermatogonia, were densely packed. Rickettsiae were found in the cytoplasm. The initial morphological change that occurred in the cells was the condensation of the nuclei, after which the cells were released from the packed zone to another matrix area of the testis, as shown in Fig. 8. The cell seen at the top right of this figure is just being released from the cell cluster to the neighboring extracellular matrix. Interestingly, this cell seems to be in the stage of binary fission, probably meiosis, since the nuclear membrane is not seen

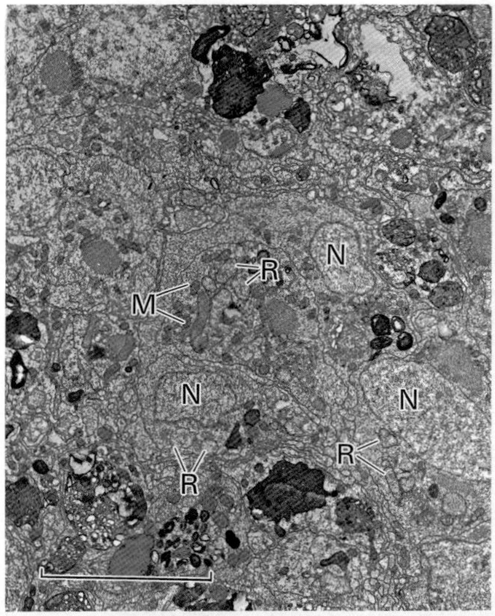

4

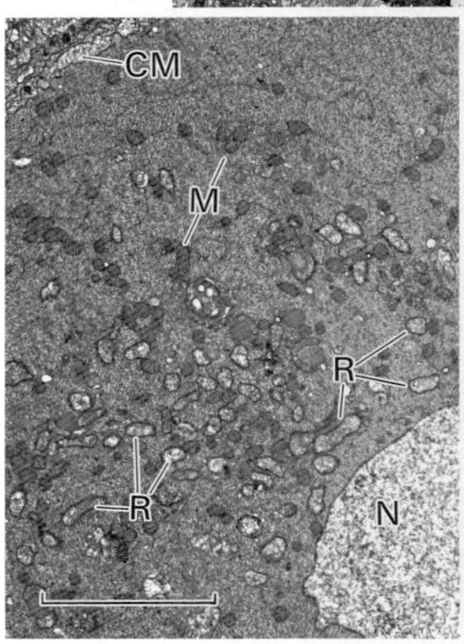

5

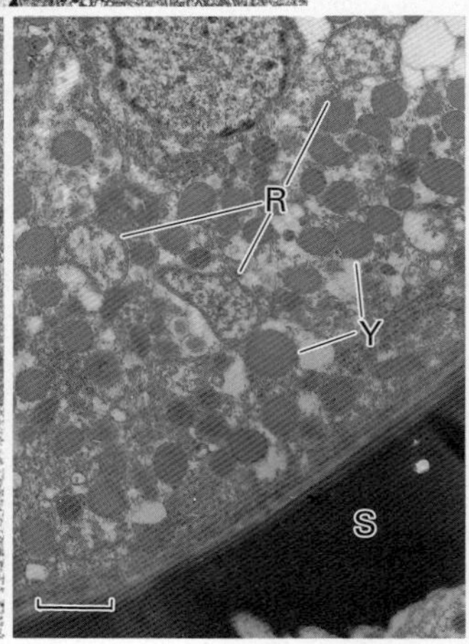

6

Figs. 4–6. *R. tsutsugamushi* in oogenesis in *L. pallidum*.

Fig. 4. Oogonia in ovary. Rickettsiae (R) are seen in the cytoplasm. M: Mitochondria; N: Nucleus. Bar = 5 μm.

Fig. 5. Developing oocyte. A number of bacillary rickettsiae (R) are observed in the cytoplasm. CM: Cytoplasmic membrane of oocyte; M: Mitochondria; N: Nucleus. Bar = 5 μm.

Fig. 6. Part of an egg after oviposition. Rickettsiae (R) are found in the cytoplasm. S: Egg shell; Y: Yolk granules. Bar = 1 μm.

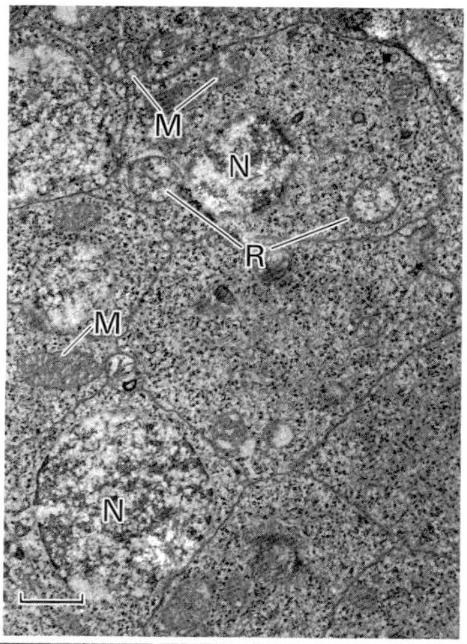

7

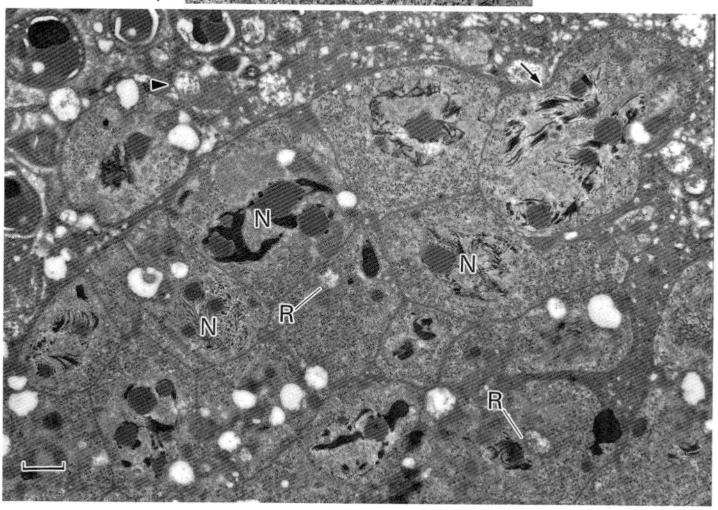

8

Figs. 7–11. Spermatogenesis in *L. pallidum* infected with *R. tsutsugamushi*.

Fig. 7. Clumping cells in a part of the testis. Cells are considered to be spermatogonia or spermatocytes. Rickettsiae (R) are seen in the cytoplasm. M: Mitochondria; N: Nucleus. Bar = 1 μm.

Fig. 8. Initiation of spermatogenesis and release of the cells from the cell cluster. The nucleus (N) lose the nuclear membrane and begin to condense, and rickettsiae (R) are found in these cells. At the top right of this figure, a cell (arrow) in meiosis is being released from the cell cluster. A cell after release (arrowhead) is migrating at the outside of the cell cluster. Bar = 1 μm.

9
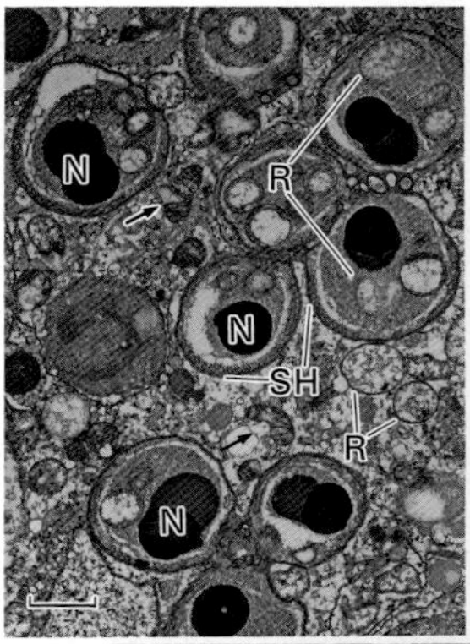

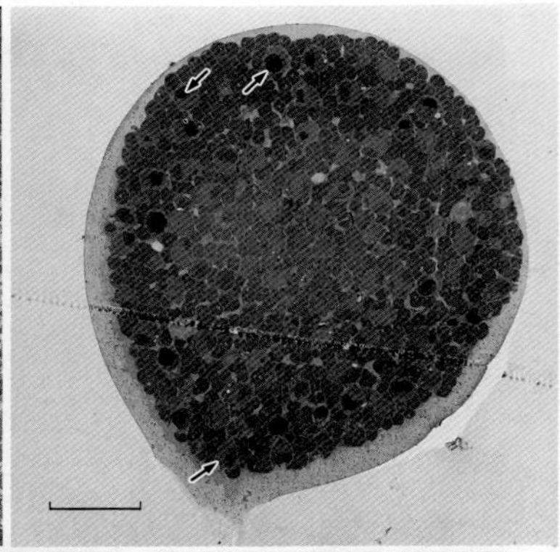
11

10
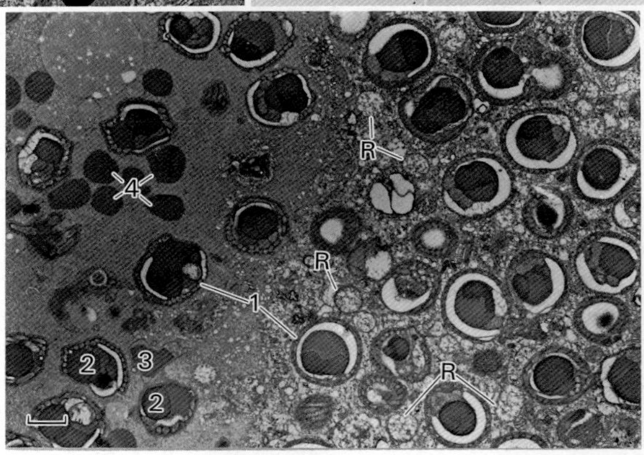

Fig. 9. Intermediate stage of spermatogenesis. Spermatids in a matrix area of the testis decrease in size, and the nuclei (N) take a more condensed form. A shell structure (SH) is formed under the cytoplasmic membrane of spermatids. Rickettsiae (R) and the content of cell cytoplasm are partially eliminated from the cells. Some rickettsiae and cell organelles (arrows) eliminated from the spermatids are observed at the outside of cells in the matrix. Bar = 1 μm.

Fig. 10. Final stage of spermatogenesis. The spermatids with a shell structure (1) change to mature sperms consisting only of a condensed nucleus (4). Intermediate forms of the spermatids (2, 3) are also seen. During spermatogenesis, the spermatids migrate from a part of the testis (right half of the figure) to another part containing smaller spermatids and mature sperms (left half of the figure). Rickettsiae (R) and organelles eliminated from the cells are observed only in the former part. Bar = 1 μm.

Fig. 11. Sperm sac of a spermatophore deposited by an infected male. Mature sperms and immature sperms (arrows) with the shell structure are seen in the sperm sac. No rickettsia is found. Bar = 5 μm.

and the chromatids appear to be separating. The cells that have been released from the cell cluster are in the spermatid stage. These spermatids have shrunk by reduction in the cytoplasmic volume and condensation of the nuclei, and a shell-like structure has been formed under the cytoplasmic membrane (Fig. 9). At this stage, some organelles and rickettsiae in the cytoplasm have been eliminated from the cells and extracellular rickettsiae are observed in the matrix, although some rickettsiae still remain in a few such shrunken spermatids.

The shrunken spermatids, which have almost completely lost their cytoplasmic components and are surrounded by a shell structure, are seen at the right side in Fig. 10. Almost all the rickettsiae are located in the extracellular matrix. The spermatids then migrate again into a neighboring area of the testis, which is seen at the left side in Fig. 10, but the eliminated cytoplasmic components and rickettsiae never migrate to this area. The spermatids in this area completely lose their shell and cytoplasm and differentiate into mature spermatozoa, which are observed as homogeneous, electron-dense, naked nuclei. The mature spermatozoa tend to aggregate to form spermatophores. The spermatophore deposited by an infected male (Fig. 11) consists of many mature and some immature spermatozoa, but never contains rickettsiae.

Thus, it was clearly demonstrated that rickettsiae in the spermatogonia, spermatocytes, and spermatids in the early stage of spermatogenesis were eliminated from these cells during the maturation process. Only the spermatids still carry rickettsiae, and they migrate to another rickettsia-free area of the testis during the final maturation process, resulting in the separation of spermatids from rickettsiae and in the production of rickettsia-free spermatophores.

2. Transmission from Mammals to Mites

a. Acquisition of rickettsiae in mites from mammals

The transovarian transmission of *Rickettsia tsutsugamushi* was elucidated after the establishment of infected laboratory colonies of *Leptotrombidium fletcheri* (Rapmund, 1984; Rapmund *et al.*, 1969; Shirai *et al.*, 1982c), *L. arenicola* (Rapmund *et al.*, 1972; Roberts and Robinson, 1977; Shirai *et al.*, 1982c), *L. deliense* (Davis, 1947; Krishnan *et al.*, 1949; Mackie *et al.*, 1946a,b; Rai and Bandopadhyay, 1978; Yu and Wu, 1959), *L. pallidum* (Takahashi, 1990; Takahashi *et al.*, 1988b), *L. gaohuensis* (Wei *et al.*, 1987), *L.*

imphalum and *Leptotrombidium* sp. (Tanskul *et al.*, 1994).

Nevertheless, since these colonies were isolated from chiggers collected from the natural environment, it is still not known how and where *R. tsutsugamushi* was introduced into these infected colonies.

In regard to the transmission dynamics of *R. tsutsugamushi*, a concept widely accepted in the past held that wild rodents were the reservoir animal for *R. tsutsugamushi* in the natural environment and that chiggers acquired the infection while feeding on the infected rodents (Harrison and Audy, 1951; Philip, 1949; Traub and Wisseman, 1968a,b; Walker *et al.*, 1973).

However, Fukuzumi (1953) found that in attempting to isolate rickttsiae from larvae 5–12 days after they were collected from eight infected rodents (*Microtus montebelli*), only one pool of 82 engorged larvae of *L. akamushi* from one host was positive for rickettsiae. The other engorged larvae, 478 *L. akamushi* and 34 *L. pallidum*, collected from the other seven rodents, were all negative. It was not possible to determine whether the positive mites acquired the infection while feeding on an infected rodent or whether the rickettsiae were transmitted by transovarian infection prior to feeding.

Fukuzumi believed that mites did not acquire infection because of the low levels of rickettsia in wild rodents. In an attempt to elucidate this question, he caught five *M. montebelli*, infested with a large number of chiggers, in an endemic area, and subcutaneously injected a concentrated rickettsial suspension prepared from infected laboratory mice into the ear lobes of these *M. montebelli*. Mites (202 *L. akamushi* and 32 *L. pallidum*) were then collected from these rodents, but no infection was confirmed in these mites. In another experiment, *M. montebelli* were collected from non-endemic areas and injected with rickettsial suspensions in the ear lobes, after which *L. akamushi* were placed on the ear lobes. Fifty-seven engorged larvae were recovered from six rodents, and all these larvae were also negative for *R. tsutsugamushi*. A series of these experiments led Fukuzumi to the conclusion that trombiculid mites seldom acquire the infection while feeding on infected wild rodents.

Kitaoka (1959) attempted to isolate *R. tsutsugamushi* from 77 pools of 4,855 mites belonging to 12 species, including *L. scutellare* and *L. pallidum* obtained from the rodents and soil in various endemic areas in Japan in the period from 1956 to 1958: none of the mites were positive for *R. tsutsugamushi*. Although 70–100% of wild rodents in endemic areas were found to be infected with *R. tsutsugamushi* in the prevalent season, the isolation of *R. tsutsugamushi* from mites infesting these rodents was difficult. These findings led Kitaoka to support Fukuzumi's conclusion. In a later experiment, Miura and Kawai (1968) placed infected mice in endemic areas for 6–24 h. Engorged larvae recovered from these infected mice were stored at 4°C for 7–14 days to reduce the mechanical transmission of *R. tsutsugamushi*, and a suspension of these mites was injected into a mouse to detect rickettsiae by the passage method. The rickettsiae were isolated from *L. pallidum*, *L. scutellare*, *L. akamushi*, and *N. japonica* during their feeding on rickettsemic mice (Table 6).

As a control, naive mice were exposed to trombiculid mites in the same experimental areas; rickettsiae were isolated, but at low rates, from the collected engorged larvae of *L. akamushi* and *L. pallidum*. The difference in *R. tsutsugamushi*-positive rates in the two groups of mites — *i.e.*, fed on infected and on naive mice — showed clearly that the mites of those two species were infected while feeding on rickettsemic mice.

Kitaoka (1959) exposed infected mice and rabbits in an area with a dense population of *L. scutellare*, in which rickttsiae had never been

Table 6. Isolation of *R. tsutsugamushi* from Trombiculid Mites Fed on Mice with Experimental Rickettsemia Placed in the Endemic Areas in Japan

Species	No. of mites collected	No. of pools examined	No. of positive pools	MIR %
L. pallidum	182	19	4	2.2
	210	22	1	0.5
L. scutellare	350	36	18	5.1
	323	33	15	4.6
L. akamushi	34	34	14	41.2
	74	26	20	27.0
N. japonica	119	2	2	1.7
L. fuji	100	1	0	0
L. kitasatoi	9	1	0	0

MIR: Minimum infection rate.
Modified from Miura and Kawai (1968).

detected. In one pool (105 mites) out of 15, rickettsiae were positive by mouse passage, and the possibility of the acquisition of infection while feeding was thus also suggested in this species.

The infection of mites while feeding on infected mice and wild rodents was further elucidated by the establishment of a method for rearing trombiculid mites (Lipovsky, 1951; Lipovsky *et al.*, 1957) and by the use of uninfected colonies. However, the infection rates in the mites feeding on infected mice, except in the case of *L. pallidum*, were not high, being 7.6% (18/238) in *L. deliense*, 1.2% (2/164) in *L. fletcheri*, 5.2% (4/77) in *L. arenicola* (Walker *et al.*, 1975), 25.6% (21/82) in *L. pallidum*, and 4.3% (1/23) in *L. fuji* (Takahashi *et al.*, 1994a). In these findings, *L. fuji* and *L. kitasatoi*, which had never been regarded as transmitters, also acquired the infection while feeding (Kaneko *et al.*, 1987; Takahashi *et al.*, 1994a) (Table 7).

Wild rodents, such as *Apodemus speciosus* and *M. montebelli*, survived concentrated rickettsia inoculation and harbored rickettsiae for at least five months (Fukuzumi, 1953; Suzuki, 1959; Takahashi *et al.*, 1990c). Experimental results confirmed that trombiculid mites were infected while feeding on these wild rodents immediately after these rodents were inoculated with *R. tsutsugamushi* (Takahashi *et al.*, 1990a) (Table 7). Another possible mode of transmission indicated by experiments was that mites acquired rickettsiae while feeding on infected rodents, and then infected a second host during the second feeding (Davis *et al.*, 1947; Traub *et al.*, 1975).

b. Transtadial transmission

The fate of rickettsiae in mites after engorgement was studied in *L. scutellare* on Hachijo Island, where the mites showed a negligible positive rate for rickettsiae (Miura and Kawai, 1968). *L. scutellare* were infested on rickettsemic mice and *M. montebelli*, and the positive rate for rickettsiae was followed up. Immediately after they had fed on the mice, the positive rate in engorged mites, in pools of ten mites each, was 80%, and no positivity was shown after 20 days. Rickettsial survival in engorged larvae was also studied in five species of trombiculid mites by Traub *et al.* (1975). In *L. deliense*, the positive rate in mite pools was 100% immediately after collection, 67% on days 1–4 after detachment, and 27% after 5–15 days. Both Traub *et al.* (1975) and Miura and Kawai (1968) agreed that the density of rickettsiae acquired by mites was greatly reduced with time

Table 7. Detection of *R. tsutsugamushi* by Mouse Passage from Pooled or Individual Mites after Feeding on Rickettsemic Mice or Other Rodents

Species	Host[a]	No. of mites collected	No. of pools	No. of positive pools	References
L. pallidum	M	58	5	4	Kaneko *et al.*, 1987
	M	39	39[b]	2	Takahashi *et al.*, 1994a
	M	82	82	21	Takahashi *et al.*, 1994a
	R	20	20	1	Takahashi *et al.*, 1990a
	R	7	7	0	Takahashi *et al.*, 1990a
L. kitasatoi	M	76	4	2	Kaneko *et al.*, 1987
L. fuji	M	27	1	1	Kaneko *et al.*, 1987
	M	41	41[b]	0	Takahashi *et al.*, 1994a
	M	23	23	1	Takahashi *et al.*, 1994a
	R	26	7	1	Takahashi *et al.*, 1990a
	R	50	9	0	Takahashi *et al.*, 1990a
L. deliense	M	238	238	18	Walker *et al.*, 1975
	M	—	27[c]	15	Traub *et al.*, 1975
	R	41	41	0	Takahashi *et al.*, 1990a
L. fletcheri	M	164	164	2	Walker *et al.*, 1975
	M	—	9[c]	4	Traub *et al.*, 1975
L. arenicola	M	77	77	4	Walker *et al.*, 1975
	M	—	20[c]	15	Traub *et al.*, 1975
L. subintermedium	M	—	57[c]	23	Traub *et al.*, 1975
G. ligula	M	—	22[c]	7	Traub *et al.*, 1975

[a] M, mouse; R, rodent (*Apodemus speciosus*).
[b] Examined by direct immunofluorescence.
[c] About 150 mites per pool.

after feeding. Similar conclusions were also reached by Toyokawa (1972).

However, results differed somewhat when positive rates were followed up according to stage by the examination of individual mites of *L. deliense*, *L. fletcheri*, and *L. arenicola* (Walker *et al.*, 1975), and of *L. pallidum* and *L. fuji* (Takahashi *et al.*, 1994a). It was found that the positive rates were not reduced continuously by stage, but fluctuated randomly by stage (Table 8).

In adult *L. pallidum* and *L. fuji*, *R. tsutsugamushi* positivity was 23.4% (15/64) and 14.3% (1/7), respectively, results suggesting that

Table 8. Evidence for Transtadial Transmission in Mites with Rickettsiae Acquired from Infected Mice or Other Rodents

Species Stage[b]	Positive rate % (No. positive / Total)						Reference
	EL	PN	DN	TN	AD	Total	
L. deliense	12.1 (7/58)	13.8 (8/58)	0 (0/54)	0 (0/36)	9.4 (3/32)	7.6 (18/238)	Walker *et al.*, 1975
L. fletcheri	0 (0/38)	2.7 (1/37)	2.9 (1/34)	0 (0/28)	0 (0/27)	1.2 (2/164)	Walker *et al.*, 1975
L. arenicola	0 (0/15)	0 (0/16)	0 (0/16)	25.0 (4/16)	0 (0/14)	5.2 (4/77)	Walker *et al.*, 1975
L. pallidum			10.0[a] (1/10)	14. 3[a] (1/7)	8.1[a] (3/37)	9.3[a] (5/54)	Takahashi *et al.*, 1994a
	33.3 (6/18)				23.4 (15/64)	25.6 (21/82)	Takahashi *et al.*, 1994a
L. fuji			25.0[a] (1/4)	0[a] (0/2)	4.0[a] (1/25)	6.5[a] (2/31)	Takahashi *et al.*, 1994a
	0 (0/16)				14.3 (1/7)	4.3 (1/23)	Takahashi *et al.*, 1994a

[a] Minimum infection rate (%) due to injection with pooled mites.
[b] EL, engorged larva; PN, protonymph; DN, deutonymph; TN, tritonymph; AD, adult.

rickettsiae surviving digestion in engorged larvae remain alive in a static mode in later stages for longer than 90 days.

After mite infestation on infected wild rodent, *A. speciosus*, 10 days after the animals were inoculated with rickettsiae, the positive rates in the mites were 9.1 % (4/44) for *L. fuji*, 5.0% (1/20) for *L. pallidum*, and 0% (0/41) for *L. deliense*; in 50 *L. fuji* and 7 *L. pallidum* larvae fed on the rodents 20 days after inoculation. *R. tsutsugamushi* was negative (Takahashi *et al.*, 1990a), possibly due to early reduction of rickettsemia in *A. speciosus* (Suzuki, 1959; Takahashi *et al.*, 1990a). It is now generally agreed by researchers, in the light of the above studies, that mites acquire *R. tsutsugamushi* while feeding on infected rodents.

c. Failed vertical transmission of acquired rickettsiae

Some researches have been performed to determine whether acquired rickettsiae were transmitted to the next generation. Walker *et al.* (1975) fed the larvae of three species on infected mice and at-

Table 9. Failed Vertical Transmission of *R. tsutsugamushi* to the Next Generation in *L. pallidum* from Females That Acquired *R. tsutsugamushi* While Feeding on Rickettsemic Mice

Female no.	No. of F1 larvae examined	Detection of *R. tsutsugamushi*	Anti-*Rt* antibody titers in passage mouse	(passage no.)
1		+	320	(I)
	5	−	—	(III)
	21	−	—	(III)
2		+	160	(I)
	20	−	—	(III)
3		+	320	(II)
	12	−	—	(III)
4		+	640	(I)
	5	−	—	(III)
	35	−	—	(III)
	58	−	—	(III)
5		+	640	(I)
	5	−	—	(III)
	20	−	—	(III)
6		+	640	(I)
	31	−	—	(III)
7		+	640	(I)
	14	−	—	(III)
8		+	160	(II)
	23	−	—	(III)
Total no. of larvae	249	−	—	

Rt, Rickettsia tsutsugamushi.
Takahashi *et al.* (1994a).

tempted rickettsial detection in the next generation, without confirming the infection in females. Rickettsiae were not detected in a total of 903 larvae in the next generation, *i.e.*, in 501 larvae from 79 female *L. deliense*, in 232 larvae from 47 female *L. fletcheri*, or in 170 larvae from 22 female *L. arenicola*.

In *L. pallidum*, larvae were fed on infected mice, and the females were then reared individually in vials. After the larvae of the next generation hatched, the presence of rickettsiae in the females was examined; 8 females were found to be positive. The next generation of these 8 females was examined for the presence of rickettsiae, in 249 larvae in 12 pools consisting of 5–58 larvae; all larvae were

Table 10. Possible Transovarian Transmission of Acquired *R. tsutsugamushi* Infection in Progeny of Uninfected Chiggers That Had Fed on Mice with Experimental Rickettsemia. Results of Tests Involving Inoculation of Engorged F1 Chiggers and of the Tissues of Mice upon Which They Fed

	L. deliense	*L. arenicola*	*L. fletcheri*	*G. ligula*
Pools of 17–1000 F1 chiggers (mean no./pool: 140)	1/23[a] (4%)	0/12	0/3	0/5
Tissues of mouse hosts of these F1 chiggers	0/19	0/8	0/1	0/3

[a] Numerator, number of pools found positive; denominator, number of pools inoculated.

Source: Traub *et al.* (1975).

negative for rickettsiae (Takahashi *et al.*, 1994a, Table 9).

In contrast to the above findings, Traub *et al.* (1975) found, by mouse passage, that, in one pool of 28 larval *L. deliense* out of 23 pools (each pool consisting of 140 larvae on average), the first generation (F1) of females had acquired rickettsiae. In *L. arenicola*, *L. fletcheri*, and *Gahrliepia ligula*, however, all larvae in the first generation were negative (Table 10).

This one report showing that acquired rickettsiae were transmitted to the next generation, led some researchers to consider the possibility (although small) of vertical transmission of acquired rickettsiae and it's epidemiological importance (Audy and Harrison, 1951; Kitaoka, 1959; Walker *et al.*, 1975). If this type of transmission were to take place in the natural environment, it would play an important role in maintaining rickettsiae in an endemic area (Traub and Wisseman, 1974b). However, such vertical transmission would be expected to be very rare or, if indeed it occurred at all, caused by experimental failure in view of most other studies (Takahashi *et al.*, 1994a; Walker *et al.*, 1975).

From the results of most of the relevant experiments, it can be considered that wild rodents, like humans, are victims of infection due to the bites of trombiculid mites, and both rodents and humans are merely a necessary source of nutrients for the development of the mites. In conclusion, it is a logical and natural consideration that trombiculid mites are the reservoir of *R. tsutsugamushi* and, at the same time, act as vectors of the infection to mammals.

6

Diagnosis

1. Isolation of *Rickettsia tsutsugamushi*

The isolation of *R. tsutsugamushi* from human patients, wild rodents, and trombiculid mites has been performed mainly by inoculating laboratory mice with test material. Isolation is also performed in cultured tissue cells. Materials examined are peripheral blood samples obtained from human patients, homogenized autopsy-derived tissues, liver and spleen samples obtained from wild or laboratory animals, and tissue samples of trombiculid mites as the transmitters.

It is relatively easy to isolate *R. tsutsugamushi* from patients in mice. The majority of isolates are, however, frequently highly pathogenic to mice. Much research experience has enabled the isolation of strains of *R. tsutsugamushi* with low pathogenicity to mice, although these strains are pathogenic to humans (Kawamura *et al.*, 1980; Kobayashi *et al.*, 1978; Misao *et al.*, 1967). In addition, some strains of *R. tsutsugamushi* have been confirmed to have low pathogenicity and to manifest as inapparent infections in humans, as described in Chapters 2 and 3 (Fan *et al.*, 1987; Kawamura *et al.*, 1980; Shishido, 1962b).

Moreover, there are mouse strains that are naturally susceptible or resistant to *R. tsutsugamushi* infection, and it has been shown that this natural resistance is controlled by the *Ric* gene (Groves and Osterman, 1978; Groves *et al.*, 1980; Jerrells and Osterman, 1981). Consequently, susceptible murine strains have been used to isolate *R. tsutsugamushi*.

The efficiency of isolating *R. tsutsugamushi* by the cultured cell method, however, has not always been favorable, irrespective of the pathogenicity of *R. tsutsugamushi* type to the host animal. Methods for the isolation of *R. tsutsugamushi* have been improved; those being used now are reviewed in this section.

a. Preparation of test materials

Blood samples can be handled quite easily and are discussed below. Other test materials, such as rodent organs and biopsy and necropsy materials obtained from humans, are removed carefully under sterile conditions and homogenized with sucrose phosphate buffered glutamic acid (SPG) solution (Bovarnick *et al.*, 1950) (Chapter 2) in a closely sealed Waring blendor, taking great care to prevent the splashing of rickettsial agents in the laboratory in the form of aerosol droplets during and after homogenization. Alternatively, the materials can be ground with a pestle in a small mortar to make a 10% emulsion in SPG solution. When organs are ground in a mortar, sterile small particles of glass or sand placed in the mortar in advance allow the organs to be readily disrupted. The homogenate is allowed to stand for about 1–2 min, after which the supernatant is drawn into a syringe with a needle, and 0.2 to 0.5 ml is injected into a mouse intraperitoneally.

For the isolation of *R. tsutsugamushi* from the trombiculid mite, a mite is placed in a drop of SPG solution in the well of a depressed glass slide and is disrupted by pressing with the tip of a glass rod or with a small spatula, to make a dense emulsion, and the entire emulsion is injected into a mouse intraperitoneally.

For isolation of *R. tsutsugamushi* in cultured cells, medium for cell culture (*e.g.* Eagle's minimum essential medium) is used in place of SPG solution as inoculum solution. The medium is supplemented with 200–400 U/ml of penicillin G and 200–400 μg/ml of streptomycin to suppress bacterial growth (Chapter 2). SPG solution is also supplemented with the same doses of these antibiotics.

b. Isolation in mice

To isolate *R. tsutsugamushi* from patients or from wild and laboratory animals, a common method has been to perform intraperitoneal injections of samples in mice. However, recent studies have demonstrated the existence of avirulent strains in mice; these avirulent strains do not show significant symptoms in hairy mice and have resulted in unsuccessful rickettsial isolation in many cases

(Kawamura *et al.*, 1980; Kobayashi *et al.*, 1978; Tachibana *et al.*, 1982b). These avirulent strains have been isolated in cyclophosphamide (CY)-treated mice (Kobayashi *et al.*, 1978) and in athymic nude mice (Kawamura *et al.*, 1980). Recently, Yamamoto *et al.* (1989) reported that successful rickettsial isolation from patients was higher than 90%, using CY-treated mice (Table 1). The procedures employed by Yamamoto (1988) are described below.

1) Preparation of blood samples

Five to 10 ml of peripheral blood is withdrawn into a centrifuge tube from a patient before antibiotics treatment is initiated. If the blood is to be kept for a long period before use, it is stored frozen at −80°C. If the isolation procedure begins within 3 days of the sample taking, it is better to store the blood in an ice bath. The blood is centrifuged at 300 × *g* for 5–10 min, and the separated serum is harvested for immunological testing. The remaining blood clot in the tube is homogenized with a mortar and pestle in an equal volume of SPG (Bovarnick *et al.*, 1950), and used for injection in mice.

However, if, at blood collection, heparin is added to the blood at a concentration of 10 U/ml, the blood is centrifuged at 300 × *g* for 5–10 min, the supernatant is separated for the immunological assay, and the thin layer of leucocytes — the buffy coat which is formed at the top of the sediment — is removed, suspended in SPG, and used for injection in mice.

2) Blood inoculation and treatment of mice with cyclophosphamide (CY)

A hairy mouse is injected intraperitoneally with 0.5 ml suspension of the blood clot homogenate or the buffy coat. Endoxan (vial containing 100 mg CY and 45 mg NaCl; Shionogi Pharmaceutical Co. Ltd.) is dissolved in sterilized distilled water at a concentration of 20 mg of CY per ml, and 0.2 mg CY per g body weight is injected intraperitoneally in the mice on the first, second, and fourth days after the inoculation of test materials. If the mice do not show any signs of illness, the CY injection is repeated once more on the seventh day.

In a modification of this procedure (Kawamori *et al.*, 1992; Kobayashi *et al.*, 1978), mice were injected subcutaneously or intraperitoneally with three doses of 0.25 mg CY per g body weight per day on days 0, 4, 5, 9, and 10 after inoculation with the test material.

The mice are sacrificed on the 10th–14th day after inoculation. At autopsy, the presence of slight splenomegaly and a heavy viscous exudate in the peritoneal cavity are carefully noted at first as the signs of infection; the spleen and liver are then harvested and, at the same time, peritoneal smears are prepared for the detection of rickettsia. The smears are stained with Giemsa or used for immunofluorescence (IF) microscopy.

The presence of the viscous abdominal exudate suggests the successful isolation of rickettsia. If rickettsiae are seen in the peritoneal smears, the isolation is judged successful. If rickettsia are not observed in the preparations, the 10% homogenate of spleen and liver in SPG is injected in other CY-treated mice for blind passage. Even if rickettsia is negative in the first passage mouse, blind passages are continued up to the third passage. Mouse sera should be retained at each passage for the detection of anti- *R. tsutsugamushi* antibodies.

c. Isolation in cultured cells

The growth of *R. tsutsugamushi* can be observed in various cultured cells, some of which are used for the isolation of *R. tsutsugamushi* from the blood of patients. Yamamoto *et al.* (1989) used the cell lines L-929 (derived from mouse fibroblast cells) and BS-C40 (derived from African greenmonkey kidney cells) for rickettsial isolation from patients. The procedures used are described briefly below.

If the homogenate of the blood clot from a patient is inoculated directly onto cultured cells, the cells will be damaged due to the high concentration of the substances in the hemolysate. Therefore, it is a good idea to separate leucocytes from heparinized blood and to inoculate the leucocyte homogenate onto the cell layers.

For the separation of leucocytes, heparinized blood from a patient is mixed with an equal amount of culture medium, and 5 ml of the mixture is layered onto 3.5 ml of Ficoll-Conray mixture (density: 1.114) and centrifuged at 500 rpm for 30 min. Leucocytes accumulated into a layer by centrifugation are homogenized with a Potter or Dounce homogenizer in 0.3 ml of culture medium containing 2% calf serum; 0.1 ml of this homogenate is then inoculated onto cell layers cultivated in Leighton tubes.

After incubation at 35–37°C for 60–90 min, to allow rickettsial adsorption to cells, the inoculum is removed and replaced with fresh culture medium containing 2% calf serum, and the cells are cultured at 35–37°C. This procedure can also be replaced by another technique in which the homogenate is inoculated on a cell layer on a flat-bottomed centrifuge tube and centrifuged at 1,500 rpm for 60 min at room temperature; rickettsial adsorption to cells should be enhanced by this procedure.

The incubation of cells is continued, with exchange of the culture medium taking place every 3–4 days until rickettsial growth is seen in the cell smears stained with Giemsa or examined by IF. If necessary, the cells are transferred to new culture bottles without homogenization. If no rickettsial growth is observed in the culture after 45 days, rickettsial isolation is regarded as unsuccessful.

Yamamoto (1988) compared the efficiency of methods for the isolation of rickettsia from the blood of patients using CY-treated mice and cultured BS-C40 and L cells (Table 1). The patients examined in this experiment were residents of Miyazaki Prefecture, in Kyushu Island, Japan, where the Kawasaki and Kuroki types are predominantly distributed.

The serum antibody titers of these patients were first assayed by IF against Gilliam, Karp, Kato, Kawasaki, and Kuroki antigens, and all sera reacted most strongly to either Kawasaki or Kuroki antigens. All blood samples positive for antibody were provided for the rickettsial isolation. As shown in Table 1, isolation of the Kawasaki type with CY-treated mice showed the highest efficiency, and the efficiency with BS-C40 cells with Kuroki type was similar. With L cells, the efficiency was low, particularly for the Kawasaki type.

It should be noted that even though the Kawasaki and Kuroki types are avirulent in hairy mice, these strains were successfully and efficiently isolated using CY-treated mice.

Table 1. Efficiency of Isolation of Kawasaki and Kuroki Types of Rickettsia from Patients

Isolation in	Kawasaki type			Kuroki type		
	No. of samples	No. of successful isolations	Efficiency (%)	No. of samples	No. of successful isolations	Efficiency (%)
CY-treated mice	22	22	100	11	10	91
BS-C cells	20	16	80	11	11	100
L cells	20	7	35	11	9	82

[a] Samples were obtained from patients detected from October, 1985 to March, 1986 in Miyazaki Prefecture. CY, Cyclophosphamide.

d. Identification and typing

1) Identification of isolated rickettsiae

(a) Direct immunofluorescence (IF)

Antibodies used for direct IF are produced by immunizing rabbits or guinea pigs with various types of *R. tsutsugamushi*, or monoclonal type-specific antibodies of each *R. tsutsugamushi* are used. The antibodies produced are labeled with fluorescein isothiocyanate (FITC), a fluorescent dye, and after the specificities of purified conjugates against each type are examined, the conjugates are stored. These are anti-*R. tsutsugamushi* type-specific labeled antibodies. Infected mouse peritoneal smears or cultured cell lines are used as antigens and are allowed to react with these labeled antibodies. Under a fluorescence microscope, *R. tsutsugamushi* that exhibit greenish-yellow fluorescence are observed inside and outside the infected cells, and thus the identificaton and typing of *R. tsutsugamushi* are performed simultaneously (Iida *et al.*, 1966a; Murata *et al.*, 1986). However, since the conventional antibodies produced may cross-react with other types of *R. tsutsugamushi*, depending on the type-specificity of the antibodies, sometimes typing is difficult. To avoid such difficulties, direct IF findings with the isolated strain should be compared to those with known *R. tsutsugamushi* type antigens. The technical procedures for direct IF are described well by Kawamura (1977).

(b) Indirect IF

Human, mouse, or other animal sera containing IgG or IgM antibodies against known types of *R. tsutsugamushi* are prepared and serve as the primary antibody. Antibodies against IgG or IgM of the same animal as that used for the primary antibody, prepared and labeled with FITC or commercial products, serve as the secondary antibody. Several spots of isolated rickettsiae in infected cells are prepared on a glass slide; these serve as the antigen and are allowed to react with different primary antibodies against different rickettsial types. After being washed, the antigenic spots are allowed to react with the corresponding labeled antibody; for example, labeled anti-mouse IgG is used if mouse IgG antibody against *R. tsutsugamushi* is used as the primary antibody. A positive reaction observed under a fluorescence microscope at any antigen spot indicates that the isolated rickettsia is *R. tsutsugamushi*; however, definite typing is usually difficult with this procedure.

(c) Indirect immunoperoxidase method

The procedures are essentially the same as those outlined above for indirect IF. Several spots of isolated rickettsiae in infected cells are placed on a glass slide. Such antigen spots are allowed to react with the primary antibody, after which reaction takes place with a peroxidase-labeled antibody instead of an FITC-labeled antibody. After color development of the peroxidase, reactions are observed under a light microscope. Rickettsiae are observed as brown particles. Efforts should be made to distinguish these brown particles from cell debris containing peroxidase (Suto, 1982; Yamamoto and Minamishima, 1982).

(d) Polymerase chain reaction

Recently, advances in the DNA analysis of *R. tsutsugamushi* have been brought about by amplifying the DNA fragment common to all types, and identification of *R. tsutsugamushi* has been made possible (see Section 3 below).

2) Typing of rickettsiae

(a) Direct IF

Antibodies are produced by immunizing rabbits or guinea pigs. Type-specific antibodies are used for labeling with FITC. Alternatively, serum with a very high titer can be used for typing after it has been sufficiently diluted to reduce cross-reactivity (Iida *et al.*, 1966a). With type-specific monoclonal antibodies, the labeled antibody is highly specific and can be used for typing by direct IF (Murata *et al.*, 1986).

(b) Indirect IF

The antibodies prepared for direct IF serve as the primary antibodies for indirect IF. However, irrespective of the specificity of the antibodies, cross-reactivity among types is unavoidable. To make use of this characteristic for typing, the type will be determined by the primary antibody that shows the clear specificity. Typing is, however, possible if monoclonal antibodies are used for the primary antibody, since they have high specificity (Murata *et al.*, 1986; Tange *et al.*, 1991, 1992).

(c) Indirect immunoperoxidase method

Indirect immunoperoxidase method is not usually used for typing, because, even though it may sometimes be a possible choice, as occurs with indirect IF, there is high cross-reactivity, and nonspecific reactions can occur, unless type-specific monoclonal antibodies are used as the primary serum (Murata *et al.*, 1986).

(d) Polymerase chain reaction

With the detailed analysis of the type-specific areas of DNA now being done, typing can readily be performed by nested PCR, in which a large fragment of DNA common to various types is amplified in the first step and a type-specific narrower fragment is multiplied in the second step. With appropriate sets of primers, more detailed typing is made possible by multiplying the different target fragments in the DNA strand. For details of this procedure see Section 3 below (Yoshida *et al.*, 1994).

2. Detection of Antibody

a. Outline

1) Development of methodology

Diagnosis of Tsutsugamushi disease in humans has usually been determined simply and rapidly by serological methods, by measuring significant increase of specific antibodies in the sera of patients.

Weil and Felix (1916) found that the *Proteus vulgaris* PX-19 strain (now named OX-19) agglutinated with the sera of patients with epidemic typhus (Weil-Felix reaction). Then Fletcher *et al.* (1929) found that some sera of tropical typhus patients in the Malay Peninsula agglutinated the *Proteus mirabilis* PX-K strain (now OX-K) that in 1923 had been isolated by Kingsbury. This was the first serological method used to diagnose Tsutsugamushi disease.

However, the Weil-Felix test is not a serological reaction between a specific antibody and antigen, but a reaction between a *Rickettsia tsutsugamushi*-specific antibody and some component of *Proteus* OX-K that is common to *R. tsutsugamushi*. Therefore, many patients with Tsutsugamushi disease have sera that show a positive reaction by IF but a negative one for agglutination with *Proteus* OX-K (Bozeman and Elisberg, 1963). The low sensitivity of the Weil-Felix test is thus a problem.

Fifteen years after the work of Fletcher *et al.* (1929), Bengtson (1945, 1946) employed a complement fixation (CF) test and made diagnosis possible by using the ethylether-treated Cox-Craigie type antigen of *R. tsutsugamushi* that had proliferated in the yolk sacs of embryonated chicken eggs (Craigie, 1945).

Soluble antigen from ether-treated rickettsiae is usually group-specific to the typhus group or the spotted fever group of rickettsiae, and the ether-insoluble particles of rickettsiae from both these groups are species-specific antigens. As early as 1945, it had already been shown that there were scarcely any *R. tsutsugamushi* group-specific soluble antigens, and strain specificity, due to species-specific particular antigens, was strongly expressed in the CF test.

Consequently, it was proposed that the Karp and Gilliam strains of *R. tsutsugamushi* ought to be used in combination as prototype strains to allow for the heterogeneity (Bengtson, 1945, 1946; Philip, 1947). However, no progress in diagnosis was made because of the low titers of yolk sac-derived CF antigens and also because of the presence of anticomplementary reactions.

Shishido (1962a, 1964) typed the isolates of *R. tsutsugamushi* in Japan using CF antigens that had been partially purified by the cation exchange resin method developed by Yamamoto *et al.* (1958) and Kawamura (1962) and treated with bovine serum albumin. He concluded that, to use the CF test for the diagnosis of Tsutsugamushi disease in patients, it was necessary to use three prototype strains, Kato, Karp, and Gilliam, as standard antigens. Shishido *et al.* (1969) succeeded in separating soluble and particulate antigens by disrupting cultured cells containing *R. tsutsugamushi* by ultrasonication; these antigens were then fractionated by sucrose density gradient centrifugation. This purified soluble antigen, however, was not used in practice, because it represented only a small proportion of the antigen and because of its low recovery rate.

Antigens used for the CF test were improved as noted above, and the CF test was widely employed not only for the diagnosis of Tsutsugamushi disease in humans (Shishido, 1962a; Tsuboi and Oyama, 1984) but also for the typing of *R. tsutsugamushi* isolated from various other sources (Elisberg *et al.*, 1967, 1968; Shishido *et al.*, 1967).

The CF test, however, has some shortcomings compared with indirect immunofluorescence (IF) and with another test, the indirect immunoperoxidase (IP) test. These are: lower sensitivity, technological complexity, difficulties due to anticomplementary activity, and difficulties in determining precise amounts of *R. tsutsugamushi*-specific IgM and IgG antibodies individually. For these reasons, indirect IF and IP have become the major diagnostic methods in place of the CF test, as recommended by the WHO/WPR Task Force meeting on the serological diagnosis of Tsutsugamushi disease (see Chapter 1).

It was Bozeman and Elisberg (1963) who first employed indirect IF for the diagnosis of Tsutsugamushi disease. Nevertheless, there were some methodological issues to be resolved in many steps of the reagent preparation at that time, such as the labeling of FITC to the anti-human immunoglobulins to be used as the secondary antibodies, the purification of FITC-conjugated anti-human immunoglobulins, and the nonspecific fluorescence that occurred when these conjugated anti-human immunoglobulins were used.

The great improvements in technical procedures made by Kawamura and associates (Iida *et al.*, 1966a, 1966b; Kawamura, 1969, 1977; Kawamura and Aoyama, 1983; Murata and Kawamura, 1980) led to the successful elimination of nonspecific fluorescence. Critical studies were made of methods employed for purifying the FITC-conjugated anti-human immunoglobulins, the appropriate fluorochrome to protein (F/P) molar ratio was determined, and the fluorescence microscope itself was improved.

The IF technique is now used worldwide, its advantages being that it has a higher sensitivity for detecting *R. tsutsugamushi*-specific antibodies than CF, and it can detect IgM and IgG individually, so that, even in the acute phase, the antibody can be detected and diagnosis can be made. In addition, *R. tsutsugamushi*-specific IgM and/or IgG in the serum of many animals can be detected with the FITC-labeled antibodies against IgG or IgM of the same animal.

However, *R. tsutsugamushi* strains show heterogeneity (Elisberg *et al.*, 1967, 1968) and the type-specific antigens of each strain often bind specifically to antibodies against each rickettsial type. In recent years, new local types of *R. tsutsugamushi* have been identified at many localities in Japan; these types have specific antigenicity different from that of the prototype strains (Kato, Karp, and Gilliam) (Ohashi *et al.*, 1990; Tamura *et al.*, 1984; Yamamoto *et al.*, 1986, 1989).

Because of this heterogeneity of *R. tsutsugamushi* strains, detection is sometimes inconclusive, as only the prototypes are used for antigens. Therefore, one or more local non-prototype antigens should be used, in addition to the prototypes, for the diagnosis of Tsutsugamushi disease in those areas in which the existence of any local type strains of *R. tsutsugamushi* is known or suspected.

With indirect IF, the type of isolated *R. tsutsugamushi* can be readily determined by using type-specific monoclonal antibodies as the primary antibody. In addition, antigen can be detected in frozen tissue sections with IF. Because of its low nonspecific reaction, direct IF, with FITC-conjugated hyperimmune sera or type-specific monoclonal antibodies of *R. tsutsugamushi*, is the most suitable method for observing the distribution of *R. tsutsugamushi* types in the tissues (Murata *et al.*, 1985).

The IP test was put to practical use for the diagnosis of Tsutsugamushi disease by Yamamoto and Minamishima (1982), Suto and Fujimiya (1980), and Suto (1982). Since the reaction of peroxidase-labeled anti-human immunoglobulin is more sensitive than fluorescence, the sensitivity for detecting specific antibodies is a few times higher than that of IF.

After the reaction in the IP test, antigen spots on the glass slide can be preserved for a long time without discoloration.

However, the IP method has some shortcomings, such as the necessity for an experienced observer to interpret which reactions are specific or nonspecific, and difficulties that arise in detecting antigens in frozen tissue sections, due to the great extent of nonspecific reactions with peroxidase contained in the tissues.

Other methods can also be employed to detect specific antibodies of *R. tsutsugamushi*, some examples being enzyme-linked immunosorbent assay (ELISA) (Eisemann and Osterman, 1981); biotin-avidin immunofluorescence (BA-IF) (Berman and Basch, 1980), established to increase the sensitivity of IF; the dot-immunoblot method (Tamura *et al.*, 1990; Urakami *et al.*, 1989), based on ELISA and performed on a nitrocellulose membrane; and inhibition ELISA (Furuya *et al.*, 1991), which is used for determining *R. tsutsugamushi* types by monoclonal antibody.

Recently, the nucleotide sequence of the DNA fragment encoding the type-specific antigen polypeptide (56 kDa) of *R. tsutsugamushi* was determined by Stover *et al.* (1990a) and Ohashi *et al.* (1990a). Furthermore, Ohashi *et al.* (1992a) clarified the homology of the DNA fragments encoding the 56-kDa polypeptides of six types of *R. tsutsugamushi*. On the basis of these studies, a polymerase chain reaction (PCR) method was developed to be used in practice for the diagnosis of human Tsutsugamushi disease and for the detection of rickettsiae in mites (Furuya *et al.*, 1991a, 1993; Kawamori *et al.*, 1993; Murai *et al.*, 1992; Sugita *et al.*, 1992, 1993).

PCR is effective, being particularly useful for diagnosis at a very early stage of the disease. However, considering the high cost and the complexity of the technique, there is an argument whether such early diagnosis is necessary. We had experience with two peculiar cases in which the patients were suspected immunodeficient and diagnosis by PCR was required. In the first patient Tsutsugamushi disease was suspected, but repeated examinations were negative for antibodies, and the patient's condition deteriorated, with disseminated intravascular coagulation (DIC) being exhibited. PCR was then used for diagnosis: results were positive, and the patient was cured with the appropriate treatment. The second patient, who died of a febrile illness, had not shown an increase in *R. tsutsugamushi* antibodies by conventional indirect IF, and was therefore not treated appropriately. *R. tsutsugamushi* DNA was detected by PCR in a necropsy sample. Thus, PCR appears to be the only method with which a diagnosis of Tsutsugamushi disease can be made in immunodeficient patients, and it is the method of choice when a patient with suspected Tsutsugamushi disease does not show positive serum reactions within 10 days of the onset of disease.

It is noteworthy that nested PCR (Furuya *et al.*, 1993) can be used to determine the type of *R. tsutsugamushi* by using several sets of inner primers, without the need to isolate *R. tsutsugamushi* from the patient. The isolation procedure takes at least a few weeks using a laboratory animal and/or cultured cells, whereas PCR takes only 1 to 2 days, including the time taken to perform the procedures for the extraction of *R. tsutsugamushi* DNA from blood samples. However, this does not mean that the isolation of *R. tsutsugamushi* is not necessary; it is still of critical importance in fundamental and practical studies of *R. tsutsugamushi*.

Great progress has been made by many investigators over the last century in serological and other methods used for the diagnosis of Tsutsugamushi disease. Patients now seldom die of Tsutsugamushi disease due to misdiagnosis. However, care should be taken in special cases; such sad results as those mentioned above will be avoided if medical staffs avail themselves of methods other than serological diagnosis.

From now on, efforts will be directed to develop simple sero-diagnostic methods using recombinant polypeptide antigens that have high sensitivity and high specificity, so that these methods can be used in practice worldwide, as the Weil-Felix and CF tests have been in the past. Genetic methods for the diagnosis of Tsutsugamushi disease will also be a possiblity; the method used for the extraction of DNA and the methods used for reading DNA fragments after DNA amplification by PCR will need to be simplified.

Details of the diagnostic methods are described and reviewed in the remainder of this chapter.

2) Aspects to be considered in diagnosis in humans

The serological methods have been well developed, and are highly sensitive and specific. However, special aspects needed to be considered for the diagnosis of human patients, even though these methods are satisfactory. These aspects are: examination of paired serum samples, differentiation of IgM and IgG, and the involvement of local types of *R. tsutsugamushi* as antigens.

(a) Paired serum samples

In Tsutsugamushi disease, an increased antibody titer is usually observed 10–14 days after infection. The latent period before the appearance of clinical manifestations is 7–10 days; therefore, the antibody titer at the time of hospitalization is usually low. For serodiagnosis, a second serum sample should be taken after a few days, and the increase in antibody titer between these paired sera should be examined to ensure a correct diagnosis, even if a satisfactory serological method is used.

(b) Differentiation of IgG and IgM

It is recommended to titrate IgG and IgM antibodies separately in paired serum samples, since most recent serodiagnostic methods can be used to analyze the titers of both antibodies. To differentiate IgG and IgM antibodies, anti-human IgG (gamma-chain-specific) and anti-human IgM (mu-chain-specific) rabbit sera are used as the secondary antibodies in indirect assays for the diagnosis of the disease in humans.

Changes in IgM and IgG titers along the time course of Tsutsugamushi disease are similar to those in other infectious disease, and the results of paired serum examinations can be interpreted in many ways:

- Absence of both IgG and IgM indicates no exposure to *R. tsutsugamushi* or a very early stage of infection.
- Low IgM positivity and negative IgG indicates an early stage of active infection. Both will become clearly positive after a few days. If there is no increase in the second sample, the presence of rheuma-

toid factor (RA) should be considered, since RA may give a false positive result for IgM titer.

- High titers of both IgG and IgM indicate active infection.
- Low IgM and high IgG titers indicate a reducing phase of IgM after a primary infection, or the early stages of reinfection.
- IgG without IgM indicates the persistence of IgG after a primary infection.

(c) Local type antigens

In serodiagnosis, it should be kept in mind that there are several different antigenic types of *R. tsutsugamushi*, as mentioned above (also see Chapter 2). In routine laboratory work, the prototypes, Gilliam, Karp, and Kato, are commonly used as the antigen. Since the local types of rickettsiae have some antigenic sites cross-reactive with one or more prototypes, the sera of patients who have a local type other than the prototypes will show some antibody titers in the reaction with prototype antigens. However, the same sera would show clearer antibody elevation if the homologous local type were to be used as antigen.

Therefore, besides using the prototypes, it is recommended that the rickettsial antigens isolated in each endemic area should also be used. There is a good example of the need for this in Japan, where the Kawasaki and Kuroki types of *R. tsutsugamushi* are distributed in the southern area of the country. Although the Kawasaki type shows some cross-reaction with Gilliam, the reactions to Kawasaki type antigen in the sera of patients are several times the order of magnitude of those shown with Gilliam. Similarly, sera from patients who have the Kuroki type of *R. tsutsugamushi* react with the antigens of Karp and Kato types to a certain degree; however, the reaction with Kuroki type antigen is 2–4 times the order of magnitude of the reaction with Karp or Kato antigens (Yamamoto *et al.*, 1989).

b. Indirect immunofluorescence

It was Bozeman and Elisberg (1963) who first used indirect IF for the diagnosis of Tsutsugamushi disease. However, there were many problems to be overcome at that time, *e.g.*, nonspecific fluorescence and problems with the labeling method and with the reading of fluorescence. By avoiding nonspecific reactions, establishing a satisfactory labeling method, and overcoming other technical difficulties, the IF method was improved satisfactorily by Kawamura and associates (Iida *et al.*, 1966a; 1966b; Kawamura, 1969, 1977; Kawamura and Aoyama, 1983; Murata and Kawamura, 1980).

The antiserum to be labeled for IF is always expected to have a high antibody titer and high specificity. However, no matter how high the titer and how highly specific the antibodies, if the fluorescein isothiocyanate (FITC)-labeled antibody is improperly purified, the product causes some nonspecific fluorescence. Therefore, to eliminate the nonspecific fluorescence, special attention should be paid to the procedure of purifying the labeled antibodies, as outlined below.

After the antibody solution is labeled with FITC, unbound free FITC is eliminated through Sephadex gel filtration. The filtrate is then fractionated by diethyl aminoethyl (DEAE) cellulose column chromatography, and fractions in which the fluorochrome to protein (F/P) molar ratio is between 1 and 2 are yielded. A highly potent specific fluorescent antibody with very weak negative charge is needed. The greater the extent of fluorochrome conjugation with the antibody, the more the negative charge on the molecule increases, resulting either in nonspecific adsorption to normal tissue or in increased nonspecific fluorescence.

Details of the production of a FITC-labeled antibody are described in monographs by Kawamura (1969, 1977) and Kawamura and Aoyama (1983).

In most laboratory work, commercial products are used widely; however, attention should still be paid to the causes of nonspecific fluorescence noted above. Determination of the appropriate dilution of the labeled antibody and careful preparation of control samples are also necessary.

1) Preparation of antigen materials for IF

(a) Smears of infected cultured cells as antigen

Cultured cells infected with *R. tsutsugamushi* are widely used as antigen at present, since the amount of available antigens is massive in such cells and since, by making dots of different antigens on a glass slide, reactions of a serum sample with different antigens can be observed simultaneously. The cultured cell lines used for this purpose are L-929, BS-C40, Vero, GMK, and others. When 80% or more of the cells are infected, the cultured cells are removed using a rubber policeman, suspended in PBS, and washed three times by centrifugation at 1,500 rpm, for 10 min each time.

After the washing, cell suspension is prepared by adding PBS, and an appropriate dilution for the antigen material is determined by IF, using a serum sample with a known titer. An appropriate concentration of suspension is smeared in dots or into printed circles on a glass slide. The antigen materials are dried in cold air, fixed with cold acetone for 10 min and then stored in a tightly sealed vinyl bag at –20°C or lower. Antigenicity is maintained for 6 months when the material is stored in the freezer, but it is lost if the slide is repeatedly thawed and frozen. Therefore, thawing of such slides should be avoided until they are required for use.

(b) Peritoneal smears of infected mouse as antigen

Mice are injected intraperitoneally with *R. tsutsugamushi*. After about 10 days, when the mouse shows signs of illness, a sample 4–5 mm^2 is removed from the inner surface of the peritoneum, placed on a glass slide, and smeared across the slide. The smears are then dried and fixed with cold acetone for 10 min. The slides are kept in a tightly sealed vinyl bag and stored at –20°C or lower. The valid period for the smeared antigen is similar to that for cultured cells.

If the mice are injected with cyclophosphamide (0.2 mg/g body weight), 2 or 3 days after the injection with rickettsia, *R. tsutsugamushi* particles in the smears proliferate, making microscopic examination for IF easy.

(c) Smears of infected yolk sac

R. tsutsugamushi is injected into the yolk sac of embryonated eggs on days 5–7; the yolk sacs are harvested 5–7 days after injection. After freezing and thawing has been carried out, the material is suspended, at a concentration of 20% in PBS and disrupted in a tightly sealed Waring blendor for 60–75 sec at 0°C. The resultant suspension is centrifuged at $400 \times g$ for 10 min; the middle layer is then removed and smeared on spots on a glass slide. These smear antigens are then dried and fixed with cold acetone for 10 min. The prepared yolk sac antigen should be kept in a freezer at –60°C or lower, since preservation of antigenicity in this preparation is regarded as poor.

2) Labeled antibody

When indirect IF is used for the detection of antibody, a labeled antibody should be prepared when necessary. The characteristics of the labeled antibody should be carefully studied following the description given above, to determine that it is suitable, and a product without nonspecific fluorescence should be selected.

When a human antibody is examined, it is necessary to use labeled anti-human IgM and IgG antibodies. In a patient at the acute stage, IgM is usually detected, and diagnosis is determined by its presence. However, if IgM is not detected, serum is taken from the patient at recovery and IgG level is determined, so that the increase in the titer from that at the acute stage can be employed for making a final serological diagnosis.

When the serum of small wild rodents is examined, in principle, antisera against antibodies of individual rodents should be prepared; however, because of the cross-reaction of anti-rat antibody with the sera of other species, anti-rat IgG antibody is usually applicable to many kinds of small rodents, such as *Rattus rattus*, *R. norvegicus*, and *Apodemus speciosus*. Since anti-rat antibody sometimes does not cross-react with the serum of some wild rodents, the reactivity of the wild rodent serum with the anti-rat antibody should be determined prior to the experiment.

Irrespective of the commercial or laboratory-prepared labeled antibody product (secondary antibody) used, the highest dilution of antibody that gives the minimal fluorescence should be determined by checkerboard titration between the known positive serum (primary antibody) and the labeled antibody. The maximum dilution of the labeled antibody required to show positive fluorescence is defined as 1 unit, and 2–4 units of labeled antibody — 2- to 4-fold the concentration of conjugate — should be used in practical testing.

3) Design of control reactions

At every examination, the potency of the antigen and the labeled antibody should be examined. To do this, standardized positive and negative sera are allowed to react with the test sera as controls. By observing the intensity of fluorescence in the control sera, any decrease of potency in the antigen and labeled antibody caused by freezing and thawing can be detected.

4) Technical procedures

(1) The test serum is diluted with PBS in serial two-fold dilutions begining at 1 : 10 dilution (1 : 10 to 1 : 1,280) on a U-bottomed microplate. When a large number of serum samples is to be examined, sera diluted at 1 : 10 are examined to screen for positive sera. In the second step, only positive sera are titrated in serial dilutions.

(2) The antigen slides are taken out of the freezer and rapidly warmed to room temperature in a stream of air.

(3) One dilution of serum sample is placed on three prototype antigen spots (plus local strain antigen spots) at about 10 μl/spot on a glass slide. The slides are kept in a moist chamber in an incubator at 37°C for 30–60 min for reaction.

(4) After the reaction is completed, each slide is rinsed quickly with PBS and placed in a glass staining dish filled with about 200 ml PBS; no more than 15 slides are placed in the dish. The dish is placed on a vibrating plate, and the slides are washed for a total of 15 min while being vibrated. The PBS is changed three times, at 3-, 5-, and 7-min intervals during washing.

(5) After the completion of washing, the slides are dried, and about 10 μl of the secondary antibody (FITC-labeled antibody), appropriately diluted, is placed on each antigen spot. The reaction is continued in a moist chamber at 37°C for 30–60 min, as in step (3).

(6) The slides are washed as in step (4).

(7) The slides are dried and a drop of buffered glycerol solution is placed on the spots, which are then covered with a cover slip.

(8) The specimen is observed under a fluorescence microscope (transmitted or incident illumination type), using an ultraviolet (UV) excitation system, at 200–400 magnifications (Fig. 1). With fluorescent images of standardized positive and negative control sera, the maximum dilution showing positive fluorescence represents the titer of the test serum against the antigen for each rickettsial type.

c. Indirect immunoperoxidase (*IP*) *test*

Indirect IF is widely used for the serodiagnosis of Tsutsugamushi disease, but the disadvantages of this method are the necessity of a fluorescence microscope and the difficulty of preserving the stained preparations. The indirect IP test has a higher sensitivity than IF. The specimen can be observed under an ordinary optical microscope, and, after reaction, the color is stable for long periods; this stable color makes possible repeated observations.

Suto and Fujimiya (1980) and Suto (1985) employed this technique for the diagnosis of Tsutsugamushi disease and other rickettsioses. Lewis *et al.* (1987) prepared a compact IP test kit and supplied it to hospitals throughout Malaysia, and obtained successful results not only for the diagnosis of Tsutsugamushi disease but

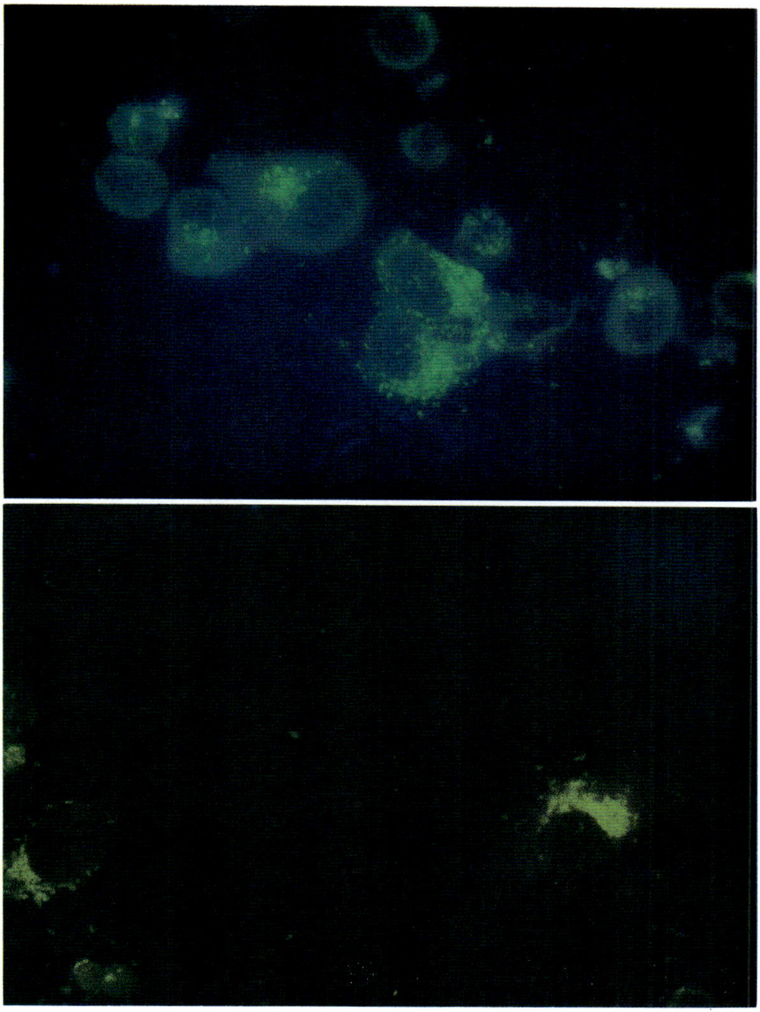

Fig. 1. Indirect (above) and direct (below) immunofluorescence observations of *R. tsutsugamushi* in mesothelial smears of DDD mouse intraperitoneally infected with Kato strain, using anti-Kato antibody (indirect) or its conjugate (direct). Specific fluorescence is observed in both figures. Magnification is ×280 (above) and ×400 (below).

also for the diagnosis of endemic typhus and tick typhus.

The principle underlying this IP technique is similar to that of indirect IF. Antigens on a glass slide are allowed to react with the patient's serum in serial two-fold dilutions and, after being washed, are allowed to react with peroxidase-conjugated anti-human IgG or IgM. A brown color is developed at the antibody-binding sites by reaction with the enzyme substrate, hydrogen peroxide and 3, 3′-diaminobenzidine tetrahydrochiloride.

Three prototypes of *R. tsutsugamushi*, the Kato, Karp, and Gilliam strains (plus local strains), grown in cultured cells such as L-929, BS-C40, Vero, and HeLa cells, usually serve as the antigens in the IP test. Because of the enzymatic reaction, the technique is highly sensitive for detecting *R. tsutsugamushi*-specific antibodies, compared to IF. On the other hand, careful attentions should be paid to differentiate whether the stained brownish particles are actually the result of a specific reaction with *R. tsutsugamushi* particles or whether they are the result of a nonspecific reaction caused by cell debris in the antigen smear. With the IP test, *R. tsutsugamushi*-specific antibodies in patients' sera can be classified as IgM and IgG.

The procedures used, based on the descriptions given by Suto and Fujimiya (1980) and by Suto (1985), are:

1) Preparation of antigen smears on glass slide

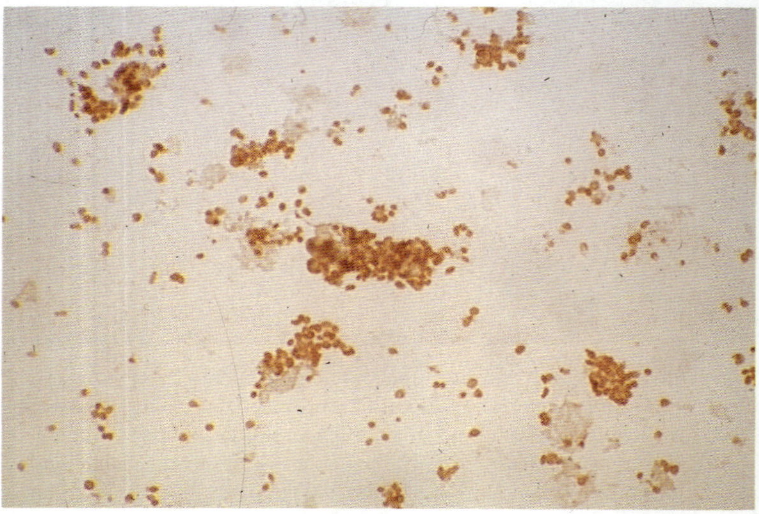

Fig. 2. Indirect immunoperoxidase test
Positive findings of *R. tsutsugamushi*
R. tsutsugamushi are observed as tiny brownish particles. Normal culture cells are stained blue with methylene blue (×400).

(1) Three strains of *R. tsutsugamushi* are cultured in cells. The growth of rickettsiae in cultured cells is confirmed with Giemsa staining. When rickettsial growth is sufficient, the cells are detached from the walls of the culture flask with a rubber policeman.

(2) The harvested cells are centrifuged at 3,000 rpm for 20 min.

(3) The resultant pellet is washed twice with PBS by centrifugation at 3,000 rpm, for 20 min each time. The PBS contains (per *l*) NaCl 8.0 g, KCl 0.2 g, KH_2PO_4 0.2 g and Na_2HPO_4 1.15 g.

(4) The pellet is resuspended in PBS and centrifuged at 700 rpm for 5min.

(5) The supernatant is centrifuged at 8,000 rpm for 5–10 min. The crude rickettsiae are obtained as a pellet.

(6) The pellet is resuspended in a small amount of PBS containing 0.3% bovine serum albumin. A small quantity of normal cultured cells is added to this suspension; this helps, as added cells are stained with methylene blue solution, to focus the microscope on an antigen smear when the rickettsiae are not stained by negative reaction.

(7) A glass slide is coated with hydrophobic paint, except for 12 round windows, 5–7 mm in diameter. A drop (2–5 μl) of each of the three prototype antigens is placed in each window and spread into a dot with a diameter of 1–1.5 mm, so that each window finally contains antigen dots of different *R. tsutsugamushi* types.

(8) The rickettsial antigens on the glass slide are dried at room temperature.

(9) The antigens on the slide are fixed with cold acetone for 10 min.

(10) The slides are dried and stored at –20°C until use. The antigens on the slide are stable for one year or more at –20°C, but the antigenicity will decrease if they are thawed and frozen repeatedly.

2) Test procedures

(1) The test serum is diluted in serial two-fold dilutions with PBS, beginning with 1 : 20, up to 1 : 40,960.

(2) The antigen slide is taken out of the freezer and warmed from –20°C to room temperature in a stream of cool air, to prevent condensation of moisture on the slide.

(3) About 10 μl of tests serum at each dilution is placed onto each window on the slide.

(4) The slide is kept in a moist chamber and incubated at 37°C for 20 min.

(5) The slide is washed with PBS, immersed in PBS in a slide staining dish, and shaken on a vibrating plate for 15–20 min to remove the unbound serum; PBS is changed three times at 5-min intervals during this process.

(6) The slide is dried in cool air, and 10 μl of secondary antibody, appropriately diluted horseradish peroxidase-conjugated anti-human IgG or IgM rabbit serum, is placed onto each window; the slide is then incubated at 37°C for 20 min in a moist chamber. The appropriate dilution of horseradish peroxidase-conjugated anti-human IgG and IgM should be determined by checkerboard titration with positive control serum prior to use.

(7) The slide is washed in the same way as in step (5).

(8) PBS remaining on the slide is rinsed with distilled water.

(9) The slide is immersed in an enzyme substrate solution in a slide staining dish for 10 min. The enzyme substrate solution contains 0.3% (w/v) 3, 3′-diaminobenzidine tetrahydrochloride ($C_{12}H_{14}N_4 \cdot 4HCl \cdot 2H_2O$), 1% sodium acetate buffer (pH 6.2), and 0.02% hydrogen peroxide. This solution is preserved at room temperature in the dark. In this condition, the solution is stable for 3 weeks, and it can be used repeatedly during this period. The solution becomes turbid with a fine precipitate within a few days, so it should be filtered through filter paper just before use.

(10) The substrate solution on the slide is rinsed off with distilled water, and the slide is immersed in methylene blue solution (Loeffler's methylene blue solution diluted 1 : 20 with distilled water) in a staining dish for 3–5 sec.

(11) The slide is washed with distilled water and dried in cool air.

(12) The antigen windows are mounted with Diatex (AB-WILH, Backer, Sweden) and covered with a cover slip.

(13) The antigens in each window are observed under an optical microscope at 400 × magnification. If the test serum contains *R. tsutsugamushi*-specific antibody, the rickettsiae are observed as tiny brownish particles (Fig. 2). Sometimes, however, the debris of cultured cells is stained brown by a nonspecific reaction. Thus, the size of the brownish particles is important for distinguishing the rickettsiae from cell debris. Confirmation that the brownish particles are rickettsiae is done with reference to the size of the rickettsia particles stained as a result of the reaction with the positive control serum. The IP titer of the test serum is the reciprocal of the highest dilution

of serum that showed a positive reaction.

With the IP technique, specific IgM antibody is first detected on day 3 or 4 after the onset of illness (shown by clinical manifestations); the IgM titer subsequently rises rapidly to 5,120 or more, on days 10–15. A few months to 1 year after the onset of the disease, IgM is undetectable.

Specific IgG antibody, on the other hand, can be detected after day 7. The titer of IgG antibody rises more slowly than the titer of IgM antibody, reaching 5,120 or more after about 3 weeks.

If, because the serum sample is collected too early, IgM antibody is not detected in a patient in whom Tsutsugamushi disease is suspected, a further serum sample should be collected a few days later for the detection of IgM.

d. Biotin-avidin immunofluorescence (*BA-IF*)

The BA-IF method (Berman and Basch, 1980) is similar to the indirect IF (Murata *et al.*, 1986; Yamamoto *et al.*, 1987). In place of the FITC-conjugated anti-immunoglobulin, biotinylated anti-immunoglobulin is used, and FITC-conjugated avidin is then allowed to react for a short time. Biotin has strong affinity to avidin at a binding constant of 10^{-5}/M, improving the reaction and making it more sensitive than routine IF. A BA-IF method for the diagnosis of Tsutsugamushi disease is described and evaluated below.

1) Procedure for BA-IF

(1) As soon as *R. tsutsugamushi* antigen is prepared, it is smeared on a glass slide, dried, and treated with cold acetone for 15 min. Thus prepared antigen slides can be preserved in a freezer. When the slide is taken out of the freezer, it is warmed quickly at room temperature just before use in a cool air stream to prevent condensation of moisture on the slide.

(2) About 10 μl of diluted test sera (starting at 1 : 10) is overlaid onto spots of *R. tsutsugamushi* smears, in the order of the highest dilution to the lowest, using the same micropipette.

(3) The slide is incubated at 37°C for 30 min in a moist chamber.

(4) The slide is washed by immersion in PBS in a slide staining dish on a vibrating plate, with gentle movement. The PBS is changed three times at 5-min intervals.

(5) The slide is dried in an air stream.

(6) The spots on the slide are overlaid with 10 μl of appropriately

diluted biotinylated anti-immunoglobulin antibody.

(7) The incubation is repeated, and washing and drying are carried out as in steps (4) and (5).

(8) The spots on the slide are overlaid with 10 μl of appropriately diluted FITC-conjugated avidin at 37°C for 10 min.

(9) Incubation, washing and drying are carried out as before (steps 3–5).

(10) The spots on the slide are mounted with buffered glycerol.

(11) The slide is observed under a transmitted illumination type fluorescence microscope at 400 × magnification.

The BA-IF reactions on both the peritoneal smear of the *R. tsutsugamushi*-infected mouse and the infected cultured cells are examined as positive controls. Specific reactions are observed in *R. tsutsugamushi* particles around and inside the cells; there are rarely nonspecific reactions.

2) Comparison of BA-IF with IP and IF

The specificity and sensitivity of BA-IF to each of the three *R. tsutsugamushi* prototypes were examined for prototype antigens and type-specific monoclonal antibodies, using IP, IF, and BA-IF techniques. The results are outlined briefly below. With all three methods, each monoclonal antibody reacted strongly to the homologous antigen, indicating high specificity. In regard to the strength of the reaction, BA-IF was slightly weaker than the IP test, but four to five times stronger than IF, and BA-IF was brighter than IF (Table 2).

Detections of IgG and IgM against *R. tsutsugamushi* were attempted in the sera of 27 patients in Kanagawa Prefecture, Japan, in whom Tsutsugamushi disease was suspected from clinical examination. The methods used for detection were BA-IF and routine IF with smeared antigens of each prototype.

As shown in Figs. 3 and 4, BA-IF reactions were always stronger than those of routine IF and showed greater brightness; BA-IF was highly correlated with IF for all prototypes. The differences between BA-IF and IF were particularly marked in the sera that had low or negligible titers by routine IF.

The BA-IF technique was evaluated in the light of these results.

The advantages of the method for the diagnosis of Tsutsugamushi disease are:

(1) Its specificity and sensitivity are satisfactory for this purpose.

(2) IgG and IgM can be detected separately.

Table 2. Comparison of Immunoperoxidase (IP), Immunofluorescence (IF), and Biotin-avidin Immunofluorescence (BA-IF) Titers of Strain-Specific Monoclonal Antibodies against Each Prototype Strain

Antigens	Anti-Gilliam (4B-6)*			Anti-Karp (I-19)*			Anti-Kato (2C-6)*		
	IP	IF	BA-IF	IP	IF	BA-IF	IP	IF	BA-I
Gilliam	163,840	20,480	81,920	<160	<10	<10	<160	<10	<10
Karp	<160	<10	<10	327,680	20,480	81,920	<160	<10	<10
Kato	<160	<10	<10	<160	<10	<10	163,840	10,240	81,920

Note: L cells infected with each prototype were used as antigen.
* Code names of monoclonal antibodies are used (see Chapter 2).

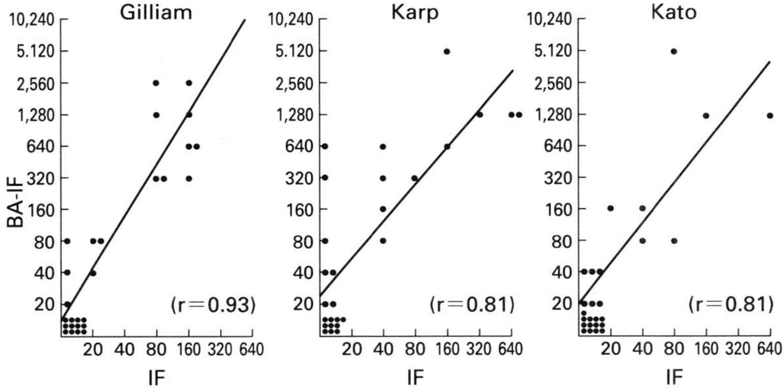

Fig. 3. Correlation between BA-IF and IF in detecting IgG with each prototype strain

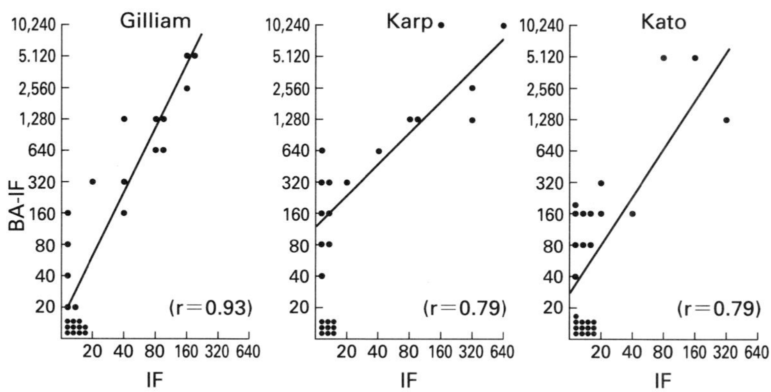

Fig. 4. Correlation between BA-IF and IF in detecting IgM with each prototype strain

(3) For clear visualization of rickettsia without background coloring, observation under the fluorescence microscope is much easier than by routine IF.

The only disadvantage in performing both IF and BA-IF is the necessity for a fluorescence microscope.

e. Dot-immunoblot method

Serodiagnosis by indirect IF (Kawamura and Aoyama, 1983) or indirect IP test (Suto, 1982) gives satisfactory results in the hands of experienced personnel, but these procedures may be troublesome for inexperienced technicians, particularly in regard to the microscope reading of the reaction in the final procedure.

The dot-immunoblot (DIB) method is based on enzyme-linked immunosorbent assay (ELISA), and nitrocellulose sheets (NCS) or nylon membranes are used for the blotting of solid phase with antigens. DIB was designed to develop a simple technique for the serodiagnosis of Tsutsugamushi disease. The principle of the procedure is the detection of anti-*R. tsutsugamushi* antibodies in test sera by reaction with antigens adhering to a solid membrane; combined human antibodies are then detected by further reactions with peroxidase-conjugated anti-human IgM or IgG rabbit serum, with diaminobenzidine serving as the enzyme substrate. The reactions are discriminated by reading the color intensity of the dots on the membrane. The advantage of this method is that no special instruments are required, and the result can be easily interpreted by untrained personnel, by comparing the color of the test dots with standardized color levels. The procedures outlined below are those described by Urakami *et al.* (1989) and Tamura *et al.* (1990).

1) Preparation of rickettsial antigens

Antigens are prepared from L 929 cell cultures infected with prototypes and local types of *R. tsutsugamushi* (Tamura *et al.*, 1984; Yamamoto *et al.*, 1986). The purified rickettsial antigens are prepared by Percoll density gradient centrifugation (Tamura *et al.*, 1982) and suspended in PBS. The suspension is irradiated with UV light (Urakami *et al.*, 1983) for inactivation before it is applied to the NCS.

2) Procedure for dot-immunoblot assay.

(1) Antigen dots on NCS are prepared with a dot-blot instrument (Bio Rad Laboratories, Hercules, Calif.), with which 8×12 dots (6-

mm diameter), containing 2 μg of purified antigen in 10 μl suspension, are applied to the NCS.

(2) The NCS is removed from the instrument, incubated in PBS (pH 7.4; 0.14 M NaCl in 0.01 M sodium phosphate buffer) containing 0.05% Tween 20 (PBS-T) for 30 min at 37°C, air-dried, and stored at −20°C until use.

(3) Before use, to prevent nonspecific reactions, the antigen dots are coated with 3% bovine serum albumin in PBS, pH 7.4, for 30 min at room temperature.

(4) The antigen-dotted NCS is immersed in PBS for 2–3 min at room temperature and then placed in 3 ml of test serum diluted 1 : 1,000 with PBS-T, where it is kept for 1 h at room temperature.

(5) The NCS is taken out and washed five times with PBS-T, with gentle shaking, replacing the washing solution 4–5 min interval.

(6) The NCS is immersed in a solution of peroxidase-conjugated anti-human IgG or IgM rabbit antibody diluted 1 : 2,000 with PBS-T for 30 min.

(7) The NCS is washed, as in step (5).

(8) Substrate solution is freshly prepared, which consists of 0.3% 3, 3′-diaminobenzidine tetrahydrochloride and 0.02% hydrogen peroxide in 75 mM sodium acetate buffer, pH 6.2.

(9) The NCS is placed in this substrate solution for 1 min at room temperature.

(10) Color development is terminated by briefly immersing the NCS in 0.2 N sulfuric acid; the NCS is then washed in distilled water, air-dried, and stored for a permanent record.

The final evaluation of antibody-positive or -negative serum is performed by comparing the color intensities of the dots with a color example which was previously prepared by the reaction with antibody-positive and -negative sera.

The NCS antigens can be stored under dry conditions at −20°C without significant loss of reactivity to antibodies for at least four months. After color development, the NCS can be stored at room temperature, and no color change occurs.

f. Enzyme-linked immunosorbent assay (*ELISA*)

Various modifications of ELISA for the detection of antigen or antibody have been reported. The dot-immunoblot method (see previous section in this chapter) performed on nitrocellulose sheets, and based on ELISA, is used for the detection of specific antibodies. Here, we briefly describe and evaluate some other modifications of ELISA.

1) Paper ELISA

Crum *et al.* (1980) developed a paper ELISA technique for the detection of antibody in human sera. A glass slide is used and substrate reactions are developed on filter paper. The three prototypes of *R. tsutsugamushi* are spotted on a glass slide and fixed with a chloroform-ethanol mixture. Human serum is placed on the spots, and the slide is incubated at 37°C for 30 min in a moist chamber. The slide is washed and dried; peroxidase-conjugated anti-human IgG rabbit serum is then dropped on the antigen spots, and the slide is incubated at 37°C for 30 min, and washed and dried again. The slide is then covered with a filter paper on which the enzyme-substrate solution has been absorbed. The color is developed on the filter paper by enzyme reaction, and the presence of antibody in the test serum is proven.

2) IgG/IgM capture ELISA

Yamamoto *et al.* (1991) developed a technique based on IgG and IgM capture ELISA. Anti-human IgM or IgG is adsorbed on the solid phase on a microplate. Reactions are followed in the order of test serum, *R. tsutsugamushi* type-specific antigen, and peroxidase-labeled anti-*R. tsutsugamushi* type-specific monoclonal antibody. Color development is performed with 2, 2′-azino-bis (3-ethylbenzthiazoline-6-sulfonic acid) diammonium salt (ABTS), the reaction is stopped with sodium fluoride, and the degree of color development represented by absorbance (optical density; OD) at a wavelength of 415 nm, is read with a spectrophotometer. The sensitivity of this method for the detection of the Kawasaki and Kuroki types of *R. tsutsugamushi* is similar to that of IF.

3) Inhibition ELISA

Furuya *et al.* (1991a) reported an inhibition ELISA using anti-*R. tsutsugamushi* type-specific monoclonal antibodies. The principle of this method is the measurement of inhibition percentage of antigen adsorption on a type-specific monoclonal antibody-coated plate by treatment of antigen with antibody-positive sera. In this system free antigen is captured between the monoclonal antibody absorbed on the solid phase and the enzyme-labeled monoclonal antibody. In the presence of the antibody, the amount of free antigen is low, the binding of the labeled monoclonal antibody is inhibited, and the final substrate reaction is inhibited.

The advantages of this test for practical use are: (1) crude antigens can be used, *i.e.*, purification of antigen is not necessary; (2) the test is more sensitive than IF; (3) the reaction is quantitative, and positive and negative reactions are determined objectively; and (4) since rickettsia type-specific antibody in individual patients can be identified, the method can be used for epidemiological surveys. The procedure is as follows:

(1) Each well of a microplate is coated with 50 μl of a type-specific monoclonal antibody, and the plate is stored overnight at 4°C.

(2) The plate is washed three times with PBS containing 0.05% Tween 20 and 0.1% bovine serum albumin (PBS-TB).

(3) PBS, containing 10% bovine serum albumin, is added to the wells, and the plate is incubated at 37°C for 2 h and again washed three times with PBS-TB.

(4) The antigen suspension (25 μl) is mixed with 25 μl of appropriately diluted test sera and 25 μl of PBS-TB in the wells of another microtiter plate, and the mixture is transferred to monoclonal antibody-coated wells.

(5) The plates are incubated at 37°C for 2 h, and the wells are washed three times with PBS-TB.

(6) Peroxidase-labeled type-specific monoclonal antibody (50 μl) is added to the wells and the plate is incubated at 37°C for 2 h, and again washed three times with PBS-TB.

(7) Freshly prepared substrate (100 μl), consisting of 0.08% ABTS and 0.0006% hydrogen peroxide in 0.05 M citrate-phosphate buffer, pH 5.0, is added to each well, and the plate is kept at room temperature for 1 h.

(8) The enzyme reaction is stopped by adding 50 μl of 1.25% sodium fluoride, and the degree of color development, represented by absorbance (optical density; OD) at 415 nm, is read with a spectrophotometer.

(9) The percent inhibition is calculated by the formula: Inhibition % = [(negative control OD – sample OD) / (negative control OD – positive control OD)] × 100, where negative, positive, and sample OD represent absorbance in the reactions with proven antibody-negative serum, type-specific monoclonal antibody, and test serum, respectively.

When Kawasaki type was the antigen and anti-Kawasaki-specific monoclonal antibodies were used, all test sera from patients in whom *R. tsutsugamushi* Kawasaki type was isolated, showed inhibition, at 70% or higher. Sera from healthy persons negative on IF and sera from patients infected with other types of *R. tsutsugamushi* showed inhibition at 30% or less. It was decided that 70% inhibition or higher represented a positive reaction, and that 30% or less was negative. The difference in color levels between positive and negative reactions can be distinguished even with the naked eye, without reading absorbance or calculating the percent inhibition. Thus, visualization of the results by this procedure clearly discriminates the presence or absence of type-specific antibody.

g. *Complement fixation (CF) test*

For the diagnosis of Tsutsugamushi disease, the CF test was the first serologic antibody detection method to employ specific antigens (Bengtson, 1945, 1946). Later, the method was used not only for the diagnosis of Tsutsugamushi disease (Shishido, 1962a; Tsuboi and Oyama, 1984) but also for typing *R. tsutsugamushi* isolates (Elisberg *et al.*, 1967, 1968; Shishido *et al.*, 1967). Even though the sensitivity of the CF test is inferior to that of indirect IF or the IP test, and the procedures are more complicated, the CF test is still being used in some clinical laboratories, since neither specific equipment nor special materials are necessary.

1) Antigens for CF test

The antigen used for the CF test has been greatly improved in several ways, and ether-treated antigens of the three prototypes, Kato, Karp, and Gilliam, are now available commercially in Japan. These products are convenient for use in routine examinations, unless local types of *R. tsutsugamushi* are to be targeted for clinical examination.

2) Comparison of indirect IF and the CF test

Tsuboi and Oyama (1984) compared indirect IF and the CF test by examining 25 paired serum samples collected from patients suspected to have Tsutsugamushi disease; the first samples were collected about one week after the onset of the disease (acute stage), and the second samples were collected at the recovery stage 2–3 weeks after the onset. Antigens derived from the three prototypes were used. At the acute stage, 24 of the 25 serum samples were positive, with a titer of 1 : 10 higher by indirect IF, whereas only 8 were positive with the CF test. By indirect IF, 21 of the 25 serum samples (84%) showed a four-fold or greater increase of antibody titer at the recovery stage compared with the titer of the first sample, whereas only 17 of the samples (68%) showed such an increase with the CF test. Of note, in one case reported in this study the serum titer of the patient had increased more than four-fold at the recovery stage, when determined by indirect IF, whereas the titer was less than 1 : 10 with the CF test. As shown in this case, at times, the CF test fails to detect the antibody not only at the acute stage but also at recovery.

The ether-treated antigens used for the CF test generally have high type specificity; however, in many areas, both in Japan and in other parts of the world, local types of *R. tsutsugamushi* have been discovered. Hence, it is very likely that, in the above case, a very specific prototype antigen for the CF test failed to detect local types of *R. tsutsugamushi.* When Tsutsugamushi disease is suspected and the patient's serum shows a negative CF test result, the serum should be re-examined by indirect IF or the IP test. The technical procedures employed for the CF test are the same as the routine methods employed to detect antibodies for other diseases, as described in many technical texts.

h. Weil-Felix (WF) reaction

Since Weil and Felix (1916) found that *Proteus vulgaris* PX-19 (OX19) strain agglutinated with the serum of a patient with epidemic typhus, the serological diagnosis of rickettsioses was made possible by their test, the WF test. Later, *Proteus mirabilis* OX-K strain was found to agglutinate with *R. tsutsugamushi* antibody (Fletcher *et al.*, 1929), and this reaction came to be used for the diagnosis of Tsutsugamushi disease.

1) Principle of WF reaction

The principle of the WF test is that *Proteus* O antigens cross-react with IgM antibody in rickettsioses. The antibody is detected by the WF test on days 5 and 6 after the onset of disease, at the earliest, but is usually detected around day 12. The aggulutinin titer is rapidly reduced after several months (Cox, 1981).

Since the test procedures are simple, and since they can be performed in any clinical laboratory with commercial *Proteus* OX-19, OX-2, and OX-K products, the test is still used at some laboratories, even though other, more specific, methods are now available. Since the WF test is not based on a specific serological reaction between antibody and antigen, its sensitivity of detection of the antibody and (if the reaction is positive) the specificity of the detected antibody are problematic particularly in patients infected with *R. tsutsugamushi*.

2) Disadvantages of WF reaction

Brown *et al.* (1983) studied the WF test in patients suspected of having Tsutsugamushi disease; they found that in 90% of the patients with a WF titer of 1 : 320 or higher, Tsutsugamushi disease was confirmed by indirect IF, but the diagnosis was questionable in the many patients whose WF titers were lower than 1 : 320. Bozeman and Elisberg (1963) reported that, in patients whose sera were positive by indirect IF, the WF test showed negative reactions, with titers lower than 1 : 20 at both the acute and recovery stages, or lower than 1 : 20 at the acute stage and remaining at from 1 : 20 to 1 : 80 at the recovery stage. Cox (1981) observed that *Proteus* OX-K also agglutinated with the sera of patients with proven urinary tract infection with *Proteus*, and with the sera of patients with relapsing fever, leptospirosis, and severe liver disease.

To use the test properly, it is necessary to examine paired sera collected at the acute and recovery stages, and to determine whether the titer has increased four-fold or more in the recovery-stage sample. In the light of the results noted above, even if the sera are negative at both stages, and even if the titer is not elevated four-fold at the recovery stage, Tsutsugamushi disease cannot be ruled out. Therefore, the WF test is regarded as inferior to indirect IF, the IP test, and ELISA for the diagnosis of Tsutsugamushi disease.

3) Antigenic agent in WF reaction

Lipopolysaccharide (LPS) and peptidoglycan (PG) in various species of rickettsiae and *Proteus* OX-19, OX-2, and OX-K have been studied in efforts to identify a common antigenic agent in rickettsiae and the *Proteus* strains used for the WF test. However, Amano *et al.* (1987) found none or only very small amounts of LPS and PG in *R. tsutsugamushi*, and they also found, in a later study (Amano *et al.*, 1990) that antibody against LPS from *Proteus* OX-K did not react with *R. tsutsugamushi*. In a more recent study, Amano *et al.* (1993) found that IgM in patients with Tsutsugamushi disease reacted with LPS from *Proteus* OX-K. Based on these results, IgM antibody rather than IgG may participate in the WF test, and *Proteus* OX-K LPS may have one of the antigenic epitopes common to the components of *R. tsutsugamushi*.

3. Detection of Rickettsial DNA by Polymerase Chain Reaction

The polymerase chain reaction (PCR) is now widely used for the diagnosis of many infectious diseases. The method is especially useful when it is difficult to perform immunological diagnosis or to isolate the causative agent. In Tsutsugamushi disease, PCR can indicate the rickettsial infection even in the early rickettsemic stage, before the antibody titer has increased. The use of PCR for the diagnosis of Tsutsugamushi disease has been reported by several research groups (Furuya *et al.*, 1991b, 1993; Kawamori *et al.*, 1993; Murai *et al.*, 1992; Sugita *et al.* 1992, 1993).

The primers used for PCR are designed on the basis of the nucleotide sequences of the gene encoding the 56-kDa protein (Ohashi *et al.*, 1992) and the 60-kDa protein (Stover *et al.*, 1990b). For identifying the rickettsial type in patients, primers have been designed from the DNA sequence of the gene encoding the 56-kDa protein (Furuya *et al.*, 1991b, 1993; Kawamori *et al.*, 1993).

The amount of rickettsial DNA in the patient's blood is usually very small even in the rickettsemic stage. Therefore, the sensitivity of the method used for the detection of rickettsial DNA is of crucial importance. Recently Yoshida *et al.* (1994) found that with nested PCR, two copies of rickettsial DNA in the specimen were sufficient for detection.

However, contamination is a problem with PCR. The increased sensitivity permitted by nested PCR can lead to increases in false positives, due to the contamination of rickettsial DNA in the sample. To avoid this contamination every step of the procedure should be performed very carefully. For example, the pipette should be changed at each step, since the inside of the syringe may often contain nucleotide fragments; the reagents used should be divided into small amounts. It is also desirable to use different rooms for the first and second PCR procedures.

a. *Type-specific amplification of* Rickettsia tsutsugamushi *DNA by nested PCR*

Furuya *et al.* (1993) reported primer pairs that detected and identified the rickettsial type in an infected patient. The primer pairs used for nested PCR were designed from the nucleotide sequence of the gene encoding the 56-kDa protein (Ohashi *et al.*, 1990), and type-specific primers were used in the second PCR amplification. Thus, this technique simultaneously permits both diagnosis of Tsutsugamushi disease and identification of the *R. tsutsugamushi* type.

1) Preparation of template DNA

(1) Homogenize blood clot corresponding to about 0.5 ml blood in 1.0 ml distilled water with a mortar and pestle.

(2) Mix the homogenate with 1/10 volume of 100 mM Tris-HCl buffer (pH 8.0), containing 10 mM EDTA, 10% SDS, and 2 mg/ml of proteinase K; incubate the mixture at 55°C for 1 h.

(3) Extract DNA in this lysate with an equal volume of phenol-chloroform-isoamylalcohol (25 : 24 : 1) mixture. Centrifuge the mixture for 5 min in a microfuge.

(4) Transfer the aqueous layer to a new tube.

(5) Repeat steps (3) and (4) two more times.

(6) Extract with an equal volume of chloroform-isoamylalcohol (24 : 1). Centrifuge for 5 min in a microfuge.

(7) Transfer the aqueous layer containing DNA to a new tube.

(8) Add 1/10 volume of 3 M sodium acetate and two volumes of cold 100% ethanol to the DNA solution and mix. Keep at –80°C for 30 min.

(9) Centrifuge the solution for 10 min in a microfuge. Carefully aspirate or decant the supernatant from the DNA pellet.

(10) Wash the pellet with cold 70% ethanol. Centrifuge for 5 min in a microfuge.

(11) Carefully aspirate or decant ethanol. Allow the pellet to air dry.

(12) Resuspend DNA pellet in a small volume of 10 mM Tris-HCl buffer (pH 8.0) containing 1 mM EDTA (TE).

2) Primers used for PCR.

The primers were designed on the basis of the nucleotide sequence of the gene encoding the 56-kDa protein.

Primer 34: 5′-TCAAGCTTATTGCTAGTGCAATGTCTGC-3′
Primer 55: 5′-AGGGATCCCTGCTGCTGTGCTTGCTGCG-3′
Primer 10: 5′-GATCAAGCTTCCTCAGCCTACTATAATGCC-3′
Primer 11: 5′-CTAGGGATCCCGACAGATGCACTATTAGGC-3′

Primer G: 5′-CTTTATATCACTATATATCTT-3′
Primer KP: 5′-ACAATATCGGATTTATAACC-3′
Primer KT: 5′-GAATATTTAATAGCACTGGA-3′
Primer KW: 5′-ATGCTGCTATTGATACAGGC-3′
Primer KR: 5′-CACCGGATTTACCATCATAT-3′

3) Amplification procedure

(1) PCR is performed with "nested" primer pairs. For this, a total volume of 50 μl of PCR amplification mixture is prepared, at final concentrations of 10 mM Tris-HCl buffer (pH 8.3), 1.5 mM $MgCl_2$, 50 mM KCl, 0.001% (w/v) gelatin, 200 μM each of dATP, dCTP, dGTP, and dTTP, 0.2 μM of outer primers 34 and 55, 1.25 units of AmpliTaq polymerase, and 5 μl of template DNA.

(2) The mixture is placed in a thermal cycler, and each temperature cycle is set at 94°C for 30 sec for denaturation, at 57°C for 2 min for annealing, and at 70°C for 2 min for chain extension. This cycle is repeated 30 times. After the first PCR with primers 34 and 55, 1003–1030 bp DNA fragments are amplified with Gilliam, Karp, Kato, Kawasaki, or Kuroki type *R. tsutsugamushi* as templates.

(3) For the second PCR amplification, a 5 μl aliquot of the first PCR product mixture is amplified by the same procedure as that outlined for step (2), except that an inner pair of primers is used.

The combination of primers 10 and 11, a universal primer pair used to detect all *R. tsutsugamushi* types, produces 481 to 507 bp DNA in the presence of the first PCR product with any type of *R. tsutsugamushi.* With different combinations of primers, as shown below, rickettsial type-specific products of DNA fragments are expected to yield:

Primers G and 10 specific to Gilliam, 407 bp DNA;
Primers KP and 10 specific to Karp, 230 bp DNA;
Primers KT and 10 specific to Kato, 242 bp DNA;
Primers KW and 11 specific to Kawasaki, 523 bp DNA; and
Primers KR and 10 specific to Kuroki, 220 bp DNA fragment.

4) Detection of PCR products

The amplified sample (5 μl) is electrophoresed in 1.5% agarose gel or 8% polyacrylamide gel, and the DNA bands are stained with 0.5 μg/ml ethidium bromide. The specificity of these products is confirmed in the hybridization test with the amplified digoxigenin-labeled probe.

This method enables the detection of rickettsial DNA from one mite and is useful for making surveys of rickettsial types in mites in endemic areas. With this method, a clear diagnosis can be made not only with blood as the template but also with sections of spleen and liver. In the light of the overall results, nested PCR is regarded as a sensitive and type-specific means of detecting *R. tsutsugamushi*.

b. Identification of rickettsial types by endonuclease fragment length polymorphism of PCR products

1) Two-step PCR for diagnosis

Kawamori *et al.* (1993) have reported a two-step PCR method for the diagnosis of Tsutsugamushi disease. The target DNA is a part of the gene producing the type-specific 56-kDa protein of *R. tsutsugamushi*. The following primers were used:

Primer a, 5′-TACATTAGCTGCGGGTATGACA-3′, which corresponds to the sequence at 225 to 246 bp downstream from the start codon of the TSA gene of the Gilliam strain (Ohashi *et al.*, 1990a);

Primer b, 5′-CCAGCATAATTCTTCAACCAAG-3′ at 536 to 557 bp;

Primer a′, 5′-GAGCAGAGCTAGGTGTTATGTA-3′ at 263 to 284 bp; and

Primer b′, 5′-TAGGCATTATAGTAGGCTGAGG-3′ at 409 to 430 bp.

For the first step of PCR, a pair of primers, a and b, is used, and polynucleotides from 306 to 339 bp are produced with the template DNAs obtained from the Gilliam, Karp, Kato, Kawasaki, Kuroki, and Shimokoshi types, but not with the DNA of *R. sibirica*.

For the second step of PCR, a pair of primers, a′ and b′, is used, and a product from 150 to 168 bp is obtained, with the template DNAs from the PCR product obtained at the first step for each type of *R. tsutsugamushi*.

2) Typing by endonuclease fragment length polymorphism of PCR products

When the products of the second-step PCR were digested with several endonucleases, *Hha*I, *Sfa*NI, *Mnl*I, *Alw*NI, *Bgl*II, and *Mbo*II, it was found that the restriction fragment profiles on polyacrylamide gel electrophoresis differed according to type, and that the rickettsial types could be identified from these profiles.

Kawamori *et al.* (1993) employed this method for the detection of DNA in both clinical specimens and naturally infected chiggers, and for the typing of rickettsia in these samples. The results were satisfactory. Rickettsia-specific amplified DNAs were derived from the patients' blood and from the mites from endemic areas by the two-step PCR, and the type of rickettsia infecting these hosts was identified from the fragment patterns of the amplified PCR products observed after endonuclease digestion.

References

Allen, A.C. and Spitz, S. 1945. A comparative study of the pathology of scrub typhus (Tsutsugamushi disease) and other rickettsial disease. *Am. J. Pathol.*, **21**: 603–681.

Allen, E.G., Bovarnick, M.R. and Snyder, J.C. 1954. The effect of irradiation with ultraviolet light on various properties of typhus rickettsiae. *J. Bacteriol.*, **67**: 718–723.

Allison, A.C. and Perkins, H.R. 1960. Presence of cell walls like those of bacteria in *Rickettsia. Nature*, **188**: 796–798.

Amano, K. and Williams, J.C. 1984a. Sensitivity of *Coxiella burnetii* peptidoglycan to lysozyme hydrolysis and correlation of sacculus rigidity with peptidoglycan-associated proteins. *J. Bacteriol.*, **160**: 989–993.

Amano, K. and Williams, J.C. 1984b. Chemical and immunological characterization of lipopolysaccharides from phase I and phase II *Coxiella burnetii. J. Bacteriol.*, **160**: 994–1002.

Amano, K., Williams, J.C., McCaul, T.F. and Peacock, M.G. 1984. Biochemical and immunological properties of *Coxiella burnetii* cell wall and peptidoglycan-protein complex fractions. *J. Bacteriol.*, **160**: 982–988.

Amano, K., Tamura, A., Ohashi, N., Urakami, H., Kaya, S. and Fukushi, K. 1987. Deficiency of peptidoglycan and lipopolysaccharide components in *Rickettsia tsutsugamushi. Infect. Immun.*, **55**: 2290–2292.

Amano, K., Mizushiri, S., Fujii, S., Fukushi, K. and Suto, T. 1990. Immunological characterization of lipopolysaccharides from *Proteus* strains used in Weil-Felix test and reactivity with patient sera of Tsutsugamushi disease. *Microbiol. Immunol.*, **34**: 135–145.

Amano, K., Suzuki, N., Fujita, M., Nakamura, Y. and Suto, T. 1993. Serological reactivity of sera from scrub typhus patients against Weil-Felix test antigens. *Microbiol. Immunol.*, **37**: 927–933.

Anacker, R.L., Pickens, E.G. and Lackman, D.B. 1967. Details of the ultrastructure of *Rickettsia prowazekii* grown in the chick yolk sac. *J. Bacteriol.*, **94**: 260–262.

Anacker, R.L., Gerloff, R.K., Thomas, L.A., Mann, R.E., Brown, W.R. and Bickel, W.D. 1974. Purification of *Rickettsia rickettsii* by density-gradient zonal centrifugation. *Canad. J. Microbiol.*, **20**: 1523–1527.

Anacker, R.L., McCaul, T.F., Burgdorfer, W. and Gerloff, R.K. 1980. Properties of selected rickettsiae of the spotted fever group. *Infect. Immun.*, **27**: 468–474.

Anderson, B.E., Regnery, R.L., Carlone, G.M., Tzianabos, T., McDade, J. E., Fu, Z. Y. and Bellini, W. J. 1987. Sequence analysis of the 17-kilodalton-antigen gene from *Rickettsia rickettsii. J. Bacteriol.*, **169**: 2385–2390.

Arai, Y. 1955. Human infesting experiments on the larvae of *Trombicula scutellaris*. pp. 23–30. In: Studies on Shichito fever. Pt. III. Dept. Hlth., Tokyo. (in Japanese.)

Arai, Y. and Komine, I. 1952. Clinical features of Shichito fever. pp. 43–49. In: Studies on Shichito fever. Pt I. Dept. Hlth., Tokyo. (in Japanese).

Asahina, S. 1952. Studies on the ecology of Trombiculid mites (II). *Jpn. J. Sanit. Zool.*, 3: 129–130. (in Japanese).

Asakawa, N. and Miyajima, M. 1905. Survey report on pathogenic agent of Tsutsugamushi disease. *Saikingaku Zasshi*, 120: 741–753. (in Japanese).

Asanuma, K. 1959. Studies on the relationship between the chigger mites and their hosts, especially birds in Japan. pp. 499–507. In: Proceedings of the 15th General Assembly of the Japan Medical Congress, Vol. 2. (in Japanese.)

Asanuma, K. 1983 . Vector trombiculid mites and their infection rates with *Rickettsia tsutsugamushi. Clin. Bacteriol.*, **10**: 174–179. (in Japanese).

Asanuma, K. 1986. Medico-zoological studies of Tsutsugamushi disease in Japan, with special reference to *Leptotrombidium pallidum*. p. 27. In: Proc. of symposium of Tsutsugamushi disease (scrub typhus) in Asia. The 28th Assembly of the Japan Tropical Medicine and Hygiene.

Asanuma, K. 1987. Transmission of *Rickettsia tsutsugamushi* by infected *Leptotrombidium pallidum* (Ab.). In: Proc. Jpn. Assoc. Acarol., **14**: 11. (in Japanese).

Asanuma, K., Kano, R., Kumada, N., Kitaoka, M. and Okubo, K. 1958. On the vector mites of Shichito fever. pp.37–40. In: Studies on Shichito fever. Pt. Sum., Dept. Hlth., Tokyo. (in Japanese).

Asanuma, K., Kumada, N., Niwayama, S., Kugoh, T., Yamamoto, H., Kitaoka, M., Kobayashi, I. Kobayashi, J., Takeda, I., Murohashi, M., Miyamoto, T. and Nakagawa, H. 1959a. Evaluation of effectiveness of BHC powder on the trombiculid mite, *Trombicula akamushi*, by bait-animal method in the endemic area of scrub typhus in Nagaoka, Niigata Pref., Japan. *Miscel. Rep. Res. Inst. Natural Resources*, **51**: 22–33. (in Japanese).

Asanuma, K., Kumada, N., Niwayama, S., Kugoh, T., Yamamoto, H., Miyamoto, T., Okubo, K., Suzuki, M., Kobayashi, I., Karasawa, T., Kobayashi, J., Takeda, I. and Murohashi, M. 1959b. Recovery of *Rickettsia orientalis* from albino rats infested with *Trombicula akamushi* and *T. pallida* after exposure in the noxious area in Niigata Prefecture, Japan. *Jpn. J. Sanit. Zool.*, **10**: 46–48. (in Japanese).

Asanuma, K., Kitaoka, M., Okubo, K., Kumada, N., Suzuki, M., Karasawa, T., Kugoh, T., Yamamoto, H., Kawamura, A. Jr., Miyamoto, T., Akiyama, J., Nakagawa, H. and Hori, S. 1959c. Evidences for *Trombicula scutellaris* to be a vector of scrub typhus in Chiba Prefecture, Japan. *Jpn. J. Sanit. Zool.*, **10**: 232–244. (in Japanese).

Asanuma, K., Kano, R., Kumada, N., Kitaoka, M., Okubo, K., Hazato, H. and Shimizu, F. 1960. Evidences for *Trombicula pallida* to be a vector of scrub typhus in Miura and Shimoda districts. *Jpn. J. Sanit. Zool.*, **11**: 59–60. (in Japanese).

Asanuma, K., Kumada, N., Okubo, K., Taniguchi, H., Kugoh, T., Kaneko, K., Karasawa, T., Akiyama, J., Miyamoto, T., Miyamoto, K., Shimizu, F., Kitaoka, M., Murohashi, M. and Sato, T. 1961. On the occurrence of *Rickettsia orientalis* in *Trombicula pallida* from Nagaoka City, one of the endemic foci of classical scrub typhus in Japan. *Miscel. Rep. Res. Inst. Natural Resources*, **54**/

55: 7–14. (in Japanese).

Asanuma, K., Kitaoka, M., Okubo, K., Kumada, N., Kugoh, T., Shimizu, F., Taniguchi, H., Hazato, H., Toyokawa, K., Yamamoto, S., Yamamoto, T., Karasawa, T., Kaneko, K., Teshigawara, M., Miyamoto, T., Akiyama, J., Miyamoto, K., Wada, T. and Nakagawa, H. 1962a. Determination of the vector mite of scrub typhus (Tsutsugamushi disease) in southern parts of Miura and Izu Peninsulas, Japan. *Miscel. Rep. Res. Inst. Natural Resources*, **58/59**: 37–55. (in Japanese).

Asanuma, K., Okubo, K., Kumada, N. and Kitaoka, M. 1962b. Determination of the vector mites of scrub typhus in Japan. *Japan. J. Med. Sci. Biol.*, **15**: 297–308.

Asanuma, K., Okubo, K., Kumada, N. and Kitaoka, M. 1962c. Determination of the vector of scrub typhus or Tsutsugamushi disease in Japan. *Miscel. Rep. Res. Inst. Natural Resources*, **58/59**: 56–63. (in Japanese).

Asanuma, K., Kitaoka, M., Taniguchi, H., Teshigawara, M., Kugoh, T., Miyamoto, T., Kumada, N., Matsuo, M., Murohashi, M. and Miyamoto, K. 1964 a. Surveys on larval trombiculid mites and positivity of *Rickettsia orientalis* of small mammals trapped at 3 selected areas in Niigata, endemic to classical scrub typhus during winter and spring, especially snow season. *Miscel. Rep. Res. Inst. Natural Resources*, **63**: 17–32. (in Japanese).

Asanuma, K., Okubo, K., Kumada, N., Kitaoka, M., Shimizu, F., Taniguchi, H., Teshigawara, M., Kugoh, T., Miyamoto, T., Yamada, K. and Murohashi, M. 1964 b. Isolation experiments of *Rickettsia orientalis* from larval trombiculid mites, *Leptotrombidium pallida* collected monthly from small mammals trapped at Kurojo, Nagaoka, one of the so-called classical scrub typhus endemic areas in Niigata, Japan. *Miscel. Rep. Res. Inst. Natural Resources*, **62**: 54–62. (in Japanese).

Asanuma, K., Kitaoka, M., Shimizu, F. and Kano, R. 1974. *Leptotrombidium scutellare* as a vector of scrub typhus at the endemic area of the foothills of Mt. Fuji, Japan. *J. Hyg. Epidemiol. Microbiol. Immunol.*, **18**: 172–184.

Audy, J.R. 1949. A summary topographical account of scrub typhus, 1908–1946. *Bull. Inst. Med. Res. Malaya*, **1**: 1–82.

Audy, J.R. 1951. Trombiculid mites and scrub-itch. *Austral. J. Sci.*, **14**: 94–96.

Audy, J.R. 1958. The role of mite vectors in the natural history of scrub typhus. Proc. 10th. Int. Congr. Ent., Montreal, 1956. **3**: 639–649.

Audy, J.R. 1961. The ecology of scrub typhus. pp. 389–432. In: Studies in disease ecology. (ed. J. M. May), Hafner Publ., New York.

Audy, J.R. 1968. Red mites and typhus. p. 191. The Athlone Press, London.

Audy, J.R. and Harrison, J.L. 1951. A review of investigations of mite typhus in Burma and Malaya, 1945–1950. *Trans. Roy. Soc. Trop. Med. Hyg.*, **44**: 371–404.

Audy, J.R., Bower, J.D., Browning, H.C., Bullock, A.A., Cockings, K.L., Ford, W., Gordon, H.T. M., Karla, S.L., Parker, M.T., Radford, C.D., Roonwal, M.L. and Thomas, H.M. 1947. Scrub typhus investigations in South East Asia; a report on investigations by G.H.Q. (India) Field Typhus Research Team, Medical Research Council Typhus Team, based on Scrub Typhus Research Laboratory, S.E. Asia Command, Imphal, India, pts. 1–3, A.M.D. 7, London, British War office.

Baca, O.G. and Paretsky, D. 1974. Some physiological and biochemical effects of a *Coxiella burnetii* lipopolysaccharide preparation on guinea pigs. *Infect. Immun.*, **9**: 939–945.

Baelz, E. and Kawakami, S. 1879. Das japanische Fluss-oder Ueberschwemmung-fieber, eine acute Infectionskrankheit. *Virchow's Arch. Path. Anat.*, **78**: 373–420.

Baker, H.J., Hubert, A.A. and Manikumaran, C. 1968. A technique for feeding larval trombiculid mites on laboratory mice. *J. Med. Entomol.*, **5**: 511–513.

Bell, E.J., Bennett, B.L. and Whitman, L. 1946. Antigenic differences between strains of scrub typhus as demonstrated by cross-neutralization test. *Proc. Soc. Exp. Biol. Med.*, **62**: 134–137.

Bengtson, I.A. 1945. Apparent serological heterogeneity among strains of Tsutsugamushi disease (scrub typhus). *Publ. Hlth. Rep.*, **60**: 1483–1488.

Bengtson, I.A. 1946. A serological study of 37 cases of Tsutsugamushi disease (scrub typhus) occurring in Burma and Philippine Islands. *Publ. Hlth. Rep.*, **61**: 887–894.

Bennett, B.L., Smadel, J.E. and Gauld, R.L. 1949. Studies on scrub typhus (Tsutsugamushi disease), IV. Heterogeneity of strains of *R. tsutsugamushi* as demonstrated by cross-neutralization tests. *J. Immunol.*, **62**: 453–461.

Bergey, D.H. 1939. Bergey's manual of determinative bacteriology. 5th ed. p. 1032. (eds. D.H. Bergey, R.S. Breed, E.G.D. Murray and A.P. Hitchens). Williams & Wilkins, Baltimore.

Bergey, D.H. 1948. Bergey's manual of determinative bacteriology. 6th ed. pp. 1089–1092. (eds. R.S. Breed, E.G.D. Murray and A.P. Hitchens). Williams & Wilkins, Baltimore.

Bergey, D.H. 1957. Bregey's manual of determinative bacteriology. 7th ed. p. 939, p.1094. (eds. R.S. Breed, E.G.D. Murray and N.R. Smith). Williams & Wilkins, Baltimore.

Berman, J.W. and Basch, R.S. 1980. Amplification of the biotin-avidin immunofluorescence techniques. *J. Immunol. Method.*, **36**: 375–378.

Binnington, K.C. and Hoffman, A.A. 1989. *Wolbachia*-like organisms and cytoplasmic incompatibility in *Drosophila simulans*. *J. Invert. Pathol.*, **54**: 344–352.

Blake, F.G., Maxcy, K.F., Sadusk, J.F. Jr., Kohls, G.M. and Bell, E.J. 1945. Studies on Tsutsugamushi disease (scrub typhus, mite-borne typhus) in New Guinea and adjacent islands: epidemiology, clinical observations and etiology in the Dobadura area. *Am. J. Hyg.*, **41**: 243–373.

Bourgeois, A.L., Olson, J.G., Fang, R.C.Y., Huang, J., Wang, C.L., Chow, L., Bechthold, D., Dennis, D.T., Coolbangh, J.C. and Weiss, E. 1982. Humoral and cellular responses in scrub typhus patients reflecting primary infection and reinfection with *Rickettsia tsutsugamushi*. *Am. J. Trop. Med. Hyg.*, **31**: 532–540.

Bovarnick, M.R. and Miller, J.C. 1950. Oxidation and transamination of glutamate by typhus rickettsiae. *J. Biol. Chem.*, **184**: 661–676.

Bovarnick, M.R. and Snyder, J.C. 1949. Respiration of typhus rickettsia. *J. Exp.*

Med., **89**: 561–565.

Bovarnick, M.R., Miller, J.C. and Snyder, J.C. 1950. The influence of certain salts, amino acids, sugars and proteins on the stability of rickettsiae. *J. Bacteriol.*, **59**: 509–522.

Bozeman, F.M. and Elisberg, B.L. 1963. Serological diagnosis of scrub typhus by indirect immunofluorescence. *Proc. Soc. Exp. Biol. Med.*, **112**: 568–573.

Breeuwer, J.A.J. and Werren, J.H. 1990. Microorganisms associated with chromosome destruction and reproductive isolation between two insect species. *Nature*, **346**: 558–560.

Breeuwer, J.A.J., Stouthamer, R., Barns, S.M., Pelletier, D.A., Weisburg, W.G. and Werren, J.H. 1992. Phylogeny of cytoplasmic incompatibility microorganisms in the parasitoid wasp genus *Nasonia* (Hymenoptera: Pteromalidae) based on 16S ribosomal DNA sequences. *Insect. Mol. Biol.*, **1**: 25–36.

Brimacombe, L.C. 1980. All-female broods in field and laboratory populations of the Egyptian cotton leafworm, *Spodoptera littoralis* (Boisduval) (Lepidoptera: Noctuidae). *Bull. Ent. Res.*, **70**: 475–481.

Brown, G.W., Saunders, J.P., Singh, S., Huxsoll, D.L. and Shirai, A. 1978. Single dose doxcycline therapy for scrub typhus. *Trans. Roy. Soc. Trop. Med. Hyg.*, **72**: 412–416.

Brown, G.W., Shirai, A., Rogers, C. and Groves, M.G. 1983. Diagnostic criteria for scrub typhus: probability values for immunofluorescent antibody and *Proteus* OXK agglutinin titers. *Am. J. Trop. Med. Hyg.*, **32**: 1101–1107.

Bulnheim, H.P. 1978. Interaction between genetic, external and parasitic factors in sex determination of the crustacean amphipod *Gammarus duebeni*. *Helgol. Wiss. Meer.*, **31**: 1–33.

Burgdorfer, W. and Varma, M.G.R. 1967. Trans-stadial and transovarian development of disease agents in arthropods. *Ann. Rev. Ent.*, **12**: 347–376.

Campbell, R.W. and Domrow, R. 1974. Rickettsiosis in Australia: isolation of *Rickettsia tsutsugamushi* and *R. australis* from naturally infected arthropods. *Trans. Roy. Soc. Trop. Med. Hyg.*, **68**: 397–402.

Carl, M., Ching, W-M. and Dasch, G.A. 1988. Recognition of typhus group rickettsia-infected targets by human lymphokine-activated killer cells. *Infect. Immun.*, **56**: 2526–2529.

Carson, H.L. 1956. A female-producing strain of *D. borealis* Patterson. *Drosophila Inform. Serv.*, **30**: 109–110.

Catanzaro, P.J., Shirai, A., Agniel, L.D. and Osterman, J.V. 1977. Host defenses in experimental scrub typhus: role of spleen and peritoneal exudate lymphocytes in cellular immunity. *Infect. Immun.*, **18**: 118–123.

Cavalcanti, A.G.L., Falcao, D.W. and Castro, L.E. 1957. Sex-ratio in *D. prosaltans*, a character due to interaction between nuclear genes and cytoplasmic factor. *Amer. Natur.*, **91**: 321–325.

Chang, W-H. and Kang, J-S. 1991. Current status of Tsutsugamushi disease in Korea. pp. 16–19. In: Abstracts of the 1st Korea-Japan International Congress of Microbiology.

Chang, W-H., Kang, J-S., Lee, W-K., Choi, M-S. and Lee, J-H. 1990. Serological classification by monoclonal antibodies of *Rickettsia tsutsugamushi* isolated in

Korea. *J. Clin. Microbiol.*, **28**: 685–688.

Chao, S-H., Chao, C-F., Hsu, C-K., Wu, C-W. and Yang, S-Y. 1953. Studies on *Rickettsia tsutsugamushi* isolated in Canton. *Acta Microbiol. Sinica*, **1**: 42–56. (in Chinese).

Ch'iu, F-H., Chung, H-L., Cheng, L-T. and Ho, L-Y. 1962. Isolation of *Rickettsia Tsutsugamushi* from patients, rats and mites. *Chinese Med. J.*, **81**: 166–169.

Clarke, C., Johnston, G. and Johnston, B. 1983. All-female broods in *Hypolimnas bolina* (L.). A re-survey of West Fiji after 60 years. *Biol. J. Linn. Soc.*, **19**: 221–236.

Clarke, C., Sheppard, P.M. and Scali, V. 1975. All-female broods in the butterfly *Hypolimnas bolina* (L.). *Proc. Roy. Soc. Ser. B.*, **189**: 29–37.

Clarke, D.H. and Fox, J.P. 1948. The phenomenon of *in vitro* hemolysis produced by the rickettsiae of typhus fever, with a note on the mechanism of rickettsial toxicity in mice. *J. Exp. Med.*, **88**: 25–41.

Clifford, E.D. Jr. 1983. Mites causing or transmitting human disease. pp. 261–283. In: Cutaneous infestations of man and animal. (eds. L.C. Parish, W.B. Nutting and R.M. Schwartzman). CBS Inc., New York., USA.

Cooper, W.G., Lien, J.C., Hsu, S-H. and Chen, W-F. 1964. Scrub typhus in the Pescadores Island: an epidemiologic and clinical study. *Am. J. Trop. Med. Hyg.*, **13**: 833–838.

Cox, H.R. 1981. Rickettsia. pp.165–182. In: Principles of immunological diagnosis in medicine. (eds. F. Milgnom, C.J. Abeyounis and K. Kano). Lea & Febiger, Philadelphia.

Craigie, J. 1945. Application and control of ethyl-ether-water interface effects to the separation of rickettsiae from yolk sac suspensions. *Canad. J. Res.*, **23**: 104–114.

Crum, J.W., Hanchalay, S. and Eamsila, C. 1980. New paper enzyme-linked immunosorbent technique compared with microimmunofluorescence for detection of human serum antibodies to *Rickettsia tsutsugamushi*. *J. Clin. Microbiol.* **11**: 584–588.

Dasch, G.A. and Weiss, E. 1977. Characterization of the Madrid E strain of *Rickettsia prowazekii* purified by Renografin density gradient centrifugation. *Infect. Immunol.*, **15**: 280–286.

Davis, G.R., Austrian, R.C. and Bell, E.J. 1947. Observations on Tsutsugamushi disease (scrub typhus) in Assam and Burma. The recovery of strains of *Rickettsia orientalis*. *Am. J. Hyg.*, **46**: 268–286.

Dennis, D.T., Hadi, T.R., Brown, R.J., Sukaeri, S., Leksana, B. and Cholid, R. 1981. A survey of scrub and murine typhus in the Ancol section of Jakarta, Indonesia. *Southeast Asian J. Trop. Med. Publ. Hlth.*, **12**: 574–580.

Dohany, A.L. and Mat, Y.B. 1970. A comparison of the male and female genitalia of *Leptotrombidium* (*Leptotrombidium*) *akamushi* (Brumpt) 1910 (Acarina: Trombiculidae). *Southeast Asian J. Trop. Med. Publ. Hlth.*, **1**: 431–432.

Dohany, A.L., Upham, R.W. Jr., Manikumaran, C., Rapmund, G. and Saunders, J.P. 1977. The life history of a colony of *Leptotrombidium* (*Leptotrombidium*) *fletcheri* (Womersley and Heaslip) infected with *Rickettsia tsutsugamushi*. *Southeast Asian J. Trop. Med. Publ. Hlth.*, **8**: 221–226.

Dohany, A.L., Shirai, A., Robinson, D.M., Ram, S. and Huxsoll, D.L. 1978. Identification and antigenic typing of *Rickettsia tsutsugamushi* in naturally infected chiggers (Acarina: Trombiculidae) by direct immunofluorescence. *Am. J. Trop. Med. Hyg.*, **27**: 1261–1264.

Dohany, A.L., Lim, B.L. and Huxsoll, D.L. 1979. Vectors of scrub typhus and their hosts on a mature oil palm estate. *Southeast Asian J. Trop. Med. Publ. Hlth.*, **10**: 510–513.

Dohany, A.L., Shirai, A., Lim, B.L. and Huxsoll, D.L. 1980. Variation in populations of chigger vectors of scrub typhus in developing oil palm area of different ages. *Japan. J. Med. Sci. Biol.*, **33**: 263–270.

Domrow, R. and Lester, L.N. 1985. Chiggers of Australia (Acari: Trombiculidae): an annotated checklist, keys and bibliography. *Austral. J. Zool.*, **114**: 1–111.

Earle, N.W. and MacFarlane, J. 1968. A unisexual strain of the salt-marsh caterpillar, *Estigmene acrea. Ann. Entomol. Soc. Amer.*, **61**: 949–953.

Ebbert, M. A. 1991. The interaction phenotype in the *Drosophila willistoni*-spiroplasm symbiosis. *Evolution*, **45**: 971–988.

Ebbert, M. A. 1993. Endosymbiotic sex ratio distorters in insects and mites. pp. 150–191. In: Evolution and diversity of sex ratio in insects and mites. (eds. M.A. Ebbert and D.L. Wrench). Chapman and Hall., New York.

Eisemann, C.S. and Osterman, J.V. 1981. Antigens of scrub typhus rickettsiae: separation by polyacrylamide gel electorophoresis and identification by enzyme-linked immunosorbent assay. *Infect. Immun.*, **32**: 525–533.

Eisemann, C.S. and Osterman, J.V. 1985. Identification of strain-specific and group-reactive antigenic determinants on the Karp, Gilliam and Kato strains of *Rickettsia tsutsugamushi. Am. J. Trop. Med. Hyg.*, **34**: 1173–1178.

Elisberg, B.L., Sangkasuvana, V., Campbell, J.M., Bozeman, F.M., Boahidatta, P. and Rapmund, G. 1967. Physiographic distribution of scrub typhus in Thailand. *Acta Medica et Biologica*, **15** (Suppl.): 61–67.

Elisberg, B.L., Campbell, J.M. and Bozeman, F.M. 1968. Antigenic diversity of *Rickettsia tsutsugamushi*: epidemiologic and ecologic significance. *J. Hyg. Epidemiol. Microbiol. Immunol.*, **12**: 18–25.

Elisberg, B.L., Needy, C.F. and Bozeman, F.M. 1978. Antigenic inter-relationships among strains of *Rickettsia tsutsugamushi*. pp. 253–262. In: Rickettsiae and rickettsial diseases. (eds. J. Kazár, R.A. Ormsbee and I.N. Tarasevich). VEDA Publ. House Slovak. Acad. Sci., Bratislava.

Elsson-Dew, R. 1943. Relapsing fever and *B. proteus* Kingsbury. *Nature*, **152**: 565.

Ewing, H.E. 1944. The trombiculid mites (chigger mites) and their relation to disease. *J. Parasitol.*, **30**: 339–365.

Ewing, E.P. Jr., Takeuchi, A., Shirai, A. and Osterman, J.V. 1978. Experimental infection of mouse peritoneal mesothelium with scrub typhus rickettsiae: an ultrastructural study. *Infect. Immun.*, **19**: 1068–1075.

Fan, M-Y., Walker, D.H., Yu, S-R. and Liu, Q-H. 1987. Epidemiology and ecology of rickettsial diseases in the People's Republic of China. *Rev. Infect. Dig.*, **9**: 823–840.

Farrell, C.E. and Wharton, G.W. 1948. A successful method for shipping larval trombiculids (Chiggers). *J. Parasitol.*, **34**: 71.

Farrell, C.E. and Wharton, G.W. 1949. A culture medium for chiggers (Trombiculidae). *J. Parasitol.*, **35**: 435.

Felix, A. and Rhodes, M. 1931. Serological varieties of typhus fever. *J. Hyg.* **31**: 226–246.

Fetisova, N.F., Reshetnikov, P.P. and Tarasevich, I.V. 1968. In: III nauchnoe soveshchanie po problemam meditsinskoi geografii, Leningrad 1968. p. 115.

Fine, P.E.M., Ellis, D.S. and Curtis, C.F. 1977. Further studies of *Wolbachia* and cytoplasmic incompatibility in *Culex pipiens*. *Trans. Roy. Soc. Trop. Med. Hyg.*, **71**: 382.

Fletcher, W., Lesslar, J.E. and Lewthwaite, R. 1929. The etiology of the Tsutsugamushi disease and tropical typhus in the Federated Malay States. Part II. *Trans. Roy. Soc. Trop. Med. Hyg.*, **23**: 57–70.

406th Medical General Laboratory Professional Report U.S. Army. January 1961 through June 1962. 1962. Rickettsial infection. pp. 157–159.

Fox, J.P. 1948. The long persistence of *Rickettsia orientalis* in the blood and tissue of infected animals. *J. Immunol.*, **54**: 109–114.

Fox, J.P. 1949. The neutralization technique in Tsutsugamushi disease (scrub typhus) and the antigenic differentiation of rickettsial strains. *J. Immunol.*, **62**: 341–352.

Fukuzumi, S. 1953. The route of infection of scrub typhus. *Japan. J. Bacteriol.*, **8**: 149–156. (in Japanese).

Fukuzumi, S., Obata, Y. and Owada, H. 1950. Studies on Tsutsugamushi disease and Trombicula in the vicinity of Yokohama. *Trans. Soc. Pathol. Japan.*, **39**: 40–42. (in Japanese).

Fuller, H.S. 1952. The mite larvae of the family Trombiculidae in the Oudemans Collection. Taxonomy and medical importance. *Zool. Verhandl. Leiden.*, **18**: 1–261.

Furuya, Y. and Yoshida, Y. 1992. Detection of *Rickettsia tsutsugamushi* DNA by polymerase chain reaction. *Nippon Rinsho*, **642**: 422–426. (in Japanese).

Furuya, Y., Yoshida, Y., Katayama, T., Kawamori, F., Yamamoto, S., Ohashi, N., Tamura, A. and Kawamura, A. Jr. 1991a. Specific amplification of *Rickettsia tsutsugamushi* DNA from clinical specimens by polymerase chain reaction. *J. Clin. Microbiol.*, **29**: 2628–2630.

Furuya, Y., Yamamoto, S., Otsu, M., Yoshida, Y., Ohashi, N., Murata, M., Kawabata, N., Tamura, A. and Kawamura, A. Jr. 1991b. Use of monoclonal antibodies against *Rickettsia tsutsugamushi* Kawasaki for serodiagnosis by enzyme-linked immunosorbent assay. *J. Clin. Microbiol.*, **29**: 340–345.

Furuya, Y., Yoshida, Y., Katayama, T., Yamamoto, S. and Kawamura, A. Jr. 1993. Serotype-specific amplification of *Rickettsia tsutsugamushi* DNA by nested polymerase chain reaction. *J. Clin. Microbiol.*, **31**: 1637–1640.

Geier, P.W. and Briese, D.T. 1978. The light-brown apple moth *Epiphias postvittana* (Walker). 2. Uneven sex ratios and a condition contributing to them in the field. *Austr. J. Ecol.*, **3**: 467–488.

Gherna, R.L., Werren, J.H., Weisburg, W., Cote, R., Woese, C.R., Mandelco, L. and Brenner, D.J. 1991. *Arsenophonus nasoniae*, gen. nov., sp. nov., the causative agent of the "son-killer trait" in the parasitic wasp *Nasonia vitripennis*.

Int. J. Syst. Bacteriol., **41**: 563–565.

Gildemeister, E. and Haagen, E. 1940. Fleckfieberstudien. 1. Mitteilung: Nackweis eines Toxins in Rickettsien-Eiculturen (*Rickettsia mooseri*). *Deuts. Med. Wochschr.*, **66**: 878–880.

Ginsburger-Vogel, T. and Desportes, I. 1979. Etude ultrastructural de la sporulation de *Paramarteilia orchestiae*, Gen. N., Sp. N., Parasite de I'Amphipode *Orchestia gammarellus* (Pallas). *J. Protozool.*, **26**: 390–403.

Gispen, R. 1950. The role of rats and mites in the spread of endemic scrub typhus in Batavia. *Med. Maandbl.*, **3**: 45–58.

Goff, M.L., Loomis, R.B., Welbourn, W.C. and Wrenn, W.J. 1982. A glossary of chigger terminology (Acari: Trombiculidae). *J. Med. Entomol.*, **19**: 221–238.

Gojobori, T., Ishii, K. and Nei, M. 1982. Estimation of average number of nucleotide substitutions when the rate of substitution varies with nucleotide. *J. Mol. Evol.*, **18**: 414–423.

Gotoh, T. and Niijima, K. 1986. Characteristics and agent(s) of abnormal sex ratio (SR) in two aphidophagous coccinellid species. pp. 545–550. In: Ecology of Aphidophaga. (ed. I. Hodek). Academia, Prague.

Gotoh, A. 1968. Immunofluorescent studies on the type-specific antigen of the Tsutsugamushi disease rickettsia. *Japan. J. Bacteriol.*, **23**: 437–446. (in Japanese).

Greisman, S.E. and Wisseman, C.L. Jr. 1958. Studies of rickettsial toxins. IV. Cardiovascular functional abnormalities induced by *Rickettsia mooseri* toxin in the white rat. *J. Immunol.*, **81**: 345–354.

Groves, M. G. and Kelly, D. J. 1989. Characterization of factors determining *Rickettsia tsutsugamushi* pathogenicity for mice. *Infect. Immun.*, **57**: 1476–1482.

Groves, M.G. and Osterman, J.V. 1978. Host defenses in experimental scrub typhus: genetics of natural resistance to infection. *Infect. Immun.*, **19**: 583–588.

Groves, M.G., Rosenstreich, D.L., Taylor, B.A. and Osterman, J.V. 1980. Host defenses in experimental scrub typhus: mapping the gene that controls natural resistance in mice. *J. Immunol.*, **125**: 1395–1399.

Guo, H-B., Yu, M-M., Xu, M-H., Tang, J-G. and Wu, G-G. 1993. Studies on serological typing of anti-*Rickettsia tsutsugamushi* antibody in Jiangsu. *Chinese J. Microbiol. Immunol.*, **13**: 316–317.

Hackett, K.J., Lynn, D.E., Williamson, D.L., Ginsberg, A.S. and Whitcomb, R.F. 1986. Cultivation of the *Drosophila* sex-ratio spiroplasma. *Science*, **232**: 1253–1255.

Hadi, T.R., Stafford, E.E. and Irsiana, R. 1979. The occurrence of *Leptotrombidium (Leptotrombidium) arenicola* in Indonesia. In: Proc. BIOTROP Symp. Ectoparasite Biol., 21–23. Jun. 1976. Bogor, Indonesia, Vol. 6: 61–66, Biotrop. Spec. Publ.

Hamada, T. 1954. Studies on so-called Umayado disease in Kagawa Prefecture. *Bull. Kagawa. Pref. Inst. Publ. Hlth.*, **15**: 1–9. (in Japanese).

Hanaichi, T., Suto, T. and Iwamoto, T. 1986. A stable lead by modification of Suto's method. *J. Electron Microsc.*, **35**: 304–306.

Hanson, B. 1984. Characterization of *Rickettsia tsutsugamushi* outer membrane protein. pp. 240–243. In: Microbiology-1984. (eds. L. Leive and D.

Schlessinger). American Society for Microbiolgy. Washington, D.C.

Hanson, B. 1985. Identification and partial characterization of *Rickettsia tsutsugamushi* major protein immunogens. *Infect. Immun.*, **50**: 603–609.

Hanson, B. 1987. Improved plaque assay for *Rickettsia tsutsugamushi*. *Am. J. Trop. Med. Hyg.*, **36**: 631–638.

Hanson, B. and Wisseman, C.L. Jr. 1981. Heterogeneity among *Rickettsia tsutsugamushi* isolates: a protein analysis. pp. 503–514. In: Rickettsiae and rickettsial diseases. (eds. W. Burgdorfer and R.L. Anacker). Academic Press, New York, London, Tront, Sydney, San Francisco.

Hanson, B.A. 1983. Effect of immune serum on infectivity of *Rickettsia tsutsugamushi*. *Infect. Immun.*, **42**: 341–349.

Harrison, J.L. and Audy, J.R. 1951. Hosts of the mite vector of scrub typhus. II. An analysis of the list of recorded hosts. *Ann. Trop. Med. Parasitol.*, **45**: 186–194.

Hase, T. 1983a. Growth pattern of *Rickettsia tsutsugamushi* in irradiated L cells. *J. Bacteriol.*, **154**: 879–892.

Hase, T. 1983b. Assembly of *Rickettsia tsutsugamushi* progeny in irradiated L cells. *J. Bacteriol.*, **154**: 976–979.

Hase, T., Roberts, L.W., Hildebrandt, P.K. and Cavanough, D.C. 1978. Stylostome formation by *Leptotrombidium* mite (Acari: Trombiculidae). *J. Parasitol.*, **64**: 712–718.

Hatori, J. 1919–20. On the endemic Tsutsugamushi disease in Formosa. *Ann. Trop. Med. Parasitol*, **13**: 233–354. (in Japanese).

Hatori, J. 1920. Studies on Tsutsugamushi disease in Formosa (Part 5). *J. Med. Assoc. Formosa.*, **209**: 317–352. (in Japanese).

Hayashi, N. 1906. Preliminary report on studies on Tsutsugamushi disease. *Hokuetsu Med. J.*, **156**: 358–368. (in Japanese).

Hayashi, N. 1907. Preliminary report on 2nd year studies on Tsutsugamushi disease. *Hokuetsu Med. J.*, **162**: 225–232. (in Japanese).

Hayashi, N. 1909. On Tsutsugamushi disease. *Hokuetsu Med. J.*, **168**: 1–69. (in Japanese).

Hayashi, N. 1920. Etiology of Tsutsugamushi disease. *J. Parasitol.*, **7**: 53–68.

Hayashi, N. 1924. On Ricketts' corpuscles. *Trans. Japan. Pathol. Soc.*, **22**: 569–576. (in Japanese).

Hayashi, N. 1932. On Tsutsugamushi disease. *Trans. Japan. Pathol. Soc.*, **22**: 689–690. (in Japanese).

Hayashi, N., Mukoyama, K. and Oshima, F. 1919. Results of studies on Tsutsugamushi disease, 1918 (Kuhara's grant, second year). *Central Med. J.*, **26**: 106–144. (in Japanese).

Hayashi, N., Oshima, F., Eguchi, N. and Hozumi, K. 1924. Relationship between Tsutsugamushi disease and birds (I). *Trans. Japan. Pathol. Soc.*, **1**: 461–493. (in Japanese).

Hayashi, N., Oshima, F., Eguchi, N. and Hozumi, K. 1925. Relationship between Tsutsugamushi disease and birds (II). A note on a constructive preventive measure against Tsutsugamushi disease. *Trans. Japan. Pathol. Soc.*, **2**: 1079–1092. (in Japanese).

Hayashi, S. and Suzuki, T. 1954. Studies on the ecology of trombiculid mites in

Japan (II). Studies on the surface distribution of *Trombicula scutellaris* Nagayo *et al.* 1921. *Jpn. J. Sanit. Zool.*, **5**: 93–100. (in Japanese).

Hayashi, S. and Tanaka, H. 1955. A large number of feeding larvae of *T. scutellaris* Nagayo *et al.* collected from a man. pp. 52–53. In: Studies on Shichito fever. Pt. III. Dept. Hlth., Tokyo. (in Japanese).

Hayashi, S., Suzuki, T., Tanaka, H., Teramura, S., Ueno, Y. and Sasa, M. 1955. Distribution of unfed larvae of *L. scutellare, E. wichmanni* and *L. akamushi* on soil surface. pp. 61–74. In: Studies on Shichito fever. Pt. III. Dept. Hlth., Tokyo. (in Japanese).

Hayes, S.F. and Burgdorfer, W. 1979. Ultrastructure of *Rickettsia rhipicephali*, a new member of the spotted fever group rickettsiae in tissues of the host vector *Rhipicephalus sanguineus*. *J. Bacteriol.*, **137**: 605–613.

Hayes, S.F. and Burgdorfer, W. 1982. Reactivation of *Rickettsia rickettsii* in *Dermacentor andersoni* ticks : an ultrastructural analysis. *Infect. Immun.*, **37**: 779–785.

Hemmingsen, S.M., Woolfold, C., van der Vies, S.M., Tilly, K., Dennis, D.T., Georgopoulos, C.P., Hendrix, R.W. and Ellis, R.J. 1988. Homologous plant and bacterial proteins chaperone oligomeric protein assembly. *Nature*, **333**: 330–334.

Hickman, C.J., Stover, C.K., Joseph, S.W. and Oaks, E.V. 1991. Molecular cloning and sequence analysis of a *Rickettsia tsutsugamushi* 22 kDa antigen containing B- and T-cell epitopes. *Microb. Pathog.*, **11**: 19–31.

Hickman, C.J., Stover, C.K., Joseph, S.W. and Oaks, E.V. 1993. Murine T-cell response to native and recombinant protein antigens of *Rickettsia tsutsugamushi*. *Infect. Immun.*, **61**: 1674–1681.

Higashi, N. 1959. Electron microscopic studies on the organization in the bacterial cell and on the intracellular rickettsial cell. *Ann. Rept. Inst. Virus Res., Kyoto Univ.*, **2**: 167–186.

Higashi, N. 1962. Electron microscopic studies of *Rickettsia orientalis*. pp. 145–156. Recent advances in studies of Tsutsugamushi disease in Japan. (ed. T. Tamiya). Medical Culture Inc., Tokyo.

Hoffmann, A.A., Turelli, M. and Simmons, G.M. 1986. Unidirectional incompatibility between populations of *Drosophila simulans*. *Evolution*, **40**: 692–701.

Hopps, H.E., Jackson, E.B., Danauskas, J.X. and Smadel, J.E. 1959. Study on the growth of rickettsiae. IV. Effect of chloramphenicol and several metabolic inhibitors on the multiplication of *Rickettsia tsutsugamushi* in tissue culture cells. *J. Immunol.*, **82**: 172–181.

Hsiao, C. and Hsiao, T.H. 1985. Rickettsia as the cause of cytoplasmic incompatibility in the alfalfa weevil, *Hypera postica*. *J. Invert. Pathol.*, **45**: 244–246.

Hsu, P-K., Su, K-C. and Chen, H-T. 1959. Larvae of *Trombicula akamushi* var. *deliensis* as related to the epidemiology of tsutsugamushi. *Acta Microbiol. Sinica.*, **7**: 1–9. (in Chinese).

Hsu, Y-C. 1959. Studies on the life history of chigger mites. *Acta Entomol. Sinica.*, **9**: 452–459. (in Chinese).

Hubert, A.A. and Baker, H.J. 1963a. Studies on the habitats and population of *Leptotrombidium* (*Leptotrombidium*) *akamushi* and *Leptotrombidium*

(*Leptotrombidium*) *deliensis* in Malaya (Acarina: Trombiculidae). *Am. J. Hyg.*, **78**: 131–142.

Hubert, A.A. and Baker, H.J. 1963b. The persistence of foci of *Leptotrombidium* (*Leptotrombidium*) *akamushi* along a transect in Malaya (Acarina: Trombiculidae). *Am. J. Hyg.*, **78**: 143–149.

Huger, A.M., Skinner, S.W. and Werren, J.H. 1985. Bacteria infections associated with the son-killer trait in the parasitoid wasp *Nasonia* (= *Mormoniella*) *vitripennis* (Hymenoptera: Pteromalidae). *J. Invert. Pathol.*, **46**: 272–280.

Hyland, K.E. Jr. 1951. Observations on the chigger mite *Trombicula* (*Eutrombicula*) *splendens* Ewing (Acarina: Trombiculidae). *Ann. Ent. Soc. Amer.*, **44**: 297–301.

Hyland, K.E. 1961. Parasitic phase of chigger mite, *Hannemania hegeneri*, on experimentally infected amphibians. *Exp. Parasitol.*, **11**: 212–225.

Iida, T., Kawashima, H. and Kawamura, A. Jr. 1966a. Direct immunofluorescence for typing of Tsutsugamushi disease rickettsia. *J. Immunol.*, **95**: 1129–1133.

Iida, T., Okubo, K. and Ishimaru, M., 1966b. Immunofluorescene for sero-epidemiological study of Tsutsugamushi disease rickettsia. *Jpn. J. Exp. Med.*, **36**: 435–447.

Ikeda, H. 1970. The cytoplasmic-inherited "sex-ratio" condition in natural and experimental populations of *D. bifasciata. Genetics*, **65**: 311–333.

Ishikura, M., Watanabe, M., Morita, O. and Uetake, H. 1985. Epidemiological studies on the background of the endemic occurrence of Tsutsugamushi disease in Toyama Prefecture. 1. Epidemiology of infection with *Rickettsia tsutsugamushi* among field rodents in endemic and nonendemic areas. *Microbiol. Immunol.*, **29**: 859–872.

Ito, S. and Rikihisa, Y. 1981. Techniques for electron microscopy of rickettsia. pp. 213–227. In: Rickettsiae and rickettsial diseases. (eds. W. Bergdorfer and R.L. Anacker) Academic Press, New York, London, Tront, Sydney, San Francisco.

Ito, S., Vinson, J.W. and McGuire, T.J. Jr. 1975. Murine typhus rickettsiae in the oriental rat flea. *Ann. N.Y. Acad. Sci.*, **266**: 35–60.

Ito, S., Vinson, J.W. and Whitescarver, J. 1978. Ultrastructural observations of *Rickettsia typhi* in the human body louse. pp. 53–64. In: Rickettsiae and rickettsial diseases. (eds. J. Kazár, R.A. Ormsbee and I.N. Tarasevich). VEDA Publ. House, Slovak Acad. Sci., Brastilava.

Ito, T. and Obata, Y. 1961. Trombiculid mites and Tsutsugamushi disease in Niigata Prefecture. pp.1–213. *Dept. Hlth. Niigata Pref.*, (in Japanese).

Ito, T., Obata, Y. and Ono, M. 1957. Eggs of dragon-fly as new food for trombiculid mites. *Acta Med. Biol.*, **5**: 169–199.

Iwasa, M., Kasuya, S., Noda, N., Hioki, A., Ito, A. and Ohtomo, H. 1990. Trombicuilid mites (Acari: Trombiculidae) and *Rickettsia tsutsugamushi* isolated from wild rodents in a new endemic area of Japan. *J. Med. Entomol.*, 27: 501–508.

Jackson, E.B., Donauskas, J.X., Smadel, J.E., Fuller, H.S., Coale, M.C. and Bozeman, F.M. 1957. Occurrence of *Rickettsia tsutsugamushi* in Korean rodents and chiggers. *Am. J. Hyg.*, **66**: 309–320.

Jameson, E.W. Jr. 1968. Experimental rearing of some Japanese trombiculid mites.

Jpn. J. Exp. Med., **38**: 279–288.

Jayewickreme, S.H. and Niles, W.I. 1946. Successful feeding experiments with an adult trombiculid mite (Order, Acarina). *Nature*, 157: 878.

Jenkins, D.W. 1947. A labolatory method of rearing chiggers affecting man. *Ann. Ent. Soc. Amer.*, **40**: 56–68.

Jenkins, D.W. 1949. Trombiculid mites affecting man. Ⅳ. Revision of *Eutrombicula* in the American hemisphere. *Ann. Ent. Soc. Amer.*, **42**: 289–318.

Jerrells, T.R. 1983. Association of an inflammatory I region-associated antigen-positive macrophage influx and genetic resistance of inbred mice to *Rickettsia tsutsugamushi*. *Infect. Immun.*, **42**: 549–557.

Jerrells, T.R. 1985. Immunosuppression associated with the development of chronic infections with *Rickettsia tsutsugamushi*: adherent suppressor cell activity and macrophage activation. *Infect. Immun.*, **50**: 175–182.

Jerrells, T.R. and Eisemann, C.S. 1983. Role of T-lymphocytes in production of antibody to antigens of *Rickettsia tsutsugamushi* and other *Rickettsia* species. *Infect. Immun.*, **41**: 666–674.

Jerrells, T.R. and Osterman, J.V. 1981. Host defenses in experimental scrub typhus: inflammatory response of congenic C3H mice differing at the *Ric* gene. *Infect. Immun.*, **31**: 1014–1022.

Jerrells, T.R. and Osterman, J.V. 1982a. Host defenses in experimental scrub typhus: delayed-type hypersensitivity responses of inbred mice. *Infect. Immun.*, **35**: 117–123.

Jerrells, T.R. and Osterman, J.V. 1982b. Role of macrophages in innate and acquired host resistance to experimental scrub typhus infection of inbred mice. *Infect. Immun.*, **37**: 1066–1073.

Jerrells, T.R. and Osterman, J.V. 1983a. Development of specific and cross-reactive lymphocyte proliferative responses during chronic immunizing infections with *Rickettsia tsutsugamushi*. *Infect. Immun.*, **40**: 147–156.

Jerrells, T.R. and Osterman, J.V. 1983b. Parameters of cellular immunity in acute and chronic *Rickettsia tsutsugamushi* infections of inbred mice. *Adv. Exp. Med. Biol.*, **162**: 355–360.

Jerrells, T.R., Palmer, B.A. and Osterman, J.V. 1983. Gamma-irradiated scrub typhus immunogens: development of cell-mediated immunity after vaccination of inbred mice. *Infect. Immun.*, **39**: 262–269.

Jones, B.M. 1950. Experimental rearing of the British harvest mite to the adult stage. *Nature*, **166**: 823.

Jones, B.M. 1951. The growth of the harvest mites, *Trombicula autumnalis* Shaw. *Parasitol.*, **41**: 229–248.

Kadosaka, T. and Kaneko, K. 1987. Comparative histopathology of styostome formation by three species of trombiculid mites (Ab.). *Japan. J. Trop. Med. Hyg.*, **15**: 253. (in Japanese).

Kaiho, I., Tokieda, M., Yoshida, Y., Furuya, Y., Murata, M., Tanaka, H. and Kawamura, A. Jr. 1993. Epidemiology of Tsutsugamushi disease and typing of isolated *Rickettsia* in Chiba Prefecture. *J. Japan. Assoc. Infect. Dis.*, **67**: 196–201. (in Japanese).

Kalra, S.L. 1959. Progress in the knowledge of rickettsial disease in India. *Indian. J.*

Med. Res., **47**: 477–483.

Kamimura, K., Watanabe, M., Katori, K., Suzuki, H., Wada, Y., Shirasaka, A., Tsuboi, Y. and Kubota, K. 1972. Seasonal occurrence of trombiculid mites and its epidemiological aspects in a mountain village of Toyama Prefecture. *Jpn. J. Sanit. Zool.*, **23**: 83–87. (in Japanese).

Kamiya, H. 1983. Trombiculid mites and Tsutsugamushi disease — epidemiological consideration in Akita Prefecture. *J. Akita Clin. Lab. Assoc.*, **No.21**: 8–14. (in Japanese).

Kamo, H. 1954. Records of trombiculid mites from Aves in Kyushu. *Jpn. J. Sanit. Zool.*, **5**: 50–51. (in Japanese).

Kamo, H. 1956. Records of trombiculid mites from Aves in Kyushu. *Kyushu J. Med. Sci.*, **8**: 209–216.

Kane, M.D. and Pierce, N.E. 1994. Diversity within diversity: molecular approaches to studying microbial interactions with insects. pp. 1–17. In: Molecular methods in ecology and evolution. (eds. B. Schierwater, B. Streit, G. Wagner and R. DeSalle). A volume to be published by Birkhauser Verlag in 1994.

Kaneko, K., Shiwaku, K., Kadosaka, T. and Chigusa, Y. 1987. Transmission of *Rickettsia tsutsugamushi* from experimentally infected mice to three species of *Leptotrombidium* mites (Ab.). *Japan. J. Trop. Med. Hyg.*, **15**: 254.

Kaneko, S., Feinstone, S.M. and Miller, R.N. 1989. Rapid and sensitive method for the detection of serum hepatitis B virus DNA using the polymerase chain reaction technique. *J. Clin. Microbiol.*, **27**: 1930–1933.

Kanemitsu, N. 1987. Production and characterization of the monoclonal antibodies to *Rickettsia tsutsugamushi. J. Japan. Assoc. Infect. Dis.*, **61**: 819–829. (in Japanese).

Karasawa, T. 1956. Geographical distribution of Tsutsugamushi disease and rickettsia harboring hosts along the Shinano and Agano Rivers. *J. Niigata Med. Assoc.*, **70**: 52–77. (in Japanese).

Kasuya, S., Hioki, A., Ito, A. and Ohtomo, H. 1985. Studies on Tsutsugamushi disease in Gifu Prefecture. 2. A speculation on the vector. *J. Japan. Assoc. Infect. Dis.*, **59**: 1142–1148. (in Japanese).

Katsura, S. 1953. Clinical studies on Tsutsugamushi disease. *J. Japan. Assoc. Infect. Dis.*, **27**: 1–19. (in Japanese).

Kaufman, T. and Traub, R. 1966. Preliminary notes parthenogenesis in a species of trombiculid mite, *Leptotrombidium arenicola* Traub, 1960 (Acarina: Trombiculidae). *J. Med. Entomol.*, **3**: 256–258.

Kawamori, F., Akiyama, M., Sugieda, M., Kanda, T., Akahane, S., Uchikawa, K., Yamada, Y., Kumada, N., Furuya, Y., Yoshida, Y., Yamamoto, S., Ohashi, N. and Tamura, A. 1992. Epidemiology of Tsutsugamushi disease in relation to the serotypes of *Rickettsia tsutsugamushi* isolated from patients, field mice, and unfed chiggers on the eastern slope of Mount Fuji, Shizuoka Prefecture, Japan. *J. Clin. Miclobiol.*, **30**: 2842–2846.

Kawamori, F., Akiyama, M., Sugieda, M., Kanda, T., Akahane, S., Yamamoto, S., Ohashi, N. and Tamura, A. 1993. Two-step polymerase chain reaction for diagnosis of scrub typhus and identification of antigenic variants of *Rickettsia tsutsugamushi*. *J. Vet. Med. Sci.*, **55**: 749–755.

Kawamura, A. Jr. 1953. On the causative agent of Shichito fever. II. pp. 34–37. In: Studies on Shichito fever. Pt. II. Dept. Hlth., Tokyo. (in Japanese).

Kawamura, A. Jr. 1958. Present status of rickettsiosis in Japan and diagnostic techniques. *Eisei Kensa*, **7**: 1–8. (in Japanese).

Kawamura, A. Jr. 1962. A study on the antigen analysis of *Rickettsia orientalis*. *Japan. J. Med. Sci. Biol.*, **15**: 322–330.

Kawamura, A. Jr. 1969. Fluorescent antibody techniques and their applications. pp. 1–203. University of Tokyo Press, Tokyo and University Park Press, Baltimore and Manchester.

Kawamura, A. Jr. 1977. Fluorescent antibody techniques and their application. 2nd Ed. pp. 1–292. University of Tokyo Press, Tokyo and University Park Press, Baltimore and London.

Kawamura, A. Jr. 1984. Rickettsiosis — especially Tsutsugamushi disease. *Modern Media*, **30**: 310–339. (in Japanese).

Kawamura, A. Jr. and Aoyama, Y., 1983. Immunofluorescence in medical science. pp. 1–262. University of Tokyo Press, Tokyo.

Kawamura, A. Jr. and Takigami, T. 1957. Rickettsiosis in Japan. *Sogo Igaku*, **14**: 4–10. (in Japanese).

Kawamura, A. Jr. and Tanaka, H. 1988. Rickettsiosis in Japan. (a review). *Jpn. J. Exp. Med.*, **58**: 169–184.

Kawamura, A. Jr., Suzuki, K., Oda, A., Iwasaki, T., Sasa, M., Nakaya, I., Ohara, R., Kawashima, F. and Kawashima, H. 1952. Studies on Tsutsugamushi disease in Kochi Prefecture (I). The causative agent isolated from rodents from endemic area. *Tokyo Med. J.*, **69**: 495–498. (in Japanese).

Kawamura, A. Jr., Murata, M., Osono, M., Nogami, S., Shirasaka, A., Tanaka, H., Sudo, K., Suzuki, K., Miyairi, T. and Kijima, H. 1980. Studies on inapparent infection of Tsutsugamushi disease in Izu Shichito Islands; seroepidemiology and demonstration of an avirulent rickettsia strain for mice. *Jpn. J. Exp. Med.*, **50**: 91–105.

Kawamura, R. 1925. Studies on Tsutsugamushi disease. pp. 1–329. Nanko-do, Tokyo. (in Japanese).

Kawamura, R. 1926. Studies on Tsutsugamushi disease (Japanese flood fever). *Med. Bull. Coll. Med. Univ., Cincinnati, USA*. **4**: 1–229.

Kawamura, R. 1930. Die Tsutsugamushi Krankheit. pp. 1387–1414. In: Hand. d. pathog. Microorganismen (Hg. W. Kolle und A.V. Wasserman), 3 Auft. Bd. VIII, Gustav Fischer, Jena und Urbau & Schwarzenberg, Berlin und Wien.

Kawamura, R. 1940. Ecological study of *Trombicula akamushi*, Brumpt. *Nihon Kiseichugakkai Kiji*, **12**: 40–41. (in Japanese).

Kawamura, R. and Ikeda, K. 1936. Ecological study of the tsutsugamushi, *Trombicula akamushi* (Brumpt). *Zool. Mag.*, **48**: 553–563. (in Japanese).

Kawamura, R. and Imagawa, Y., 1931. Die Feststellung des Erregers bei der Tsutsugamushikrankheit. *Zbl. f. Bakt.*, (1 Abt.), Orig., **122**: 261.

Kawamura, R. and Yamaguchi, M. 1916. The anatomy of adult Tsutsugamushi and its life cycle. *Hokuetsu Med. J.*, **31**: 439–461. (in Japanese).

Kawamura, R., Hattori, S. and Yamaguchi, M. 1920. On seasonal occurrence of

Trombicula akamushi. Japan. J. Pathol., **10**: 471–479. (in Japanese).

Kawamura, R., Hattori, S. and Yamaguchi, M. 1921. Relationship between birds and *Trombicula akamushi*, together with its significance for preventing Tsutsugamushi disease. *Tokyo Med. J.*, **No. 2213**: 259–271. (in Japanese).

Kawamura, R., Ito, T. and Imagawa, Y. 1932. *Rickettsia akamushi* in body of *Trombicula akamushi* and its relation to field rodents. *Tokyo Med. J.*, **2769**: 683–687. (in Japanese).

Kellen, W.R., Hoffmann, D.F. and Kwock, R.A. 1981. *Wolbachia* sp. (Rickettsiales: Rickettsiaceae) a symbiont of the almond moth, *Ephestia cautella*: ultrastructure and influence on host fertility. *J. Invert. Pathol.*, **37**: 273–283.

Kenmotsu, M., Sekikawa, H., Sato, Y., Watanabe, H. and Otsuru, M. 1979. Recent surveys on trombicuilid mite and Tsutsugamushi Disease. Pt. II. Results of isolating *Rickettsia tsutsugamushi. Eisei Kensa*, **28**: 562–566. (in Japanese).

Kim, I-S., Seong, S-Y., Woo, S-G., Choi, M-S. and Chang, W-H. 1993a. High-level expression of a 56-kilodalton protein gene (*bor 56*) of *Rickettsia tsutsugamushi* Boryong and its application to enzyme-linked immunosorbent assays. *J. Clin. Microbiol.*, **31**: 598–605.

Kim, I-S., Seong, S-Y., Woo, S-G., Choi, M-S., Kong, J-S. and Chang, W-H. 1993b. Rapid diagnosis of scrub typhus by a passive hemoagglutination assay using recombinant 56-kilodalton polypeptides. *J. Clin. Microbiol.*, **31**: 2057–2060.

Kitahara, K. 1952. *Trombicula wichmanni* in Kuroshima which parasites upon the lizard and bites the inhabitants. *Ann. Kagoshima Med. College*, **2**: 193–194.

Kitaoka, M., 1959. Epidemiology of scrub typhus in Japan. pp. 477–490. In: Proc. 15th General Assembly of the Japan Medical Congress Vol. 2. (in Japanese).

Kitaoka, M. and Asanuma, K. 1968. Monthly observation on rickettsia and complement fixing antibody response in *Microtus montebelli* placed once on the ground endemic of scrub typhus or inoculated experimentally with *Rickettsia orientalis. J. Hyg. Epidemiol. Microbiol. Immunol.*, **12**: 147–161.

Kitaoka, M. and Okubo, K. 1953. Studies on Shichito fever in Miyake Island — isolation of causative agent from wild birds. pp. 23–24. In: Studies on Shichito fever. Pt. II. Dept. Hlth., Tokyo. (in Japanese).

Kitaoka, M. and Okubo, K. 1958. Negative isolation of rickettsia from birds caught on Izu Seven Islands in winter season. p. 49. In: Studies on Shichito fever. Pt. Sum. Dept. Hlth., Tokyo, (in Japanese).

Kitaoka, M., Okubo, K. and Asanuma, K. 1953a. On zoophilism of *Trombicula scutellaris*, suspected as vector of Shichito-netsu, with additional notes on *T. pallida*. pp. 81–82. In: Studies on Shichito fever. Pt. II. Dept. Hlth., Tokyo. (in Japanese).

Kitaoka, M., Okubo. K., Takano, K. and Asanuma, K. 1953b. On Shichito fever — researches on reservoir animals and vectors of the pathogen. pp. 29–34. In: Studies on Shichito fever. Pt. II. Dept. Hlth., Tokyo. (in Japanese).

Kitaoka, M., Okubo, K. and Asanuma, K. 1967. Epidemiological survey by means of complement fixation test on scrub typhus in Japan. *Acta Medica et Biologica*, **15** (Suppl.): 69–85.

Kitaoka, M., Asanuma, K., Okubo, K., Taniguchi, H., Tsuboi, M. and Hattori, K. 1973. Seasonal occurrence of trombiculid mites species and *Leptotrombidium kawamurai* (Acarina, Trombiculidae) as a carrier of *Rickettsia orientalis* in the Nopporo area, Hokkaido, Japan. *J. Hyg. Epidemiol. Microbiol. Immunol.*, **17**: 478–486.

Kitaoka, M., Asanuma, K. and Otsuji, J. 1974. Transmission of *Rickettsia orientalis* to man by *Leptotrombidium akamushi* at a scrub typhus endemic area in Akita Prefecture, Japan. *Am. J. Trop. Med. Hyg.*, **23**: 993–999.

Kitaoka, M., Asanuma, K. and Otsuji, J. 1976. Experiments on chickens placed on ground endemic of classical scrub typhus in Akita Prefecture, Japan. *J. Hyg. Epidemiol. Microbiol. Immunol.*, **20**: 195–200.

Kobayashi, Y., Tachibana, N., Matsumoto, I., Oyama, T. and Kageyama, T. 1978. Isolation of very low virulent strain of *Rickettsia tsutsugamushi* by the use of cyclophosphamide-treated mice. pp. 181–188. In: Rickettsiae and rickettsial diseases. (eds. J. Kazár, R.A. Ormsbee and I.N. Tarasevich). VEDA Publ. House, Slovak Acad. Sci., Bratislava.

Kobayashi, Y., Kawamura, S. and Oyama, T. 1985. Immunological studies of experimental Tsutsugamushi disease in congenitally athymic (nude) mice. *Am. J. Trop. Med. Hyg.*, **34**: 568–577.

Kobayashi, Y., Kanemitsu, N., Tange, Y., Tachibana, N. and Tamura, A. 1987. Immunological analysis of newly isolated strains of *Rickettsia tsutsugamushi* using monoclonal antibodies. *J. Japan. Assoc. Infect. Dis.*, **61**: 1264–1269. (in Japanese)

Kodama, K., Kawamura, S., Yasukawa, M. and Kobayashi, Y. 1987. Establishment and characterization of a T-cell line specific for *Rickettsia tsutsugamushi. Infect. Immun.*, **55**: 2490–2495.

Kodama, K., Yasukawa, M. and Kobayashi, Y. 1988. Effect of rickettsia antigen-specific T-cell line on the interaction of *Rickettsia tsutsugamushi* with macrophage. *Microbiol. Immunol.*, **32**: 435–439.

Kohls, G.M., Armbrust, C.A., Irons, E.N. and Philip, C.B. 1945. Studies on Tsutsugamushi disease (scrub typhus, mite-bone typhus) in New Guinea and adjacent islands: further observations on epidemiology and etiology. *Am. J. Hyg.*, **41**: 374–399.

Krieg, N.R. and Holt, J.G. 1984. Bergey's manual of systematic bacteriology. Vol. 1. pp. 687–698, p. 964. Williams and Wilkins, Baltimore and London.

Krishnan, K.V., Smith, R.O.A., Bose, P.N., Neogy, K.N., Roy, B.K.G. and Ghosh, M. 1949. Transmission of *Rickettsia orientalis* by the bite of the larvae of *Trombicula deliensis. Indian. Med. Gaz.*, **84**: 41–43.

Kudryashova, N.I. and Tarasevich, I.V. 1964. Red mites in a natural focus of Tsutsugamushi fever in the Southern Primorye territory. *Med. Parasitol.*, **33**: 718–721. (in Russian).

Kudryashova, N.I., Tarasevich, I.V. and Plotnikova. L.F. 1967. On the methods of studying natural infection of chiggers with *Rickettsia tsutsugamushi. Parazitologya* **1**: 339–341. (in Russian).

Kudryashova, N.I., Mirolyubova, L.V., Tarasevichi, I.V., Plotnikava, L.F. and Ezorova, A.D. 1968. Natural infection of chigger mites with *R. tsutsugamushi* in the Primorye territory. *Med. Parasitol.*, **37**: 302–305.

Kulagin, S.M., Tarasevich, I.V., Kudryashova, N.I. and Gopachenko, I.M. 1967. On the natural focus of scrub typhus in the south of the Primorye areas of the USSR. *Acta Medica et Biologica*, **15** (Suppl.): 49–52.

Kulagin, S.M., Tarasevich, I.V., Kudryashova, N.I. and Plotnikova, L.F. 1968. The investigation of scrub typhus in the USSR. *J. Hyg. Epidemiol. Microbiol. Immunol.*, **12**: 257–264.

Kumada, N. 1983. Trombiculid mites. pp. 161–206, pp. 467– 469. In: Acarina. Revised Ed. (ed. M. Sasa). University of Tokyo Press, Tokyo. (in Japanese).

Kumada, N. and Oya, S. 1968. Transovarial and transtadial infections of *R. tsutsugamushi* in *L. pallidum*. *Jpn. J. Sanit. Zool.*, **19**: 127. (in Japanese).

Kumada, N., Reka, S.A., Mizuno, S., Fujioka, H. and Uchikawa, K. 1986. Positive isolation of *Rickettsia tsutsugamushi* from field mice and larvae of *Leptotrombidium pallidum* collected in Iida City, Nagano Prefecture. *Bull. Environ. Conserv. Shinshu Univ.*, **8**: 6–11. (in Japanese).

Kumura, K., Minamishima, Y., Yamamoto, S., Ohashi, N. and Tamura, A. 1991. DNA base composition of *Rickettsia tsutsugamushi* determined by reversed-phase high-performance liquid chromatography. *Int. J. Syst. Bacteriol.*, **41**: 247–248.

Kundin, W.D., Liu, C., Harmon, P. and Rodina, P. 1964. Pathogenesis of scrub typhus infection (*Rickettsia tsutsugamushi*) as studied by immunofluorescence. *J. Immunol.*, **93**: 772–781.

Kunitomo, F. 1956. Studies on the trombiculid mites and Tsutsugamushi disease in Kochi Prefecture. III. The relationship between birds and trombiculid mites. *Ochanomize Med. J.*, **4**: 441–443. (in Japanese).

Kuwabara, Y. 1990. Gathering pheromon and Sex pheromon. pp. 145–152. (ed. S. Ehara). Stories of mites and ticks 1. From behavior up to control. Gihoudo, Tokyo. (in Japanese).

Kuwata, T. 1952. Analysis of immunity in experimental Tsutsugamushi disease. *J. Immunol.*, **68**: 115–120.

Kyte, J. and Doolittle, R.F. 1982. A simple method for displaying the hydropathic character of a protein. *J. Mol. Biol.*, **157**: 105–132.

Lachumanan, R., Devi, S., Cheong, Y-M., Rodda, S.J. and Pang, T. 1993. Epitope mapping of the *sta 58* major outer membrane protein of *Rickettsia tsutsugamushi*. *Infect. Immun.*, **61**: 4527–4531.

Lanier, G.N. and Oliver, J.H. Jr. 1966. "Sex-ratio" condition: unusual mechanisms in bark beetles. *Science*, **153**: 208–209.

Leslie, J.F. 1984. A "sex-ratio" condition in *Oncopeltus fasciatus*. *J. Hered.*, **75**: 260–264.

Lewis, G.E. Jr., Kelly, D.J., Lim, P. and Gan, E. 1987. Modification and evaluation of an indirect immunoperoxidase technique for the serodiagnosis of scrub typhus, endemic typhus and tick typhus. pp. 34–35. In: Report of meeting of the task force on the serological diagnosis of Tsutsugamushi disease (scrub typhus). Regional Office for the Western Pacific of the WHO, Okinawa, Japan.

Liao, H-R., Lin, Z-H. and Wang, D-Q. 1981. On the life history of *Leptotrombidium pallidum* and *Leptotrombidium scutellare*. *Zoological Research*, **2**: 137–143.

(in Chinese).

Lien, J-C., Liu, S-Y. and Lin, H-M. 1967. Field observation on the bionomics of *L. deliense*, the vector of scrub typhus in the Pescadores. *Acta Medica et Biologica*, **15** (Suppl.): 27–31.

Lim, T.S., Twartz, J.C. and Groves, M.G. 1986. Suppression of lymphocyte responsiveness during acute *Rickettsia tsutsugamushi* infection in mice. *Japan. J. Med. Sci. Biol.*, **39**: 129–138.

Lipovsky, L.J. 1951. Collembola as food for chiggers (Acarina: Trombiculidae). *J. Parasitol.*, **37**: 324–326.

Lipovsky, L.J., Byers, G.W. and Kardos, E.H. 1957. Spermatophores — the mode of insemination of chiggers (Acarina: Trombiculidae). *J. Parasitol.*, **44**: 256–262.

Login, G.R. and Dvorak, A.M. 1985. Microwave energy fixation for electron microscopy. *Am. J. Pathol.*, **120**: 230–243.

Lopage, S.P., Sneath, P.H.A., Lessel, E.F., Skerman, V.B.D., Seelinger, H.P.R. and Clark, W.A. 1976. International code of nomenclature of bacteria. p. 180. American Society for Microbiology, Washington, D.C.

Louis, C. and Nigro, L. 1989. Ultrastructual evidence of *Wolbachia* rickettsiales in *Drosophila simulans* and their relationships with unidirectional cross-incompatibility. *J. Invert. Pathol.*, **54**: 39–44.

Luft, J.H. 1961. Improvements in epoxy resin embedding methods. *Biophys. Biochem. Cytol.*, **9**: 409–414.

Lyle, P.B. and Burgdorfer, W. 1971. Fine structure of *Rickettsia canada* in tissues of *Dermacentor andersoni* stiles. *J. Bacteriol.*, **105**: 1149–1159.

Mackie, T.T., Davis, G.E., Fuller, H.S., Knapp, J.A., Steinacker, M.L., Stager, K.E., Traub, R., Jellison, W.L., Millspaugh, D.D., Austrian, R.C., Bell, E.J., Kohls, G.M., Hsi, W. and Girsham, J.A.V. 1946a. Observations on Tsutsugamushi disease (scrub typhus) in Assam and Burma. Preliminaly report. *Am. J. Hyg.*, **43**: 195–218.

Mackie, T.T., Davis, G.E., Fuller, H.S., Knapp, J.A., Steinacker, M.L., Stager, K.E., Traub, R., Jellison, W. L., Millspaugh, D.D., Austrian, R.C., Bell, E.J., Kohls, G.M., Hsi, W. and Girsham, J.A.V. 1946b. Observations on Tsutsugamushi disease (scrub typhus) in Assam and Burma. Preliminary report. *Trans. Roy. Soc. Trop. Med. Hyg.*, **40**: 15–46.

MacMillan, J.G., Rice, R.M. and Jerrells, T.R. 1985. Development of antigen-specific cell-mediated immune responses after infection of Cynomolgus monkeys (*Macaca fascicularis*) with *Rickettsia tsutsugamushi*. *J. Infect. Dis.*, **152**: 739–749.

Martin, G., Juchault, P. and Legrand, J.J. 1973. Mise en evidence d'uu microorganisme intracytoplasmique symbiote de I'oniscoide *Armadillidium vulgare* Latr. dont la presence accompagne I'intersexualite ou la feminisation totale des males genetiques de la lignee thelygene. *C. R. Acad. Sci. Paris*, **276**: 2313–2316.

Matsuno, K., Nakajima, S., Adachi, M., Ueda, Y., Ebina, J. and Yoshida, Y. 1990. Isolation of *Rickettsia tsutsugamushi* from wild rodents and tsutsugamushi mites, and its drug susceptibility in mice. *Ann. Rept. Kyoto Pref. Inst. Hyg.*

Environ. Sci., **35**: 66–71. (in Japanese).

McClure, W. 1985. Mechanism and control of transcription initiation in prokaryotes. *Ann. Rev. Biochem.*, **54**: 171–204.

McCulloch, R.N. 1946. Studies in the control of scrub typhus. *Med. J. Australia*, **1**: 717–738.

McDade, J.E. and Gerone, P.J. 1970. Plaque assay for Q fever and scrub typhus rickettsiae. *Applied Microboil.*, **19**: 963–965.

Melvin, R. 1946. A note on the culturing of chiggers. *Ann. Entomol. Soc. Amer.*, **39**: 143–144.

Michener, C.D. 1946a. A method of rearing chigger mites. *Am. J. Trop. Med.*, **26**: 251–256.

Michener, C.D. 1946b. Observations on the habits and life history of a chigger mite, *Eutrombicula batatas* (Acarina: Trombiculinae). *Ann. Ent. Soc. Amer.*, **39**: 101–118.

Michener, C.D. 1946c. The taxonomy and bionomics of a new subgenus (Megatrombicula) of chigger mites (Acarina: Trombicula). *Ann. Ent. Soc. Amer.*, **39**: 431–445.

Misao, T., Kobayashi, Y., Kageyama, T., Ikeda, O., Fujimoto, T., Hirano, T., Tachibana, N., Fukiyama, K., Ichiki, T., Shirahama, S., Nagai, K., Ohya, I., Kusaba, T., Miyazaki, K. and Ueki, R. 1967. Etiological, clinical and epidemiological studies of Tsutsugamushi disease in Takahara-machi, Miyazaki Prefecture, Kyushu, Japan. *Med. J. Mutual Aid Assoc.*, **16**: 1–17. (in Japanese).

Mitchell, R. and Nadchatram, M. 1969. Schzeckenosy: the substitute for defecation in chigger mites. *J. Natur. Hirst.*, **3**: 121–124.

Miura, A. 1960. Studies on the life history of tsutsugamushi (trombiculid mites) by laboratory rearings. Part I. Descriptions of improved techniques and their results. *Jpn. J. Sanit. Zool.*, **11**: 1–5. (in Japanese).

Miura, T. and Kawai, K. 1968. Mode of transmission of Tsutsugamushi disease. *Japan. J. Trop. Med. Hyg.*, **9**: 13–15. (in Japanese).

Miyajima, M. 1908. Zoological studies of Tsutsugamushi disease. *J. Zool. Sci.*, **238**: 293–297. (in Japanese).

Miyajima, M. and Okumura, T. 1916. The life cycle of Akamushi. *Saikingaku Zasshi*, **253**: 1091–1106. (in Japanese).

Miyajima, M. and Okumura, T. 1917. On the life cycle of the 'Akamushi' carrier of Nippon River Fever. *Kitasato Arch. Exp. Med.*, **1**: 1–14.

Miyamura, S. and Ohta, T. 1991. *In vitro* susceptibility of rickettsial strains from patients with Japanese spotted fever to quinolones, penicillins and other selected chemotherapeutic agents. *Chemotherapy*, **39**: 258–260. (in Japanese).

Miyamura, S., Sato, N. and Tamura, A. 1985. *In vitro* susceptibility of recent clinical isolates of *Rickettsia tsutsugamushi* to chemotherapeutic agents. *J. Japan. Assoc. Infect. Dis.*, **59**: 486–488. (in Japanese).

Miyamura, S., Ohta, T. and Tamura, A. 1989. Comparison of *in vitro* susceptibilities of *Rickettsia prowazakii*, *R. rickettsii*, *R. sibirica*, and *R. tsutsugamushi* to antimicrobial agents. *Japan. J. Bacteriol.*, **44**: 717–721. (in Japanese).

Miyata, Y. 1960. Observations on the internal morphology of the adult mites of *Trombicula akamushi* (Brumpt). *Niigata Igakkai Zasshi*, **74**: 961–972. (in Japa-

nese).
Morishita, K. 1934. The distribution and epidemiology of Tsutsugamushi disease in Formosa. *Taiwan Sotokufu Chuokenkyusho Eiseibuyoho*, **216**: 1–76. (in Japanese).
Motoda, S. and Shibata, M. 1990. Preservation of *Rickettsia tsutsugamushi* smear for serodiagnosis and try of kit for immunoperoxidase (IP) reagents. *Clin. Virol.*, **18**: 433–438. (in Japanese).
Murai, K., Tachibana, N., Okayama, A., Shishime, E., Tsuda, K. and Oshikawa, T. 1992. Sensitivity of polymerase chain reaction assay for *Rickettsia tsutsugamushi* in patients' blood samples. *Microbiol. Immunol.*, **36**: 1145–1153.
Murata, M. and Kawamura, A. Jr. 1977. Restoration of the infectivity of *Rickettsia tsutsugamushi* to susceptible animals by passage in athymic nude mice. *Jpn. J. Exp. Med.*, **47**: 385–391.
Murata, M. and Kawamura, A. Jr. 1980. Effect of molar ratio of fluorescent dye to IgG on the detection of lymphocyte surface immunoglobulins by immunofluorescence. *Microbiol. Immunol.*, **24**: 65–78.
Murata, M., Nogami, S., Shirasaka, A., Tanaka, H., Kawamura, A. Jr. Mochizuki, H. and Oyama, H. 1980. Tsutsugamushi disease at the foothill of Mt. Fuji. *J. Japan. Assoc. Infect. Dis.,* **54**: 291–298. (in Japanese).
Murata, M., Sudo, K., Suzuki, K., Aoyama, Y., Nogami, S., Tanaka, H. and Kawamura, A. Jr. 1985. Proliferating sites of *Rickettsia tsutsugamushi* in mice by different routes of inoculation evidenced with immunofluorescence. *Jpn. J. Exp. Med.*, **55**: 193–199.
Murata, M., Yoshida, Y., Osono, M., Ohashi, N., Oyanagi, M., Urakami, H., Tamura, A., Nogami, S., Tanaka, H. and Kawamura, A. Jr. 1986. Production and characterization of monoclonal strain-specific antibodies against prototype strains of *Rickettsia tsutsugamushi*. *Microbiol. Immunol.*, **30**: 599–610.
Muur, I., Lim, B.L. and Walker, J.S. 1975. Mammals and scrub typhus ecology in peninsular Malaysia. *Trans. Roy. Soc. Trop. Med. Hyg.*, **69**: 121–130.
Myers, W.F. and Wisseman, C.L. Jr. 1980. Genetic relatedness among the typhus group of rickettsiae. *Int. J. Syst. Bacteriol.*, **30**: 143–150.
Myers, W.F. and Wisseman, C.L. Jr. 1981. The taxonomic relationship of *Rickettsia canada* to the typhus and spotted fever groups of the genus *Rickettsia*. pp. 313–325. In: Rickettsiae and rickettsial diseases. (eds. W. Burgdorfer and R.L. Anacker). Academic Press, New York, London, Tront, Sydney, San Francisco.
Myers, W.F., Ormsbee, R.A., Osterman, J.V. and Wisseman, C.L. Jr. 1967. The presence of diaminopimelic acid in the rickettsiae. *Proc. Soc. Exp. Biol. Med.*, **125**: 459–462.
Myers, W.F., Wisseman, C.L. Jr., Fiset, P., Oaks, E.V. and Smith, J.F. 1979. Taxonomic relationship of vole agent to *Rochalimaea quintana*. *Infect. Immun.*, **26**: 976–983.
Myers, W.F., Baca, O.G. and Wisseman, C.L. Jr. 1980. Genomic size of the rickettsia *Coxiella burnetii*. *J. Bacteriol.*, **144**: 460–461.
Nacy, C.A. and Groves, M.G. 1981. Macrophages in resistance to rickettsial infections: early host defence mechanisms in experimental scrub typhus. *Infect.*

Immun., **31**: 1239–1250.

Nacy, C.A. and Meltzer, M.S. 1984. Macrophages in resistance to rickettsial infection : protection against lethal *Rickettsia tsutsugamushi* infection by treatment of mice with macrophage-activating agents. *J. Leukoc. Biol.*, **35**: 385–396.

Nacy, C.A. Osterman, J.V. 1979. Host defenses in experimental scrub typhus : role of normal and activated macrophages. *Infect. Immun.*, **26**: 744–750.

Nacy, C.A., Meltzer, M.S., Leonard, E.J., Stevenson, M.M. and Skamene, E. 1983. Activation of macrophages for killing of rickettsiae : analysis of macrophage effector function after rickettsial inoculation of inbred mouse strains. *Adv. Exp. Med. Biol.*, **162**: 335–353.

Nadchatram, M. 1968. A technique for rearing trombiculid mites (Acarina) developed in a tropical laboratory. *J. Med. Entomol.*, **5**: 465–469.

Nadchatram, M. 1970. Correlation of habitat, environment and color of chiggers, and their potential significance in the epidemiology of scrub typhus in Malaya (Prostigmata: Trombiculidae). *J. Med. Entomol.*, **7**: 131–144.

Nadchatram, M. and Audy, J.R. 1965. The unusual life cycle of *Vatacarus ipoides* Southcott. *Med. J. Malaya.*, **20**: 80–81.

Nagayo, M., Miyagawa, Y., Mitamura, T. and Imamura, A. 1916. Succeeding report on *Trombidium* and Akamushi (trombiculid mite). Two new species of *Trombidium*, discovery of mobile nymphs and adults and nomenclature with morphological indicators. *Japan. J. Zool.*, **28**: 379–394. (in Japanese).

Nagayo, M., Mitamura, T. and Tamiya, T. 1919. On three species of tsutsugamushi. *Jpn. J. Exp. Med.*, **3**: 265–290. (in Japanese).

Nagayo, M., Mitamura, T. and Tamiya, T. 1920. On species of trombiculid mites. Its association with Tsutsugamushi disease. *J. Japan. Soc. Pathol.*, **10**: 503–508. (in Japanese).

Nagayo, M., Miyagawa, Y., Mitamura, T., Tamiya, T. and Tenjin, S. 1921. Five species of tsutsugamushi (the carrier of Japanese river fever) and their relation to the Tsutsugamushi disease. *Am. J. Hyg.*, **1**: 569–591.

Nagayo, M., Miyagawa, Y., Mitamura, T., Imamura, A., Tamiya, T. and Sato, K. 1923. On the experimental Tsutsugamushi disease in monkeys by intracutaneous inoculation of the virus. Scientific Reports from the Government Institute for Infectious Diseases, **2**: 371–373. (in Japanese).

Nagayo, M., Tamiya, T., Mitamura, T. and Sato, K. 1930. On the virus of Tsutsugamushi disease and its demonstration by a new method. *Trans. Japan. Pathol. Soc.*, **20**: 556–566.

Nakaya, I. 1957. Studies on Tsutsugamushi disease in Kouchi Prefecture (II). The causative agent isolated from trombiculid mites from endemic area and its epidemiological relation. *Tokyo Med. J.*, **74**: 581–588. (in Japanese).

Neal, T.J. and Barnett, H.C. 1961. The life cycle of the scrub typhus chigger mite, *Trombicula akamushi*. *Ann. Entomol. Soc. Amer.*, **54**: 196–203.

Nei, M. 1987. Molecular evolutionary genetics. pp. 293–298. Columbia Univ. Press, New York.

Neva, F.C. and Snyder, J.C. 1955. Studies on the toxicity of typhus rickettsiae. III. Observations on the mechanisms of toxic death in white mice and white rats. *J. Infect. Dis.*, **97**: 73–87.

Nigro, L. and Louis, C. 1989. *Wolbachia* endosymbiotes as putative agents of unidirectional cross-incompatibility in *Drosophila*, pp. 429–432. In: Endocytobiology. (eds. J.P. Nardon, V. Gianinazzi, A.M. Grenier, L. Margulis and D.C. Smith). Institut National de la Recherche Agronomique, Paris.

Noguchi, T., Mochizuki, H., Kitaoka, M., Okubo, K., Takano, K., Jo, K., Fukuzumi, S., Sasa, M., Obata, Y. and Takagi, M. 1953. Tsutsugamushi disease at Gotenba area in a foothill of Mt. Fuji. *Rep. Hyg. Lab. Shizuoka Pref.*, **3**: 7–10. (in Japanese).

Nokihara, S. 1955. Studies on Umayado disease in Kagawa Prefecture. *J. Okayama Med. Soc.*, **67**: 1105–1143, 1145–1193. (in Japanese).

Nur Ahmad, N. and Burney, M.I. 1962. A preliminary report on field studies and isolation of strains from Sialkot area. *Pakistan Armed Forces Med. J.*, **12**: 102–107.

Oaks, E.V., Stover, C.K. and Rice, R.M. 1987. Molecular cloning and expression of *Rickettsia tsutsugamushi* genes for two major protein antigens in *Escherichia coli*. *Infect. Immun.*, **55**: 1156–1162.

Oaks, E.V., Rice, R.M., Kelly, D.J. and Stover, C.K. 1989. Antigenic and genetic relatedness of eight *Rickettsia tsutsugamushi* antigens. *Infect. Immun.*, **57**: 3116–3122.

Oaks, S.C. Jr., Osterman, J.V. and Hetrick, F.M. 1977. Plaque assay and cloning of scrub typhus rickettsiae in irradiated L-929 cells. *J. Clin. Microbiol.*, **6**: 76–80.

Obata, Y. 1954. Anatomical studies on *Trombicula akamushi* (Brumpt), the vector of Tsutsugamushi disease. *Jpn. J. Sanit. Zool.*, **5**: 111–145. (in Japanese).

Obata, Y. and Aoki, T. 1958. Human infesting experiments on the larva of *Trombicula akamushi*. *Jpn. J. Sanit. Zool.*, **9**: 149–152. (in Japanese).

Obata, Y., Fukuzumi, S. and Ohnishi, T. 1952. On the trombiculid mites in Kanagawa Prefecture. *Rep. Hyg. Lab. Kanagawa Pref.*, II–2: 48–71. (in Japanese).

Ogata, N. 1931. Aetiologie der Tsutsugamushikrankheit: *Rickettsia tsutsugamushi*. *Zbl. f. Bakt.*, (1 Abt.), Orig., **122**: 249–253.

Ogata, N. 1958. *Rickettsia tsutsugamushi* (scrub typhus). pp. 1–167. Ishiyaku-shuppan Ltd., Tokyo. (in Japanese).

Ogata, N. and Unno, Y. 1929. On the transfer of causative agent of Tsutsugamushi disease to the rabbit testis and microorganisms appearing in the testis. *J. Chiba Med. Soc.*, **7**: 1215–1222. (in Japanese).

Ogata, N., Nakajima, G. and Kajima, S. 1932. Animals employed for experimental infection by pathogenic rickettsiae in laboratory — especially recommendation to use mouse for the detection of *Rickettsia tsutsugamushi*. *Tokyo Med. J.*, **2760**: 155–160. (in Japanese).

Ohashi, N., Tamura, A. and Suto, T. 1988. Immunoblotting analysis of anti-rickettsial antibodies produced in patients of Tsutsugamushi disease. *Microbiol. Immunol.*, **32**: 1085–1092.

Ohashi, N., Tamura, A., Ohta, M. and Hayashi, K. 1989. Purification and partial characterization of a type-specific antigen of *Rickettsia tsutsugamushi*. *Infect. Immun.*, **57**: 1427–1431.

Ohashi, N., Nashimoto, H., Ikeda, H. and Tamura, A. 1990a. Cloning and sequencing of the gene (*tsg 56*) encoding a type-specific antigen from *Rickettsia tsutsugamushi*. *Gene*, **91**: 119–122.

Ohashi, N., Tamura, A., Sakurai, H. and Yamamoto, S. 1990b. Characterization of a new antigenic type, Kuroki, of *Rickettsia tsutsugamushi* isolated from a patient in Japan. *J. Clin. Microbiol.*, **28**: 2111–2113.

Ohashi, N., Nashimoto, H., Ikeda, H. and Tamura, A. 1992a. Diversity of immunodominant 56-kDa type-specific antigen (TSA) of *Rickettsia tsutsugamushi*. Sequence and comparative analyses of the genes encoding TSA homologous from four antigenic variants. *J. Biol. Chem.*, **267**: 12728–12735.

Ohashi, N., Urakami, H., Fukuhara, M. and Tamura, A. 1992b. Analysis of type-specific antigen genes of *Rickettsia tsutsugamushi* by PCR method (Ab.). *Japan. J. Bacteriol.*, **47**: 302. (in Japanese)

Ohashi, N., Koyama, Y., Urakami, H., Higo, M. and Tamura, A. 1994. Characterization of *Rickettsia tsutsugamushi* isolated from rodents and chiggers in Taiwan (Ab.). *Japan. J. Bacteriol.*, **49**: 270. (in Japanese).

Ohashi, N., Fukuhara, M., Shimada, M. and Tamura, A. 1995. Phylogenetic position of *Rickettsia tsutsugamushi* and the relationship among its antigenic variants by analyses of 16S rRNA gene sequences. *FEMS Microbiol. Letters*, **125**: 299–304.

Ohse, T., Tada, T., Maeda, K., Obara, Y. and Fukushima, T. 1958. Trombiculid fauna of Fukui Prefecture. *Jpn. J. Sanit. Zool.*, **9**: 284–289. (in Japanese).

Olson, J.G., Ho, C-M., Peenen, P.F.D.V. and Santana, F.J. 1978. Isolation of *Rickettsia tsutsugamushi* from mammals and chiggers (Fam. Trombiculidae) in the Pescadores Islands, Taiwan. *Trans. Roy. Soc. Trop. Med. Hyg.*, **72**: 192–194.

Oliver, D. 1985. Protein secretion in *Escherichia coli*. *Ann. Rev. Microbiol.*, **39**: 615–648.

O'Neill, S.L. 1989. Cytoplasmic symbionts in *Tribolium confusum*. *J. Invert. Pathol.*, **53**: 132–134.

O'Neill, S.L. and Karr, T.L. 1990. Bidirectional incompatibility between conspecific populations of *Drosophila simulans*. *Nature*, **348**: 178–180.

O'Neill, S.L., Giordano, R., Colbert, A.M.E., Karr, T.L. and Robertson, H.M. 1992. 16S rRNA phylogenetic analysis of the bacterial endosymbionts associated with cytoplasmic incompatibility in insects. *Proc. Natl. Acad. Sci.*, **89**: 2699–2702.

Ono, Y. 1956. Studies on trombiculid mites in Kagawa Prefecture. *J. Okayama. Med. Soc.*, **68**: 1517–1534, 1821–1837. (in Japanese).

Osterman, J.V. 1985. Rickettsiae and hosts. *Acta Virol.*, **29**: 166–173.

Osuga, K., Kimura, M., Goto, H., Shimada, K. and Suto, T. 1991. A case of Tsutsugamushi disease probably contracted in Africa. *Eur. J. Clin. Microbiol. Infect. Dis.*, **10**: 95–96.

Otsuru, M. 1992. Recent advances in knowledges of Tsutsugamushi disease. *J. Niigata Med. Soc.*, **106**: 473–478. (in Japanese).

Oyama, T., Akugawa, T., Ootani, H., Nakajima, A., Ishikura, K., Ujiie, A., Hanyu, I. and Asahina, T. 1982. Tsutsugamushi disease in Gumma Prefecture Ⅳ. *Ann. Rep. Gumma Inst. Publ. Hlth.*, **14**: 25–30. (in Japanese).

Oyama, T., Ootani, H., Akuzawa, T., Machida. H., Ishikura, K., Saito, T., Ujiie, A.,

Saito, A., Hanyu, I., Tsuboi, Y. and Takeda, H. 1983. Tsutsugamushi disease in Gumma Prefecture V. *Ann. Rep. Gumma Inst. Publ. Hlth.*, **15**: 35–41. (in Japanese).

Palmer, B.A., Hetrick, F.M. and Jerrells, T.R. 1984. Production of gamma interferon in mice immune to *Rickettsia tsutsugamushi. Infect. Immun.*, **42**: 59–65.

Palmer, E.L., Mallavia, L.P., Tzianabos, T. and Obijeski, J.F. 1974. Electron microscopy of the cell wall of *Rickettsia prowazekii. J. Bacteriol.*, **118**: 1158–1166.

Paterson, P.Y., Wisseman, C.L. Jr. and Smadel, J.E. 1954. Studies of rickettsial toxins. I. Role of hemolysis in fatal toxemia of rabbits and rats. *J. Immunol.*, **72**: 12–23.

Philip, C.B. 1947. Observation on Tsutsugamushi disease (mite-borne or scrub typhus) in Northwest Honshu Island, Japan in the fall of 1945. I. Epidemiological and ecological data. *Am. J. Hyg.*, **46**: 45–59.

Philip, C.B. 1948a. Tsutsugamushi disease (scrub typhus) in the World War II. *J. Parasitol.*, **34**: 169–191.

Philip, C.B. 1948b. *Rickettsia tsutsugamushi.* In: Bergey's manual of determinative bacteriology. 6th ed., pp. 1089–1092. (eds. R.B. Breed, E.G.D. Murray and A.P. Hitchens). Williams & Wilkins, Baltimore.

Philip, C.B. 1949. Scrub typhus, or Tsutsugamushi disease. *Sci. Monthly*, **69**: 281–289.

Philip, C.B. and Kohls, G.M. 1945. Studies on Tsutsugamushi disease (scrub typhus, mite-borne typhus) in New Guinea and adjacent islands: Tsutsugamushi disease with high endemicity on a small South Sea Island. *Am. J. Hyg.*, **42**: 195–202.

Philip, C.B. and Kohls, G.M. 1948. Mites and scrub typhus. pp. 1656–1662. In: Proc. 4th Int. Congr. Trop. Med. Malar., Washington, D.C.

Philip, C.B., Woodward, T.E. and Sullivan, R.R. 1946. Tsutsugamushi disease (scrub or mite-borne typhus) in the Philippine Islands during American reoccupation in 1944–45. *Am. J. Trop. Med.*, **26**: 229–242.

Philip, C.B., Traub, R. and Smadel, J.E. 1949. Chloramphenicol (Chloromycetin) in the chemoprophylaxis of scrub typhus (Tsutsugamushi disease). 1. Epidemiological observations on hyperendemic areas of scrub typhus in Malaya. *Am. J. Hyg.*, **50**: 63–74.

Pontecorvo, G. 1975. Production of mammalian somatic cell hybrids by means of polyethylene glycol treatment. *Somatic Cell Genetics.*, **1**: 397–400.

Popov, V.L. and Ignatovich, V.F. 1976. Electron microscopy of surface structures of *Rickettsia prowazekii* stained with ruthenium red. *Acta Virol.*, **20**: 424–428.

Popov, V.L., Dyuisalieva, R.G., Smirnova, N.S., Tarasevich, I, V. and Rybkin, N.N. 1986. Ultrastructure of *Rickettsia sibirica* during interaction with the host cell. *Acta Virol.*, **30**: 494– 498.

Popov, V.L., Prozorovsky, S.V., Vovk, O.A., Kekcheeva, N.K., Smirnova, N.S. and Barkhatova, O.I. 1987. Electron microscopic analysis of *in vitro* interaction of *Rickettsia prowazekii* with guinea pig macrophages. I. Macrophages from nonimmune animals. *Acta Virol.*, **31**: 53–58.

Portaro, J.K. and Barr, A.R. 1975. "Curing" Wolbachia infections in *Culex pipiens.*

J. Med. Entomol., **12**: 265.

Poulson, D.F. 1968. Nature, stability, and expression of hereditary SR infections in *Drosophila*. *Proc. XII Int. Congr. Genet.*, **2**: 91–92.

Price, W.H. 1953. The epidemiology of Rocky Mountain spotted fever. I. The characterization of strain virulence of *Rickettsia rickettsii*. *Am. J. Hyg.*, **58**: 248–268.

Rai, J. and Bandopadhyay, D. 1978. Vertical transmission in chigger-borne rickettiosis. *Indian J. Med. Res.*, **68**: 31–38.

Raoult, D., Roussellier, P., Galicher, V., Perez, R. and Tamalet, J. 1986. *In vitro* susceptibity of *Rickettsia conorii* to ciprofloxacin as determined by suppressing lethality in chicken embryos and by plaque assay. *Antimicrob. Agents Chemother.*, **29**: 424–425.

Raoult, D., Roussellier, P., Galicher, V. and Tamalet, J. 1987a. *In vitro* antibiotic susceptibility of *Rickettsia rickettsii* and *Rickettsia conorii*: plaque assay and micro-plaque colorimetric assay. *J. Infect. Dis.*, **155**: 1059–1069.

Raoult, D., Roussellier, P., Vestris, G., Galicher, V., Perez, R. and Tamalet, J. 1987b. Susceptibility of *Rickettsia conorii* and *Rickettsia rickettsii* to pefloxacin, *in vitro* and *in ovo*. *J. Antimicrob. Chemother.*, **19**: 303–305.

Raoult, D., Roussellier, P. and Tamalet, J. 1988. *In vitro* evaluation of josamycin, spiramycin and erythromycin against *Rickettsia rickettsii* and *R. conorii*. *Antimicrob. Agents Chemother.*, **32**: 255–256.

Rapmund, G. 1984. Rickettsial diseases of the Far East: new perspectives. *J. Infect. Dis.*, **149**: 330–338.

Rapmund, G., Upham, R.W. Jr., Kundin, W.D., Manikumaran, C. and Chan, T.C. 1969. Transovarial development of scrub typhus rickettsiae in a colony of vector mites. *Trans. Roy. Soc. Trop. Med. Hyg.*, **63**: 251–258.

Rapmund, G., Dohany, A.L., Manikumaran, C. and Chan, T.C. 1972. Transovarial transmission of *Rickettsia tsutsugamushi* in *Leptotrombidium* (*Leptotrombidium*) *arenicola*, Traub (Acarina: Trombiculidae). *J. Med. Entomol.*, **9**: 71–72.

Ree, H-I., Lee, I-Y. and Cho, M-K. 1991a. Determination of the vector species of Tsutsugamushi disease in Korea. *Korean J. Parasitol.*, **29**: 87–92.

Ree, H-I., Lee, M-C. and Lee, I-Y. 1991b. Study on the population density of chigger mites, the vector of Tsutsugamushi disease in Korea. *Korean J. Zool.*, **34**: 257–264. (in Korean).

Ree, H-I., Lee, H-S., Lee, I-Y. and Yoshida, Y. 1991c. Epidemiological studies on host animals of Tsutsugamushi disease in Korea. *Korean J. Parasitol.*, **29**: 181–188.

Reed, L.J. and Muench, H. 1938. A simple method of estimating fifty percent endopoints. *Am. J. Hyg.*, **17**: 493–496.

Regional Office for the Western Pacific of the WHO. 1987. Report of meeting of the task force on the serological diagnosis of Tsutsugamushi disease (scrub typhus), Manila, Philippines.

Rehacek, J. and Tarasevich, I.V. 1988. Acari-borne rickettsiae and rickettsiosis in Eurasia. VEDA Publ. House, Slovak. Acad. Sci., Bratislova.

Rights, F.L. and Smadel, J.E. 1948. Studies on scrub typhus (Tsutsugamushi disease). III. Heterogenicity of strains of *R. tsutsugamushi* as demonstrated by cross-vaccination studies. *J. Exp. Med.*, **87**: 339–351.

Rikihisa, Y. and Ito, S. 1980. Localization of electron-dense tracers during entry of *Rickettsia tsutsugamushi* into polymorphonuclear leukocytes. *Infect. Immun.*, **30**: 231–243.

Rikihisa, Y. and Ito, S. 1981. Outer membrane vesicles of *Rickettsia tsutsugamushi*. pp. 229–240. In: Rickettsiae and Rickettsial diseases. (eds. W. Burgdorfer and R.L. Anacker). Academic Press, New York, London, Toronto, Sydney, San Francisco.

Rikihisa, Y. and Ito, S. 1982. Entry of *Rickettsia tsutsugamushi* into polymorphonuclear leukocytes. *Infect. Immun.*, **38**: 343–350.

Rikihisa, Y. and Ito, S. 1983. Effect of antibody on entry of *Rickettsia tsutsugamushi* into polymorphonuclear leukocyte cytoplasm. *Infect. Immun.*, **39**: 928–938.

Rikihisa, Y., Rota, T., Lee, T.H., MacDonald, A.B. and Ito, S. 1979. Changes in immunoferritin labeling of *Rickettsia tsutsugamushi* after serial cultivation in ^{60}Co-irradiated BHK cells. *Infect. Immun.*, **26**: 638–650.

Roberts, L.W. and Ram, S. 1973. Microdissection of scrub typhus vectors. *Southeast Asian J. Trop. Med. Publ. Hlth.*, **4**: 271.

Roberts, L.W. and Robinson, D.M. 1977. Efficiency of transovarial transmission of *Rickettsia tsutsugamushi* in *Leptotrombidium arenicola* (Acari: Trombiculidae). *J. Med. Entomol.*, **13**: 493–496.

Roberts, L. Robinson, D.M. and Cavanaugh, D.C. 1982. Protection against natural infection with *Rickettsia tsutsugamushi* in mice. *J. Infect. Dis.*, **145**: 768.

Roberts, L.W., Gan, E., Rapmund, G., Chan, T.C., Ramasamy, S.M. and Walker, J.S. 1975a. Identification of *Rickettsia tsutsugamushi* in the life stages of *Leptotrombidium fletcheri* with isolation and immunofluorescence techniques. *Ann. N. Y. Acad. Sci.*, **266**: 73–79.

Roberts, L.W., Robinson, D.M., Rapmund, G., Walker, J.S. Gan, E. and Ram, S. 1975b. Distribution of *Rickettsia tsutsugamushi* in organs of *Leptotrombidium (Leptotrombidium) fletcheri* (Prostigmata: Trombiculidae). *J. Med. Entomol.*, **12**: 345–348.

Roberts, L.W., Rapmund, G. and Cadigan, F.C. Jr. 1977. Sex ratios in *Rickettsia tsutsugamushi*-infected and noinfected colonies of *Leptotrombidium* (Acari: Trombiculidae). *J. Med. Entomol.*, **14**: 89–92.

Robinson, D.M., Brown, G., Gan, E. and Huxsoll, D.L. 1976. Adaptation of a microimmunofluorescence test to the study of human *Rickettsia tsutsugamushi* antibody. *Am. J. Trop. Med. Hyg.*, **25**: 900–905.

Robinson, D.M., Roberts, L.W., Dohany, A.L., Gan, E., Chan, T.C. and Huxsoll, D.L. 1977. Virulence and antigenic properties of *Rickettsia tsutsugamushi* in a naturally infected laboratory colony of *Leptotrombidium (Leptotrombidium) arenicola*. *Southeast Asian J. Trop. Med. Publ. Hlth.*, **8**: 227–231.

Rollwagen, F.M., Dasch, G.A. and Jerrells, T.R. 1986. Mechanisms of immunity to rickettsial infection: characterization of a cytotoxic effector cell. *J. Immunol.*, **136**: 1418–1421.

Rousset, F., Bouchon, D., Pintureau, B., Juchault, P. and Solignac, M. 1992.

Wolbachia endosymbionts responsible for various alterations of sexuality in arthropods. *Proc. Roy. Soc. Lond. B.*, **250**: 91–98.

Saito, H., Sekikawa, H. and Kenmotsu, M. 1981. Clinical review on new type Tsutsugamushi disease — from clinical cases in Niigata Prefecture. *Nihon Iji Shinpo*, **3007**: 23–30. (in Japanese).

Saitou, N. and Nei, M. 1987. The neighbor-joining method: a new method for reconstructing phylogenetic trees. *Mol. Biol. Evol.*, **4**: 406–425.

Saito, Y. and Otsuru, M. 1959. Notes on trombiculid mites collected in Sado Island of Japan and isolation of rickettsia with a description of *Trombicula* (*Neotrombicula*) *sadoensis* n. sp. *Acta Medica et Biologica*, **7**: 65–80.

Saito, Y., Yamashita, T., Sekikawa, H. and Otsuru, M. 1977. Improvement in setting method of sentinel animals for collecting larval trombiculid mites. *Jpn. J. Sanit. Zool.*, **28**: 58. (in Japanese).

Sakita, H. 1934. A case of suspected Tsutsugamushi disease encountered at the foothills of Mt. Fuji. *Japan. Army Med. J.*, **248**: 289. (in Japanese).

Sasa, M. 1954. Studies on tsutsugamushi. *Trombicula scutellaris* Nagayo *et al.*, and its relationships to the winter scrub typhus of Japan, together with systematic accounts for the four species of tsutsugamushi described by Nagayo and others. *Jpn. J. Sanit. Zool.*, 4, Special number for Dr. H. Kobayashi's 70th birthday. 233–251. (in Japanese).

Sasa, M. 1955. Comparative epidemiology of Shichito-type Tsutsugamushi disease. pp. 45–52. In: Studies on Shichito fever. Pt. III. Dept. Hlth., Tokyo. (in Japanese).

Sasa, M. 1956. Tsutsugamushi and Tsutsugamushi disease. pp. 1–497. Igakushoin Ltd., Tokyo (in Japanese).

Sasa, M. 1959: Epidemiology of Tsutsugamushi disease. pp. 243–251. In: Proc. of 14th General Assembly of Japan Medical Congress. Vol. Special Lectures. (in Japanese).

Sasa, M. and Kano, R. 1950. Discovery of *Trombicula wichmanni* in Japan. *Tokyo Med. J.*, **67**: 9–10. (in Japanese).

Sasa, M. and Miura, A. 1953. Studies on the life history of tsutsugamushi (Trombiculid mites) of Japan in the laboratory. *Jpn. J. Exp. Med.*, **23**: 171–185.

Sasa, M., Miura, A. and Teramura, S. 1951. Successful rearing of *Trombicula akamushi* in glass vials. *Tokyo Med. J.*, **68**; 13. (in Japanese).

Sasa, M., Komine, I., Kawamura, A. Jr., Miura, A., Hayashi, S., Suzuki, T. and Tanaka, H. 1953. Zoophilism of *Trombicula scutellaris* on Hachijo Island. pp. 82–87. In: Studies on Shichito fever. Pt. II. Dept. Hlth., Tokyo. (in Japanese).

Sasa, M., Ueno, Y., Tanaka, H., Miura, A., Hayashi, S., Suzuki, T. and Tanaka, H. 1958. Studies on the bionomics of the summer chiggers (trombiculid mites) of Hachijo Island. pp. 93–101. In: Studies on Shichito fever. Pt. Sum. Dept. Hlth., Tokyo. (in Japanese).

Schluger, E.G. and Kudryashova, N.I. 1967. Red bodied mites (Trombiculidae) and *Rickettsia tsutsugamushi*. pp. 143–150. In: Biological relationships between bloodsucking arthropods and pathogens of human disease. (ed. P.A. Petrishcheva). Meditsina, Moscow. (in Russian).

Schramek, S. 1974. Deoxyribonucleic acid base composition of rickettsiae belonging to the Rocky Mountain spotted fever group isolated in Czechoslovakia. *Acta Virol.*, **18**: 173–174.

Schramek, S. and Mayer, H. 1982. Different sugar compositions of lipopolysaccharides isolated from phase I and pure phase II cells of *Coxiella burnetii. Infect. Immun.*, **38**: 53–57.

Schramek, S., Brezina, R. and Kazar, J. 1977. Some biological properties of an endotoxic lipopolysaccharide from the typhus group rickettsiae. *Acta Virol.*, **21**: 439–441.

Schumacher, H.H. and Hoeppli, R. 1963. Histochemical reactions to Trombiculid mites, with special reference to the structure and function of the "stylostome". *Z. Tropenmed. Parasitol.*, **16**: 192–208.

Sekikawa, H., Kenmotsu, M., Watanabe, H., Takai, A., Hashimoto, T. and Tazaki, T. 1984. Basic and clinical research of Tsutsugamushi disease — observation from epidemiology. *Niigata. Med. J.*, **98**: 318–324. (in Japanese).

Shibata, M., Abe, S., Nezu, H., Kamimura, K., Tamura, A., Takahashi, K., Miyamura, S., Sekikawa, H. and Kenmotsu, M. 1984. Serological properties of *Rickettsia tsutsugamushi* isolated from patients: Shimokoshi strain which shows low cross reactivity with prototype strains. *Clin. Virol.*, **12**: 294–298. (in Japanese).

Shimada, M., Ohashi, N. and Tamura, A. 1994. Analysis of genomic DNA structure in *Rickettsia tsutsugamushi* by pulse field gel electrophoresis (Ab.). *Japan. J. Bacteriol.*, **49**: 293. (in Japanese).

Shine, J. and Dalgarno, L. 1974. The 3'-terminal sequence of *Escherichia coli* 16S ribosomal RNA: complementarity to nonsense triplets and ribosomal binding sites. *Proc. Natl. Acad. Sci.*, **71**: 1342–1346.

Shirai, A. and Wisseman, C.L. Jr. 1975. Serological classification of scrub typhus isolates from Pakistan. *Am. J. Trop. Med. Hyg.*, **24**: 145–153.

Shirai, A., Catanzaro, P.J., Phillips, S.M. and Osterman, J.V. 1976. Host defenses in experimental scrub typhus: role of cellular immunity in heterologous protection. *Infect. Immun.*, **14**: 39–46.

Shirai, A., Robinson, D.M., Lim. B.L., Dohany, A.L. and Huxsoll, D.L. 1978. *Rickettsia tsutsugamushi* infection in chiggers and small mammals on a natural oil palm estate. *Southeast Asian J. Trop. Med. Publ. Hlth.*, **9**: 356–360.

Shirai, A., Chan, T.C., Gan, E. and Huksoll, D.L. 1979a. Presistence and reactivation of *Rickettsia tsutsugamushi* infections in laboratory mice. *Japan. J. Med. Sci. Biol.*, **32**: 179–184.

Shirai, A., Robinson, D.M., Brown, G.W., Gan, E. and Huxsoll, D.L. 1979b. Antigenic analysis by direct immunofluorescence of 114 isolates of *Rickettsia tsutsugamushi* recovered from febrile patients in rural Malaysia. *Japan. J. Med. Sci. Biol.*, **32**: 337–344.

Shirai, A., Dohany, A.L., Gan, E., Chan, T.C. and Huxsoll, D.L. 1980. Antigenic classification of *Rickettsia tsutsugamushi* isolated from small mammals trapped in developing oil palm complex in Peninsula Malaysia. *Japan. J. Med. Sci. Biol.*, **33**: 231–234.

Shirai, A., Brown, G.W., Gan, E., Huxsoll, D.L. and Groves, M.G. 1981a. *Rickett-*

sia tsutsugamushi antibody in mother / cord pairs of sera. *Japan. J. Med. Sci. Biol.*, **34**: 37–39.

Shirai, A., Dohany, A.L., Ram, S., Chiang, G.L. and Huxsoll, D.L. 1981b. Serological classification of *Rickettsia tsutsugamushi* organisms found in chiggers (Acarina: Trombiculidae) collected in Peninsular Malaysia. *Trans. Roy. Soc. Trop. Med. Hyg.*, **75**: 580–582.

Shirai, A., Gan, E., Huxsoll, D.L. and Miles, J.A.R. 1981c. Serologic classification of scrub typhus isolates from Malaysia. *Southeast Asian J. Trop. Med. Publ. Hlth.*, **12**: 148–150.

Shirai, A., Tanskul, P.L., Andre, R.G., Dohany, A.L. and Huxsoll, D.L. 1981d. *Rickettsia tsutsugamushi* strains found in chiggers collected in Thailand. *Southeast Asian J. Trop. Med. Publ. Hlth.*, **12**: 1–6.

Shirai, A., Campbell, R.W., Gan, E., Chan, T.C. and Huxsoll, D.L. 1982a. Serological analysis of *Rickettsia tsutsugamushi* isolates from North Queensland. *Aust. J. Exp. Biol. Med. Sci.*, **60**: 203–205.

Shirai, A., Coolbaugh, J.C., Gan, E., Chan, T.C., Huxsoll, D.L. and Groves, M.G. 1982b. Serological analysis of scrub typhus isolates from the Pescadores and Philippine Islands. *Japan. J. Med. Sci. Biol.*, **35**: 255–259.

Shirai, A., Huxsoll, D.L., Dohany, A.L., Montrey, R.D., Werner, R.M. and Gan, E. 1982c. Characterization of *Rickettsia tsutsugamushi* strains in two species of naturally infected laboratory-reared chiggers. *Am. J. Trop. Med. Hyg.*, **31**: 395–402.

Shirai, A., Saunders, J.P., Dohany, A.L., Huxsoll, D.L. and Groves, M.G. 1982d. Transmission of scrub typhus to human volunteers by laboratory-reared chiggers. *Japan. J. Med. Sci. Biol.*, **35**: 9–16.

Shirai, A., Chan, T.C., Gan, E. and Groves, M.G. 1984a. Lack of transplacental infection with scrub typhus organisms in laboratory mice. *Am. J. Trop. Med. Hyg.*, **33**: 285–287.

Shirai, A., Ram, S., Gan, E., Lewis, G.E. Jr., Kanda, T., Chiang, G.L. and Groves, M.G. 1984b. Comparative studies on the karyotypes of *Leptotrombidium deliense, L. fletcheri* and *L. arenicola* (Acari: Trombiculidae). *J. Med. Entomol.*, **21**: 616–617.

Shirasaka, A. and Sasa, M. 1967. Observations on the life history in the laboratory of some Japanese and Thai trombiculid mites. *Jpn. J. Exp. Med.*, **37**: 129–140.

Shishido, A. 1962a. Identification and serological classification of the causative agents of scrub typhus in Japan. *Japan. J. Med. Sci. Biol.*, **15**: 308–321.

Shishido, A. 1962b. Inapparent infection of scrub typhus in Japan. *Japan. J. Med. Sci. Biol.*, **15**: 330–335.

Shishido, A. 1964. Strain variation of *Rickettsia orientalis* in the complement fixation test. *Japan. J. Med. Sci. Biol.*, **17**: 59–72.

Shishido, A., Ohtawara, M., Tateno, S., Mizuno, S., Ogura, M. and Kitaoka, M. 1958. The nature of immunity against scrub typhus in mice. I. The resistance of mice, surviving subcutaneous infection of scrub typhus rickettsia, to intraperitoneal reinfection of the same agent. *Japan. J. Med. Sci. Biol.*, **11**: 383–399.

Shishido, A., Ohtawara, M., Hikita, M. and Kitaoka, M. 1959. The nature of immunity against scrub typhus in mice. II . The cross-protection test with mice for identification and differentiation of several strains of *Rickettsia orientalis* newly isolated in Japan. *Japan. J. Med. Sci. Biol.*, **12**: 391–404.

Shishido, A., Kohno, S., Hikita, M., Iida, T., Kawashima, H. and Kawamura, A. Jr. 1967. Complement fixation and direct immunofluorescence for typing of Tsutsugamushi disease rickettsia. *Acta Medica et Biologica*, **15** (Suppl.): 87–95.

Shishido, A., Hikita, M., Sato, T. and Kohno, S. 1969. Particulate and soluble antigens of *Rickettsia tsutsugamushi* in the complement fixation test. *J. Immunol.* **103**: 480–490.

Shubin, F.N., Natsky, K.V. and Somov, G.P. 1970. Concerning the vector of Tsutsugamushi fever in the Far East. *Zh. Mikrobiol. Epidemiol. Immunol.*, **47**: 112–115. (in Russian).

Shull, A.F. 1948. An all-female strain of lady beetles with reversions to normal sex rations. *Amer. Natur.*, **82**: 241–251.

Silverman, D.J. and Wisseman, C.L. Jr. 1978. Comparative ultrastructural study on the cell envelopes of *Rickettsia prowazekii, Rickettsia rickettsii* and *Rickettsia tsutsugamushi. Infect. Immun.*, **21**: 1020–1023.

Silverman, D.J. and Wisseman, C. L. Jr. 1979. *In vitro* studies of rickettsia-host cell interactions: ultrastructural changes induced by *Rickettsia rickettsii* infection of chicken embryo fibroblasts. *Infect. Immun.*, **26**: 714–727.

Silverman, D.J., Wisseman, C.L. Jr., Waddell, A.D. and Jones, M. 1978. External layers of *Rickettsia prowazekii* and *Rickettsia rickettsii*: occurrence of a slime layer. *Infect. Immun.*, **22**: 233–246.

Silverman, D.J., Wisseman, C.L. Jr. and Waddell, A. 1980. *In vitro* studies of rickettsia-host cell interactions: ultrastructural study of *Rickettsia prowazekii*-infected chicken embryo fibroblasts. *Infect. Immun.*, **29**: 778–790.

Skerman, V.B.D., McGowan, V. and Sneath, P.H.A. 1980. Approved list of bacterial names. *Int. J. Syst. Bacteriol.*, **30**: 225–420.

Skinner, S.W. 1982. Maternally inherited sex ratio in the parasitoid wasp *Nasonia vitripennis. Science*, **215**: 1133–1134.

Skinner, S.W. 1985. Son-killer: a third extrachromosomal factor affecting the sex ratio of the parasitoid wasp, *Nasonia vitripennis. Genetics*, **109**: 745–759.

Smadel, J.E., Jackson, E.B., Bennett, B.L. and Rights, F.L. 1946. A toxic substance associated with Gilliam strain of *R. orientalis. Proc. Soc. Exp. Biol. Med.*, **62**: 138–140.

Smadel, J.E., Traub, R., Ley, H.L. Jr., Philip, C.B., Woodward, T.E. and Lewthwaite, R. 1949. Chloramphenicol (chloromycetin) in the chemoprophylaxis of scrub typhus (Tsutsugamushi disease). II. Results with volunteers exposed in hyperendemic area of scrub typhus. *Am. J. Hyg.*, **50**: 75–91.

Smadel, J.E., Traub, R., Frick, L.P., Diercks, F.H. and Bailey, C.A. 1950. Chloramphenicol (chloromycetin) in the chemoprophylaxis of scrub typhus (Tsutsugamushi disease). III. Suppression of overt disease among volunteers by prophylactic regimens of four-weeks duration. *Am. J. Hyg.*, **51**: 216–228.

Smirnova, N.S., Popov, V.L. and Kokorin, I.N. 1986. Peculiarities of *Rickettsia prowazekii* in the cell culture as revealed by cryoultramicrotomy. *Acta Virol.*,

30: 436–439.

Snyder, J.C., Bovarnick, M.R., Miller, J.C. and Chang, R.S-M. 1954. Observation on the hemolytic properties of typhus rickettsiae. *J. Bacteriol.*, **67**: 724–730.

Stouthamer, R. 1991. Effectiveness of several antibiotics in reverting thelytoky to arrhenotoky in *Trichogramma* spp. pp. 119–122. In: *Trichogramma* and other egg parasitoids. Paris: INRA.

Stouthamer, R. 1993. The use of sexual versus asexual wasps in biological control. *Entomophaga*, **38**: 3–6.

Stouthamer, R., Luck, R.F . and Hamilton, W.D. 1990a. Antibiotics cause parthenogenetic *Trichogramma* (Hymenoptera / Trichogrammatidae) to revert to sex. *Proc. Natl. Acad. Soc.*, **87**: 2424–2427.

Stouthamer, R., Pinto, J.D., Platner, G.R. and Luck, R.F. 1990b. Taxonomic status of thelytocous forms of *Trichogramma* (Hymenoptera: Trichogrammatidae). *Ann. Ent. Soc. Amer.*, **83**: 475–481.

Stouthamer, R., Breeuwer, J.A.J., Luc, R.F. and Werren, J,H. 1993. Molecular identification of microorganisms associated with parthenogenesis. *Nature*, **361**: 66–68.

Stover, C.K., Vodkin, M.H. and Oaks, E.V. 1987. Use of conversion adaptors to clone antigen gene in λgt11. *Anal. Biochem.*, **163**: 398–407.

Stover, C.K., Marana, D.P., Carter, J.M., Roe, B.A., Mardis, E. and Oaks, E.V. 1990a. The 56-kilodalton major protein antigen of *Rickettsia tsutsugamushi*: molecular cloning and sequence analysis of the *sta 56* gene and precise identification of a strain-specific epitope. *Infect. Immun.*, **58**: 2076–2084.

Stover, C.K., Marana, D.P., Dasch, G.A. and Oaks, E.V. 1990b. Molecular cloning and sequence analysis of the *sta-58* major antigen gene of *Rickettsia tsutsugamushi*: sequence homology and antigenic comparison of *sta-58* to the 60-kilodalton family of stress proteins. *Infect. Immun.*, **58**: 1360–1368.

Suenaga, O. 1982. Treatment of *Wolbachia pipientis* infection with tetracycline hydrochloride and the change of compatibility in a strain of *Culex pipiens* complex. *Trop. Med.*, **24**: 9–15. (in Japanese).

Suenaga, O. 1992. Treatment of *Wolbachia pipientis* infection with tetracycline hydrochloride and the change of cytoplasmic incompatibility in a strain of *Culex pipiens quinquefasciatus* from Bangkok, Thailand. *Trop. Med.*, **34**: 15–19.

Sugita, Y., Nagatani, T., Okuda, K., Yoshida, Y. and Nakajima, H. 1992. Diagnosis of typhus infection with *Rickettsia tsutsugamushi* by polymerase chain reaction. *J. Med. Microbiol.*, **37**: 357–360.

Sugita, Y., Yamakawa, Y., Takahashi, K., Nagatani, T., Okuda, K. and Nakajima, H. 1993. A polymerase chain reaction system for rapid diagnosis of scrub typhus within six hours. *Am. J. Trop. Med. Hyg.*, **49**: 636–640.

Suto, T. 1982. Rapid and sensitive serodiagnosis of Tsutsugamushi disease by means of indirect immunoperoxidase reaction. *Clin. Pathol.*, **30**: 10–17. (in Japanese).

Suto, T. 1985. Rapid and accurate serologic diagnosis of Tsutsugamushi disease in Japan employing the immunoperoxidase reaction. pp. 444–452. In: Rickettsiae and rickettsial diseases. (ed. J. Kazár). VEDA Publ. House of the Slovak Acad.

of Sci. Bratislava.
Suto, T. 1986. Present states of Tsutsugamushi disease, especially its epidemiology, clinical features and etiological diagnosis in Japan. *Virus*, **36**: 55–70. (in Japanese).
Suto, T. 1987. Indirect immunoperoxidase technique. pp. 32–33. In: Report of meeting of the task force on the serological diagnosis of Tsutsugamushi disease (scrub typhus). Regional Office for the Western Pacific of the WHO, Okinawa, Japan.
Suto, T. 1991a. A ten years experience on diagnosis of rickettsial diseases using the indirect immunoperoxidase methods. *Acta Virol.*, **35**: 580–586.
Suto, T. 1991b. New story of Tsutsugamushi disease. pp. 1–277. Mumeisha Press, Akita, Japan. (in Japanese).
Suto, T. 1993. Laboratory manual of immuno-peroxidase antibody titration for rapid serologic diagnosis of rickettsial diseases. Personal communication.
Suto, T. and Fujimiya, Y. 1980. Rapid serodiagnosis of Tsutsugamushi disease by immunoperoxidase reaction by using rickettsiae in cultured cells as antigen. *Clin. Virol.*, **8**: 425–429. (in Japanese).
Suto, T. and Hatakeyama, H. 1990. Stabilization of *Rickettsia tsutsugamushi* antigen in high molar sodium chloride solution. *Clin. Virol.*, **18**: 582–584. (in Japanese).
Suzuki, H. 1976. Reports of medico-zoological investigations in the Nansei Islands. Part V. Six new species of chiggers from the Amami Islands (Prostigmata; Trombiculidae). *Jpn. J. Sanit. Zool.*, **27**: 271–282. (in Japanese).
Suzuki, K. 1951. Studies on the toxicity of *Rickettsia mooseri* for mice especially on the effects of enzymatic inhibitor and accelerator. *Jpn. J. Exp. Med.*, **21**: 291–298.
Suzuki, M. 1959. On the persistence of *Rickettsia orientalis* in the body of albino rats and field rodents (*Microtus montebelli* and *Apodemus speciosus speciosus*) following experimental infection. *Japan. J. Hyg.*, **14**: 917–926. (in Japanese).
Suzuki, N. 1992. A serological study of common antigens between *Rickettsia tsutsugamushi* and Weil-Felix test antigens. *Akita. J. Med.*, **19**: 769–779. (in Japanese).
Suzuki, T. 1953. Studies on the bionomics and chemical control of tsutsugamushi (scrub-typhus mites). Part I. *Trombicula akamushi* (Brumpt) in Northwestern Honshu, Japan. *Jpn. J. Exp. Med.*, **23**: 487–516.
Suzuki, T. 1954. Studies on the bionomics and chemical control of tsutsugamushi (scrub-typhus mites). Part II. *Trombicula scutellaris* Nagayo *et al.* in Southern Kanto of Japan. *Jpn. J. Exp. Med.*, **24**: 181–197.
Suzuki, T. and Sekikawa, H. 1981. Four cases of Tsutsugamushi disease (scrub typhus) complicated with disseminated intervescular coagulation. *J. Japan. Assoc. Infect. Dis.*, **55**: 642–648. (in Japanese).
Suzuki, T., Tanaka, H., Kaneko, K., Kumada, N. and Sasa, M. 1953. Studies on the distribution of larval trombiculid mites on the soil surface of Hachijo and Oshima Islands. pp. 65–78. In: Studies on Shichito fever Pt. II. Dept. Hlth., Tokyo. (in Japanese).
Suzuki, T., Hayashi, S. and Teramura, S. 1955. Studies on the bionomics of

tsutsugamushi. Pt. I. Collecting method of unengorged larvae of trombiculid mites by bakelite-plate. *Tokyo Med. J.*, **72**: 93–95. (in Japanese).

Suzuki, T., Sasa, M., Tanaka, H., Hayashi, S. and Ueno, Y. 1958. Notes on the species of trombiculid mites collected by the bakelite plate method (Studies on Tsutsugamushi, 99). pp. 102–106. In: Studies on Shichito fever. Pt. Sum. Dept. Hlth., Tokyo. (in Japanese).

Tachibana, N. 1985. Recent medical topics: Tsutsugamushi disease in special relation to the new type disease. *Japan. J. Internal Med.*, **74**: 1218–1222. (in Japanese).

Tachibana, N. 1987. Clinical aspects of diagnosis. pp. 40–41. In: Report of meeting of the task force on the serological diagnosis of Tsutsugamushi disease (scrub typhus), Manila, Philippines. Regional Office for the Western Pacific of the WHO.

Tachibana, N. 1989. Clinics of Tsutsugamushi Disease. pp. 60–73. In: Recent topics of infectious diseases by obligatory intracellular parasitic bacteriae. (eds. R. Fukushima and A. Matsumoto). Medicinal J. Press. Tokyo. (in Japanese).

Tachibana, N. and Kobayashi, Y. 1975. Effect of cyclophosphamide on the growth of *Rickettsia sennetsu* in experimentally infected mice. *Infect. Immun.*, **12**: 625–629.

Tachibana, N., Kusune, E., Yokata, T., Shishime, E., Tsuda, K. and Kobayashi, Y. 1982a. Growth of *Rickettsia tsutsugamushi*, isolated in Miyazaki distinct, in BSC-1 cell. *J. Japan. Assoc. Infect. Dis.*, **56**: 664–670. (in Japanese).

Tachibana, N., Kusune, E., Yokota, T., Shishime, E., Tsuda, K. and Oshikawa, T. 1982b. Epidemiological, immunological and etiological study on Tsutsugamushi disease in Miyazaki district. *J. Japan. Assoc. Infect. Dis.*, **56**: 655–663. (in Japanese).

Takada, N. 1976. Studies on trombiculid mites in Tohoku district. *Hirosaki Med. J.*, **28**: 391–426. (in Japanese).

Takada, N. 1982. Epidemiology of Tsutsugamushi disease in Aomori Prefecture. *Jpn. J. Sanit. Zool.*, **33**: 309–317. (in Japanese).

Takada, N. 1990. A pictorial review of medical acarology in Japan. pp. 1–216. Kinpodo, Kyoto, Japan. (in Japanese).

Takahashi, K., Arai, J. and Murata, M. 1981. Study on Tsutsugamushi disease in Hokkaido. Isolation of *Rickettsia tsutsugamushi* from small mammals in Nopporo area near Sapporo. *Rep. Hokkaido Inst. Publ. Hlth.*, **31**: 30–34. (in Japanese).

Takahashi, K., Urakami, H. and Tamura, A. 1985. Purification of cell envelopes of *Rickettsia tsutsugamushi*. *Microbiol. Immunol.*, **29**: 475–478.

Takahashi, M. 1987. Ecological study of *Leptotrombidium* (*Leptotrombidium*) *pallidum*. 1. Morphological observations of external genital openings and spermatophores deposited by male. *J. Saitama Med. School*, **14**: 383–392. (in Japanese).

Takahashi, M. 1988a. Ecological study of *Leptotrombidium* (*Leptotrombidium*) *pallidum*. 3. A seasonal change of fluctuation in number of larval trombiculid mite *L.* (*L.*) *pullidum* in the area of Hitsujiyama, Chichibu City, Saitama Prefecture. *J. Saitama Med. School*, **15**: 253–260. (in Japanese).

Takahashi, M. 1988b. Ecological study of *Leptotrombidium* (*Leptotorombidium*) *pallidum*. 4. Distribution of larval trombiculid mites depending on different vegetations and parasitized localizations of larvae on the body of host *Apodemus speciosus* captured in the area of Hitsujiyama, Chichibu City, Saitama Prefecture. *J. Saitama Med. School*, **15**: 277–284. (in Japanese).

Takahashi, M. 1988c. Ecological study of *Leptotrombidium* (*Leptotrombidium*) *pallidum*. 5. Effect of relative humidity on life cycle of the chigger mite, *L.* (*L.*) *pallidum*. *Ann. Rep. Ohara Hosp.*, **31**: 7–12.

Takahashi, M. 1989. Ecological study of *Leptotrombidium* (*Leptotrombidium*) *pallidum*. 6. Morphological observations and ecological features of each developmental stage of *Leptotrombidium* (*Leptotrombidium*) *pallidum*, and its life history observed in the containers placed in the field. *Bull. Saitama Mus. Nat. Hist.*, **7**: 7–24. (in Japanese).

Takahashi, M. 1990. Vertical transmission of *Rickettsia tsutsugamushi* in *Leptotrombidium* (*Leptotrombidium*) *pallidum*. *Jpn. J. Sanit. Zool.*, **41**: 389–403. (in Japanese).

Takahashi, M. and Sekine, M. 1983. Studies on ectoparasites on mammals and birds in Saitama Prefecture. Part III-1. Ectoparasites from small mammals on the embankment along the Irumagawa River, Kawagoe City: seasonal fluctuation of larval trombiculid mites. *Animal. Nature*, **13**: 30–32. (in Japanese).

Takahashi, M., Murata, M., Machida, K. and Hori, E. 1986a. The survey of larval trombicuid mites and isolation of *Rickettsia tsutsugamushi* in the area of Hitsujiyama, Chichibu City, Saitama Prefecture. *J. Saitama Med. School*, **13**: 167–174. (in Japanese).

Takahashi, M., Shirasaka, A., Machida, K. and Hori, E. 1986b. Studies on the life history of chigger mites in the laboratory. 1. Observation of the spermatophores deposition and oviposition of the chigger mite *Gahrliepia* (*Gateria*) *saduski* Womersley, 1952 in the laboratory. *Ann. Rep. Ohara Hosp.*, **29**: 13–20. (in Japanese).

Takahashi, M., Shirasaka, A. and Hori, E. 1987a. Studies on the life history of chigger mites in the laboratory II. Observation of the spermatophores deposition of the chigger mites *Leptotrombidium* (*Leptotrombidium*) *scutellare* and *L.* (*L.*) *fuji*. *Ann. Rep. Ohara Hosp.*, **30**: 7–11. (in Japanese).

Takahashi, M., Murata, M., Machida, K. and Hori, E. 1987b. Ectoparasite fauna of small mammals in the area of Hitsujiyama, Chichibu City, Saitama Prefecture. *Ann. Rep. Ohara Hosp.*, **30**: 13–20. (in Japanese).

Takahashi, M., Murata, M. and Hori, E. 1988a. Ecological study of *Leptotrombidium* (*Leptotrombidium*) *pallidum* Nagayo, Mitamura et Tamiya, 1919. 2. Existence of adult males in *Rickettsia tsutsugamushi*-infected colony. *Jpn. J. Sanit. Zool.*, **39**: 63–65. (in Japanese).

Takahashi, M., Murata, M., Nogami, S., Hori, E., Kawamura, A. Jr. and Tanaka, H. 1988b. Transovarial transmission of *Rickettsia tsutsugamushi* in *Leptotrombidium pallidum* successively reared in the laboratory. *Jpn. J. Exp. Med.*, **58**: 213–218.

Takahashi, M., Takahashi, K., Machida, K., Nishina, M. and Hori, E. 1988c. Studies on the life history of chigger mites in the laboratory. 3. Observations of the spermatophores deposition of the chigger mites *Leptotrombidium (Leptotrombidium) miyazakii* and *L. (L.) intermedium*. *Bull. Saitama Mus. Nat. Hist.*, **6**: 1–10. (in Japanese).

Takahashi, M., Murata, M., Hori, E., Tanaka, H. and Kawamura, A. Jr. 1990a. Transmission of *Rickettsia tsutsugamushi* from *Apodemus speciosus*, a wild rodent, to larval trombiculid mites during the feeding process. *Jpn. J. Exp. Med.*, **60**: 203–208.

Takahashi, M., Murata, M., Machida, K., Hori, E., Kawamura, A. Jr. and Tanaka, H. 1990b. Aggregated distribution of infective spots composed of *Leptotrombidium pallidum*, highly prevalent with *Rickettsia tsutsugamushi*, demonstrated by sentinel voles, *Microtus montebelli*, on the ground. *Jpn. J. Exp. Med.*, **60**: 325–335.

Takahashi, M., Murata, M., Sasaki, M., Saito, T., Machida, K., Hori, E., Tanaka, H. and Kawamura, A. Jr. 1990c. Resistance to *Rickettsia tsutsugamushi* and persistence of infection in different wild rodents. *Jpn. J. Exp. Med.*, **60**: 241–245.

Takahashi, M., Murata, M., Misumi, H. and Hori, E. 1991a. Change of the eschar observed in a case of Tsutsugamushi disease. *Ann. Rep. Ohara Hosp.*, **34**: 7–10. (in Japanese).

Takahashi, M., Misumi, H., Matsuzawa, H., Morita, K., Tuji, O., Ootsuji, J. and Hori, E. 1991b. Dermatitises caused by *Leptotrombidium akamushi*. *Ann. Rep. Ohara Hosp.*, **34**: 11–14. (in Japanese).

Takahashi, M., Murata, M., Machida, K., Saito, T., Sasaki, M., Misumi, H., Nogami, S., Hori, E., Tanaka, H. and Kawamura, A. Jr. 1992. Effect of *Rickettsia tsutsugamushi* to pregnancy of *Microtus* voles and isolation of *Rickettsia* from litters. *J. Tokyo Vet. Anim. Sci.*, **38**: 89–92. (in Japanese).

Takahashi, M., Machida, K., Murata, M., Misumi, H., Hori, E., Kawamura, A. Jr. and Tanaka, H. 1993a. Seasonal development of *Leptotrombidium pallidum* (Acari: Trombiculidae) observed by experimental rearing in the natural environment. *J. Med. Entomol.*, **30**: 320–325.

Takahashi, M., Murata, M., Machida, K., Misumi, H. Hori, E., Kawamura, A. Jr. and Tanaka, H. 1993b. Trombiculid mites and *Rickettsia tsutsugamushi* isolated from wild rodents and mites in an endemic area of Saitama Prefecture, Japan. *Jpn. J. Sanit. Zool.*, **44**: 7–14. (in Japanese).

Takahashi, M., Urakami, H., Murata, M., Misumi, H., Tsuji, O., Morita, K. and Hori, E. 1993c. Sex ratio of *Rickettsia tsutsugamushi* uninfected colony and infected colony of *Leptotrombidium fletcheri* treated with minocycline. *Jpn. J. Sanit. Zool.*, **44**: 91–96. (in Japanese).

Takahashi, M., Murata, M., Misumi, H., Hori, E., Kawamura, A. Jr. and Tanaka, H. 1994a. Failed vertical transmission of *Rickettsia tsutsugamushi* (Rickettsiales: Rickettsiaceae) acquired from rickettsemic mice by *Leptotrombidium pallidum* (Acari, Trombiculidae). *J. Med. Entomol.*, **31**: 212–216.

Takahashi, M., Misumi, H., Matsuzawa, H., Morita, K., Tsuji,O., Hori, E., Kawamura, A. Jr. and Tanaka, H. 1994b. Seasonal development of *Leptotrombidium scutellare* (Acari: Trombiculidae) observed by experimental rearing in field conditions. *Jpn. J. Sanit. Zool.*, **45**: 113–120.

Takahashi, M., Yoshida, Y., Furuya, Y., Katayama, T., Hori, E., Murata,M.,

Misumi, H., Tanaka, H. and Kawamura, A. Jr. 1994c. Multiple *Rickettsia tsutsugamushi* types detected by polymerase chain reaction in an infected laboratory colony of *Leptotrombidium pallidum*. *Jpn. J. Sanit. Zool.*, **45**: 279–284.

Takahashi, M., Morita, K., Tsuji, O., Misumi, H., Otsuji, J., Hori, E., Kawamura, A. Jr. and Tanaka, H. 1995. Seasonal development of *Leptotrombidium akamushi* (Acari: Trombiculidae) under field temperatures. *J. Med. Entomol.*, **32**: (in Press)

Tamiya, T. 1962. Recent advances in studies of Tsutsugamushi disease in Japan. pp. 1–309. Medical Culture Inc., Tokyo.

Tamura, A. 1988a. Invasion and intracellular growth of *Rickettsia tsutsugamushi*. *Microbiol. Sci.*, **5**: 228–232.

Tamura, A. 1988b. Pathogenic factors of *Rickettsia tsutsugamushi*. *Japan. J. Bacteriol.*, **43**: 629–639. (in Japanese).

Tamura, A. and Urakami, H. 1981. Easy method for infectivity titration of *Rickettsia tsutsugamushi* by infected cell counting method. *Japan. J. Bacteriol.*, **36**: 783–785. (in Japanese).

Tamura, A., Urakami, H. and Tsuruhara, T. 1982. Purification of *Rickettsia tsutsugamushi* by Percoll density gradient centrifugation. *Microbiol. Immunol.*, **26**: 321–328.

Tamura, A., Takahashi, K., Tsuruhara, T., Urakami, H., Miyamura, S., Sekikawa, H., Kenmotsu, M., Shibata, M., Abe, S. and Nezu, H. 1984. Isolation of *Rickettsia tsutsugamushi* antigenically different from Kato, Karp, and Gilliam strains from patients. *Microbiol. Immunol.*, **28**: 873–882.

Tamura, A., Ohashi, N., Urakami, H., Takahashi, K. and Oyanagi, M. 1985. Analysis of polypeptide composition and antigenic components of *Rickettsia tsutsugamushi* by polyacrylamide gel electrophoresis and immunoblotting. *Infect. Immun.*, **48**: 671–675.

Tamura, A., Ohashi, N., Sakurai, H., Urakami, H., Yamamoto, S. and Kawamori, F. 1990a. Serodiagnosis of scrub typhus by dot-blot method. *J. Japan. Assoc. Inf. Dis.*, **64**: 704–714. (in Japanese).

Tamura, A., Urakami, H. and Ohashi, N. 1990b. A comparative view of *Rickettsia tsutsugamushi* and the other groups of rickettsiae. *Eur. J. Epidemiol.*, **7**: 259–269.

Tamura, A., Ohashi, N., Urakami, H. and Miyamura, S. 1995. Classification of *Rickettsia tsutsugamushi* in a new genus, *Orientia* gen. nov. as *Orientia tsutsugamushi* comb. nov. *Int. J. Syst. Bacteriol.*, **45**: 589–591.

Tanaka, H., Sasa, M. and Ueno, Y. 1955. Studies on the stimulation effect of CO_2 on unengorged larvae of *Trombicula scutellaris* Nagayo *et al.*, 1921. *Jpn. J. Sanit. Zool.*, **6**: 137–140. (in Japanese).

Tanaka. H., Takada, N., Tada, T., Iwasaki, H. and Inada, K. 1987. Epidemiology of parasitic infections in Fukui Prefecture 3. Present status of outbreaks and vector-pathogen relationship of Tsutsugamushi disease. *Hokuriku J. Publ. Hlth.*, **14**: 19–24. (in Japanese).

Tanaka, K. 1889. Ueber Aetiologie und Pathogenase der Kedani-krankheit. *Zbl. f. Bakt.*, (1 Abt.) **26**: 432–439.

Tange, Y., Kanemitsu, N. and Kobayashi, Y. 1991. Analysis of immunological characteristics of newly isolated strains of *Rickettsia tsutsugamushi* using monoclonal antibodies. *Am. J. Trop. Med. Hyg.*, **44**: 371–381.

Tange, Y., Kanemitsu, N., Okada, T., Kobayashi, Y. and Tsuboi, T. 1992. Characterization of *Rickettsia tsutsugamushi* strains newly isolated in Ehime Prefecture, Japan. *J. Japan. Assoc. Infect. Dis.*, **66**: 1015–1021. (in Japanese).

Tanskul, P. and Gingrich, J.B. 1986. Two new species of *Leptotrombidium* (Akari: Actinedida : Trombiculidae), probable vectors of scrub typhus in Thailand. *J. Med. Entomol.*, **23**: 661–665.

Tanskul, P., Linthicum, K.J., Rosenberg, R., Watcharapichat, P., Lueprasitasankul, D. and Eamsila, C. 1994. *Rickettsia tsutsugamushi* in a rice-agriculture ecology in Northern Thailand: new chiggers and rodent associations (Ab.). p. 147. The first international Congress of Parasitology and Tropical Medicine, Kuala Lumpur.

Tarasevich, I.V. 1960. Tsutsugamushi fever (Review). *J. Mikrobiol. Epidemiol. Immunol.*, **31**: 1581–1590.

Tarasevich, I.V. 1964. Study of the Tsutsugamushi fever causative agent. *Zh. Mikrobiol. Epidemiol. Immunol.*, **41**: 11–14. (in Russian).

Tarasevich, I.V. 1969. The world distribution and natural foci of Tsutsugamushi fever and their special features. pp. 153–170. In: Geography of human disease with natural foci and problems in their prevention. (eds. P.A. Petrishcheva and N.G.P. Olsufjev). Meditsina, Moscow. (in Russian).

Teramura, S. 1954. Studies on tsutsugamushi and Tsutsugamushi disease in Akita Prefecture. *Jpn. J. Sanit. Zool.*, **5**: 26–41. (in Japanese).

Thompson, H.A., Baca, O.G. and Paretski, D. 1971. Presence of ribosomal ribonucleic acid in the rickettsia *Coxiella burnetii. Biochem. J.*, **125**: 365–366.

Toriyama, F., Suzuki, H. and Tanaka, T. 1988. Dermal changes at biting sites by *L. scutellare. Clin. Dermatol.*, **30**: 1127–1130. (in Japanese).

Toyokawa, K. 1972. Transmission of *Rickettsia orientalis* from experimentally infected mice to vector mites (Ab.). *J. Med. Entomol.*, **9**: 593.

Traub, R. 1949. Observations on Tsutsugamushi disease (scrub typus) in Assam and Burma. The mite, *Trombicula deliensis* Walch, and its relation to scrub typhus in Assam. *Am. J. Hyg.*, **50**: 361–370.

Traub, R. 1960. Malaysian parasites XLV. Two new species of chiggers of the genus *Leptotrombidium. Stud. Inst. Med. Res. F.M.S.* **29**: 193–204.

Traub, R. 1962. Some considerations of mites and ticks as vectors of human disease. pp. 123–134. In: Proc. of the symposium on biological transmission of disease agent. Academic Press, New York, London, Toronto, Sydney, San Francisco.

Traub, R. and Frick, L.P. 1950. Chloramphenicol (chloromycetin) in the chemoprophylaxis of scrub typhus (Tsutsugamushi disease). V. Relation of number of vector mites in hyperendemic area to infection rates in exposed volunteers. *Am. J. Hyg.*, **51**: 242–247.

Traub, R. and Wisseman, C.L. Jr. 1968a. Ecological considerations in scrub typhus. 1. Emerging concepts. *Bull. WHO.*, **39**: 209–218.

Traub, R. and Wisseman C.L. Jr. 1968b. Ecological considerations in scrub typhus. 2. Vector species. *Bull. WHO.*, **39**: 219–230.

Traub, R. and Wisseman, C.L. Jr. 1974a. Current concepts of the ecology of chigger-borne rickettsiosis (scrub typhus). *Japan. J. Med. Sci. Biol.*, **27**: 1–5.

Traub, R. and Wisseman, C.L. Jr. 1974b. The ecology of chigger-borne rickettsiosis (scrub typhus). *J. Med. Entomol.*, **11**: 237–303.

Traub, R., Frick, L.P. and Diercks, F.H. 1950. Observations on the occurence of *Rickettsia tsutsugamushi* in rats and mites in the Malayan jungle. *Am. J. Hyg.*, **51**: 269–273.

Traub, R., Wisseman C.L. Jr. and Nur Ahmad. 1967. The occurence of scrub typhus infection in unusual habitats in West Pakistan. *Trans. Roy. Soc. Trop. Med. Hyg.*, **61**: 23–57.

Traub, R., Wisseman, C.L. Jr., Jones, M. R. and O'keefe, J. 1975. The acquisition of *Rickettsia tsutsugamushi* by chiggers (trombiculid mites) during the feeding process. *Ann. N.Y. Acad. Sci.*, **266**: 91–114.

Tringali, G.R., Montenegro, M.R., Walker, D.H. and Mansueto, S. 1983. Immunity and rickettsial infection: a review. *Acta Tropica.*, **40**: 311–320.

Trips, M., Perrone, J.B., Reissing, M. and Parker, K.L. 1981. Control of cytoplasmic incompatibility in the *Aedes scutellaris* complex. *J. Hered.*, **72**: 313–317.

Trishnananda, M., Vasuvat, C. and Harinasuta, C. 1964. Investigations on scrub typhus in Thailand. *J. Trop. Med. Hyg.*, **67**: 215–219.

Trishnananda, M., Harinasuta, C. and Vasuvat, C. 1966. Studies on the vector of *Rickettsia tsutsugamushi* infection in Thailand. *Ann. Trop. Med. Parasitol.*, **60**: 252–256.

Tsuboi, Y. and Oyama, T. 1984. On complement fixation and Weil-Felix tests. *Clin. Virol.*, **12**: 285–288. (in Japanese).

Tsuruhara, T., Urakami, H. and Tamura, A. 1982. Surface morphology of *Rickettsia tsutsugamushi*-infected mouse fibroblasts. *Acta Virol.*, **26**: 506–511.

Twartz, J.C., Shirai, A., Selvaraju, G., Saunders, J.P., Huxsoll, D.L. and Groves, M.G. 1982. Doxycycline prophylaxis for human scrub typhus. *J. Infect. Dis.*, **146**: 811–818.

Tyeryar, F.J. Jr. Weiss, E., Millar, D.B., Bozeman, F.M. and Ormsbee, R.A. 1973. DNA base composition of rickettsiae. *Science*, **180**: 415–417.

Uchikawa, K. and Kumada, N. 1986. Chiggers distributed in Matsumoto, a nonendemic area of Tsutsugamushi disease. *Bull. Environ. Conserv., Shinshu Univ.*, **8**: 1–5. (in Japanese).

Uchikawa, K., Kumada, N. and Yamada, Y. 1985. Chiggers parasitic on green pheasant — role of the bird as carrier of *Leptotrombidium pallidum* (Nagayo *et al.*). *Jpn. J. Sanit. Zool.*, **36**: 357–361. (in Japanese).

Ueno, Y. 1956. Studies on tsutsugamushi and Tsutsugamushi disease of Hachijo Island. *Jpn. J. Sanit. Zool.*, **7**: 231–253. (in Japanese).

Ueno, Y., Tanaka, H. and Sasa, M. 1955. Notes on the massappearance phenomenon of *Trombicula scutellaris* larvae in Hachijo Island and their mode of attaching the hosts. *Jpn. J. Sanit. Zool.*, **6**: 133–134. (in Japanese).

Ujiiye, A. 1981. Recent outbreaks of Tsutsugamushi disease in Japan. *Modern Media*, **27**: 357–365: 408–416. (in Japanese).

Ukai, J. 1906. A review on surveys of Tsutsugamushi disease. *Hokuetsu Med. J.*, 151: 1–31. (in Japanese).

Umeki, I., Hirose, S., Kurihara, H., Kato, A., Nakajima, T., Kitaoka, M. and

Asanuma, K. 1970. Occurrence of Tsutsugamushi disease patients at Takeda City areas, Oita Prefecture. *J. Oita Med. Assoc.*, **178**: 20–23. (in Japanese).

Upham, R.W. Jr., Hubert, A.A., Phang, O.W., Mat, Y.B. and Rapmund, G. 1971. Distribution of *Leptotrombidium* (*Leptotrombidium*) *arenicola* (Acarina: Trombiculidae) on the ground in West Malaysia. *J. Med. Entomol.*, **8**: 401–406.

Urakami, H., Tsuruhara, T. and Tamura, A. 1982a. Observations of the same whole cells infected with *Rickettsia tsutsugamushi* by means of transmission and scanning electron microscopy. *J. Electron Microsc.*, **31**: 212–215.

Urakami, H., Tsuruhara, T. and Tamura, A. 1982b. Intranuclear *Rickettsia tsutsugamushi* in cultured mouse fibroblasts (L cells). *Microbiol. Immunol.*, **26**: 445–447.

Urakami, H., Tsuruhara, T. and Tamura, A. 1983. Penetration of *Rickettsia tsutsugamushi* into cultured mouse fibroblasts (L cells): an electron microscopic observation. *Microbiol. Immunol.*, **27**: 251–263.

Urakami, H., Tsuruhara, T. and Tamura, A. 1984. Electron microscopic studies on intracellular multiplication of *Rickettsia tsutsugamushi* in L cells. *Microbiol. Immunol.*, **28**: 1191–1201.

Urakami, H., Ohashi, N., Tsuruhara, T. and Tamura, A. 1986. Characterization of polypeptides in *Rickettsia tsutsugamushi*: effect of preparative conditions on migration of polypeptides in polyacrylamide gel electrophoresis. *Infect. Immun.*, **51**: 948–952.

Urakami, H., Tamura, A., Miyamura, S., Yamamoto, S. and Kawabata, N. 1988a. Susceptibilities of recent clinical isolates of *Rickettsia tsutsugamushi* to chemotherapeutic agents *in vitro*. *J. Japan. Assoc. Infect. Dis.*, **62**: 931–937. (in Japanese).

Urakami, H., Takahashi, M., Tamura, A. and Hori, E. 1988b. Electron microscopic observations of the embryo *Leptotrombidium* (*Leptotrombidium*) *pallidum* naturally infected with *Rickettsia tsutsugamushi*. *Microbiol. Immunol.*, **32**: 967–972.

Urakami, H., Yamamoto, S., Tsuruhara, T., Ohashi, N. and Tamura, A. 1989. Serodiagnosis of scrub typhus with antigens immobilized on nitrocellulose sheet. *J. Clin. Microbiol.*, **27**: 1841–1846.

Urakami, H., Takahashi, M., Murata, M. and Tamura, A. 1994a. Electron microscopic study of the distribution and the vertical transmission of *Rickettsia tsutsugamushi* in *Leptotrombidium pallidum*. *Japan. J. Med. Sci. Biol.*, **47**: 127–139.

Urakami, H., Takahashi, M., Hori, E. and Tamura, A. 1994b. An ultrastructural study of vertical transmission of *Rickettsia tsutsugamushi* during oogenesis and spermatogenesis in *Leptotrombidium pallidum*. *Am. J. Trop. Med. Hyg.*, **50**: 219–228.

U.S. Army Medical Research Unit (Malaya). 1960. Annual Report. pp. 106–107. In: Ann. Rep. Inst. Med. Res. (Kuala Lumpur) for 1959.

U.S. Army Medical Research Unit (Malaya). 1969. Annual Report: scrub typhus. pp. 183–198. Ann. Rep. Inst. Res. (Kuala Lumpul) for 1968.

Van Peenen, P.F.D., Ho, C.M. and Bourgeois, A.L. 1977. Indirect immunofluorescence antibodies in natural and aquired *Rickettsia tsutsugamushi* infections of

Philippine rodents. *Infect. Immun.*, **15**: 813–816.

Vercammen-Grandjean, P.H. 1968. The chigger mites of the Far East (Acarina: Trombiculidae and Leeuwenhoekiidae). pp. 1–135. U.S. Army Med. Res. Dev. Command, Washington.

Vercammen-Grandjean, P.H. and Langston, R. 1976. The chigger mites of the world. Vol. III. p. 612. *Leptotrombidium* complex. Section A. *Leptotrombidium* s. str. George Williams Hooper Foundation University of California, San Francisco.

Vodkin, M.H. and Williams, J.C. 1988. A heat shock operon in *Coxiella burnetii* produces a major antigen homologous to a protein in both mycobacteria and *Escherichia coli*. *J. Bacteriol.*, **170**: 1227–1234.

Wade, M.J. and Stevens, L. 1985. Microorganism mediated reproductive isolation in flour beetles (genus *Triborium*). *Science*, **227**: 527–528.

Walch, E.W. and Keukenschrijver, N.C. 1924a. Einige opmerkingen aangaande de epidemiologie van de pseudotyphus. *Geneesk. Tijds. Ned. Ind.*, **64**: 247–276.

Walch, E.W. and Keukenschrijver, N.C. 1924b. On pseudotyhus of Sumatra. Part II. pp. 627–643. Some notes on epidemiology. Trans. 5th Congr. Far Eastern Assoc. Trop. Med.

Walch, E.W. and Morawa, T.D. 1924. On the trombiculae, carriers of pseudotyphus, and related species from Sumatra. *Kitasato Arch. Exp. Med.*, **6**: 235–254.

Walker, D.H. and Fishbein, D.B. 1991. Epidemiology of rickettsial disease. *Eur. J. Epidemiol.*, **7**: 237–245.

Walker, D.H., Liu, Q-H. and Feng, H-M. 1990. Update on rickettsiae and rickettsial disease in China. *Rev. Infect. Dis.*, **12**: 562–563.

Walker, J.S., Gan, E., Chan, T.C. and Muul, I. 1973. Involvement of small mammals in the transmission of scrub typhus in Malaysia: isolation and serological evidence. *Trans. Roy. Soc. Trop. Med. Hyg.*, **67**: 838–845.

Walker, J.S., Chan, T.C., Manikumaran, C. and Elisberg, B.L. 1975. Attempts to infect and demonstrate transovarial transmission of *Rickettsia tsutsugamushi* in three species of *Leptotrombidium* mites. *Ann. N. Y. Acad. Sci.*, **266**: 80–90.

Wang, D-C., Wung, S-C., Hwang, Y-M. and Yu, E-S. 1965. The transovarial transmission of *Rickettsia tsutsugamushi* in two types of *Trombicula deliensis*. *Acta Parasitol. Sinica.*, **2**: 213–217. (in Chinese).

Wang, S-Q., Liang, L-S., Guo, Y-Y., Guan, B-W., Zhuang, L-P. and He, S. 1983. The vector of scrub typus in winter in Fujian Province. *Chinese J. Epidemiol.*, **4**: 257–259. (in Chinese).

Wattenberg, L.W., Elisberg, B.L., Wisseman, C.L. Jr. and Smadel, J.E. 1955. Studies of rickettsial toxins. II. Altered vascular physiology in rickettsial toxemia of mice. *J. Immunol.*, **74**: 147–157.

Wei, J-J., Li, M., Li, C-Y. and Tong, G-Z. 1983. Isolation and identification of *Rickettsia tsutsugamushi* in Zhejiang. p. 62. In: Proceedings of the First Chinese National Symposium on Rickettsiae, Chlamydiae, and Toxoplasmae Infections. Nanjing: Chinese J. Epidemiol. Press. (in Chinese).

Wei, J-J., Tong, G-Z. and Shi, S-F. 1985a. The studies of transovarial transmission of *Rickettsia tsutsugamushi* in *Leptotrombidium gaohuensis*. *Chinese J.*

Epidemiol., **6**: 206–207. (in Chinese).

Wei, J-J., Tong, G-Z. and Shi, S-F. 1985b. The new vector of scrub typhus, *Leptotrombidium gaohuensis*, discovery and epidemiology. *Chinese J. Epidemiol.*, **6**: 277–280. (in Chinese).

Wei, J-J., Tong, G-Z. and Shi, S-F. 1985c. Volunteer (author) experimentally bitten by *Leptotrombidium gaohuensis* (Ab.). p. 54. In: Proceeding of the First Chinese National Military Symposium on Rickettsialogy. Hangzhou: Third Militaly Medical University Press.

Wei, J-J., Tong, G-Z. and Shi, S-F. 1987. Study on *Leptotrombidium gaohuensis* sp. nov. newly discovered vector of Tsutsugamushi disease. *Chinese Med. J.*, **100**: 590–594.

Weil, E. and Felix, A. 1916. Zur serologischen Diagnose des Fleckfiebers. *Wien. Klin. Wochenschr.*, **29**: 33–35.

Weiss, E. and Moulder, J.W. 1984. Genus 1. Rickettsia da Rocka-Lima 1916, 567^{AL}. pp. 688–698. In: Bergey's manual of systematic bacteriology, Vol. 1. (eds. N.R. Krieg and J.G. Holt). Williams and Wilkins, Baltimore and London.

Weiss, E., Coolbaugh, J.C. and Williams, J.C. 1975. Separation of viable *Rickettsia typhi* from yolk sac and L cell host components by Renografin density gradient centrifugation. *Appl. Microbiol.*, **30**: 456–463.

Wen, T-W. 1958. Observations on the mating process of *Acomatacarus yosanoi* Fukuzumi *et* Obata, 1953, with the discovery of its spermatophores (Acariformes: Trombiculidae). *Acta Zool. Sinica.*, **10**: 221–224. (in Chinese).

Wen, T-W. 1959. Observations on the process of transferring spermatophores in *Acomatacarus yosanoi* Fukuzumi *et* Obata, 1953, with a description of the male and female genitalia. *Chinese Med. J.*, **78**: 283. (in Chinese).

Wen, T-W. 1984. Sand mites of China (Acariformes: Trombiculidae and Leeuwenhoekiidae). pp. 1–370. Xue Lin Publishing House. Shanghai. (in Chinese).

Werren, J.H., Skinner, S.W. and Huger, A. 1986. Male-killing bacteria in a parasitic wasp. *Science*, **231**: 990–992.

Wharton, G.W. 1946. Observations of *Ascoschoengastia indica* (Hirst, 1915). *Ecol. Monogr.*, **16**: 151–158.

Wharton, G.W. and Carver, R.K. 1946. Food of nymphs and adults of *Neoshöngastia indica* (Hirst 1915). *Science*, **104**: 76–77.

Wharton, G.W. and Fuller, H.S. 1952. A manual of the chiggers. *Mem. Ento. Soc. Wash.*, **4**: 1–185.

Wharton, G.W. and Hardcastle, A.B. 1946. The genus Neoschöngastia (Acarna: Trombiculidae) in the western Pacific area. *J. Parasitol.*, **32**: 286–332.

WHO working group on rickettsial disease. 1982. Rickettsiosis: a continuing disease problem. *Bull. WHO.*, **60**: 157–164.

Williamson, D.L. and Poulson, D.F. 1979. Sex ratio organisms (spiroplasmas) of *Drosophila*, pp. 175–208. In: The Mycoplasmas, Vol. 3. (eds. R.F. Whitcomb and J.G. Tully). Academic Press, New York, London, Toronto, Sydney, San Francisco.

Wisseman, C.L. Jr. and Ordonez, S.V. 1986. Actions of antibiotics on *Rickettsia rickettsii*. *J. Infect. Dis.*, **153**: 626–628.

Wisseman, C.L. Jr and Waddell, A. 1982. *In vitro* susceptibility of *Rickettsia rickettsii* to doxycycline. *J. Infect. Dis.*, **145**: 584.

Wisseman, C.L. Jr, Waddell, A.D. and Walsh, W.T. 1974. *In vitro* studies of the action of antibiotics on *Rickettsia prowazekii* by two basic methods of cell culture. *J. Infect. Dis.*, **130**: 564–574.

Wisseman, C.L. Jr, Waddell, A.D. and Silverman, D.J. 1976. *In vitro* studies on rickettsia-host cell interactions: lag phase in intracellular growth cycle as a function of stage of growth of infecting *Rickettsia prowazekii*, with preliminary observations on inhibition of rickettsial uptake by host cell fragments. *Infect. Immun.*, **13**: 1749–1760.

Wisseman, C.L. Jr., Silverman, D.J., Waddell, A. and Brown, D.T. 1982. Penicillin-induced unstable intracellular formation of spheroplasts by rickettsia. *J. Infect. Dis.*, **146**: 147–158.

Wolf, J.W. 1931. Observation on Weil-Felix reaction in Tsutsugamushi disease. *J. Hyg.* , **31**: 352–360.

Wood, D.O., Williamson, L.R., Winkler, H.H. and Krause, D.C. 1987. Nucleotide sequence of the *Rickettsia prowazekii* citrate synthase gene. *J. Bacteriol.*, **169**: 3564–3572.

Woodman, D.R., Grays, R. and Weiss, E. 1977. Improved chicken embryo cell culture plaque assay for scrub typhus rickettsiae. *J. Clin. Microbiol.*, **6**: 639–641.

Wormersley, H. 1952. The scrub-typhus and scrub-itch mites (Trombiculidae, Acarina) of the Asiatic-Pacific region. *Rec. South Australian Mus.*, **10**: 1–673.

Wright, J.D., Hastriter, M.W. and Robinson, D.M. 1984. Observations on the ultrastructure and distribution of *Rickettsia tsutsugamushi* in naturally infected *Leptotrombidium (Leptotrombidium) arenicola* (Acari: Trombiculidae). *J. Med. Entomol.*, **21**: 17–27.

Xiangrui, C., Jinju, W., Yongguo, Z., Yanan, W., Chunmu, Y., Zhaoping, X., Junli, W. and Yufu, Y. 1991. Recent studies on scrub typhus and *Rickettsia tsutsugamushi* in Shandong Province — China. *Eur. J. Epidemiol.*, **7**: 304–306.

Yamaguchi, N., Hasegawa, T., Tamura, A. and Urakami, H. 1984. A morphological study on inhibition of growth of *Rickettsia tsutsugamushi* by tetracycline, chloramphenicol and erythromycin. *Med. J. Niigata Prefecture Hospitals.*, **32**: 38–40. (in Japanese).

Yamamiya, C. and Honda, S. 1933. Observation on the Tsutsugamushi disease of the Pescadores. *J. Formosan Med. Assoc.*, **32**: 1803–1804. (in Japanese).

Yamamoto, S. 1961. An investigation on trombiculid mites in the Tojinwara area of Kaseda City, Kagoshima Prefecture. *Jpn. J. Sanit. Zool.*, **12**: 169–173. (in Japanese).

Yamamoto, S. 1984. Clinics and diagnosis of Tsutsugamushi disease: specificity and evaluation of serodiagnosis — fluorescence. *Clin. Virol.*, **12**: 270–274. (in Japanese).

Yamamoto, S. 1988. *Rickettsia tsutsugamushi. Clinics and Microorganisms*, **15**: 603–607. (in Japanese).

Yamamoto, S. and Minamishina, Y. 1982. Serodiagnosis of Tsutsugamushi fever (scrub typhus) by the indirect immunoperoxidase technique. *J. Clin. Microbiol.*, **15**: 1128–1132.

Yamamoto, S., Kawabata, N., Tamura, A., Urakami, H., Ohashi, N., Murata, M., Yoshida, Y. and Kawamura, A. Jr. 1986. Immunological properties of *Rickettsia tsutsugamushi*, Kawasaki strain, isolated from a patient in Kyushu. *Microbiol. Immunol.*, **30**: 611–620.

Yamamoto, S., Murata, M. and Nogami, S. 1987. Indirect immunofluorescence and avidin-biotin complex method. pp. 30–31. In: Report of meeting of the task force on the serological diagnosis of Tsutsugamushi diseases (scrub typhus). Regional office for the Western Pacific, WHO., Manila, Philippines.

Yamamoto, S., Kawabata, N., Ooura, K., Murata, M. and Minamishima, Y. 1989. Antigenic types of *Rickettsia tsutsugamushi* isolated from patients with Tsutsugamushi fever and their distribution in Miyazaki Prefecture. *J. Japan. Assoc. Infect. Dis.*, **63**: 109–117. (in Japanese).

Yamamoto, S., Ooura, K., Kawabata, N., Furuya, Y., Yoshida, Y., Otsu, M. and Minamishima, Y. 1991. Serologic diagnosis of Tsutsugamushi disease by enzyme-linked immunosorbent assay (ELISA): development of an indirect sandwich and capture methods. pp. 44–64. In: Report on development of simple and specific diagnostic kits for Tsutsugamushi disease. (in Japanese).

Yamamoto, T., Kawamura, A. Jr., Hara, H. and Aikawa, K. 1958. Partial purification of rickettsiae with a cation exchange resin, 1. Method of purification. *Jpn. J. Exp. Med.*, **28**: 329–336.

Yamané, K. 1955. Effect of pregnancy on the distribution of *Rickettsia orientalis* in the mice recovered from the infection. *Japan. J. Bacteriol.*, **10**: 745–748. (in Japanese).

Yamashita, T., Kasuya, S., Nagano, I. and Ohtomo, H. 1992. Studies on Tsutsugamushi disease in Gifu Prefecture. 5. Characterization of monoclonal antibodies to prototype strains of *Rickettsia tsutsugamushi* and immunological grouping of newly isolated strains using the antibodies. *J. Japan. Assoc. Infect. Dis.*, **66**: 1262–1269. (in Japanese).

Yen, J.H. and Barr, A.R. 1973. The etiological agent of cytoplasmic incompatibility in *Culex pipens*. *J. Invert. Pathol.*, **22**: 242–250.

Yoshida, Y., Matsushima, A., Furuya, Y. and Oda, K. 1985. Immunological and serological diagnosis of Tsutsugamushi disease patients in Kanagawa Prefecture. *Bull. Kanagawa Publ. Hlth. Lab.*, **15**: 7–11. (in Japanese).

Yoshida, Y., Furuya, Y., Katayama, T., Kaiho, I. and Yamamoto, S. 1994. Serotype-specific amplification of *Rickettsia tsutsugamushi* DNA from clinical specimens by nested polymerase chain reaction. *J. Japan. Assoc. Inf. Dis.*, **68**: 601–606. (in Japanese).

Yu, E-S. and Lin, S-J. 1957. Study on the condition of natural infection with *R. tsutsugamushi* among mites and domestic animals in Fukien. *Acta Microbiol. Sinica*, **5**: 425–432. (in Chinese).

Yu, E-S. and Wu, H-Y. 1959. Further study on the different types of *Trombicula deliensis* and transovarian transmission of *Rickettsia orientalis*. *Acta Microbiol. Sinica*, **7**: 10–15. (in Chinese).

Index